Qualitative Inquiry—Past, Present, and Future

This title is sponsored by the

INTERNATIONAL CONGRESS OF QUALITATIVE INQUIRY

The International Congress of Qualitative Inquiry has been hosted each May since 2005 by the International Center for Qualitative Inquiry at the University of Illinois, Urbana-Champaign. This volume, as well as preceding ones, are products of plenary sessions from these international congresses. All of these volumes are edited by Norman K. Denzin and Michael D. Giardina and are available from Left Coast Press, Inc. Main series volumes include

10. **Qualitative Inquiry and the Politics of Research**
    2015, based on the 2014 Congress
9. **Qualitative Inquiry Outside the Academy**
    2014, based on the 2013 Congress
8. **Global Dimensions of Qualitative Inquiry**
    2013, based on the 2012 Congress
7. **Qualitative Inquiry and the Politics of Advocacy**
    2012, based on the 2011 Congress
6. **Qualitative Inquiry and Global Crises**
    2011, based on the 2010 Congress
5. **Qualitative Inquiry and Human Rights**
    2010, based on the 2009 Congress
4. **Qualitative Inquiry and Social Justice**
    2009, based on the 2008 Congress
3. **Qualitative Inquiry and the Politics of Evidence**
    2008, based on the 2007 Congress
2. **Ethical Futures in Qualitative Research**
    2007, based on the 2006 Congress
1. **Qualitative Inquiry and the Conservative Challenge**
    2006, based on the 2005 Congress

Qualitative Inquiry—Past, Present, and Future

A Critical Reader

Norman K. Denzin & Michael D. Giardina
Editors

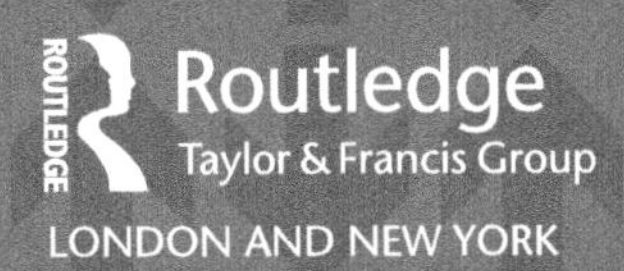

LONDON AND NEW YORK

First published 2015 by Left Coast Press, Inc.

Published 2016 by Routledge
2 Park Square, Milton Park, Abingdon, Oxon OX14 4RN
711 Third Avenue, New York, NY 10017, USA

Routledge is an imprint of the Taylor & Francis Group, an informa business

Library of Congress Cataloging-in-Publication Data:
Qualitative inquiry—past, present, and future : a critical reader / edited by Norman K. Denzin & Michael D. Giardina.
pages cm
Includes bibliographical references and index.
ISBN 978-1-62958-187-3 (paperback)—ISBN 978-1-62958-188-0 (institutional eBook)—ISBN 978-1-62958-189-7 (consumer eBook)
1. Qualitative research—Study and teaching. 2. Research. 3. Social sciences—Research. I. Denzin, Norman K. II. Giardina, Michael D., 1976-
H62.Q3474 2015
001.4'2—dc23
2014045503

ISBN 978-1-62958-187-3 paperback

Contents

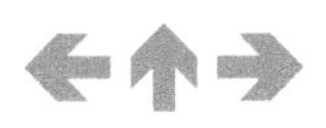

Chapter 1

Introduction

Norman K. Denzin and Michael D. Giardina

Educators need to defend what they do as political, support the university as a place to think, and create programs that nurture a culture of questioning. But there is even more at stake here. It needs to be recognized on a broad scale that the very way in which knowledge is selected, pedagogies are defined, social relations are organized, and futures imagined is always political, though these processes do not have to be politicized in a vulgar or authoritarian way.

— Henry Giroux, 2009

Proem

Ten years ago (2005), we founded and hosted the first International Congress of Qualitative Inquiry at our home university, the University of Illinois at Urbana-Champaign.[1] The theme for that very first Congress—qualitative inquiry and the conservative challenge—was positioned as a response to the political and methodological conservatism of the new millennium (circa 2005). The politics of evidence. Research Assessment Exercises (RAEs).

Qualitative Inquiry—Past, Present, and Future: A Critical Reader, edited by Norman K. Denzin and Michael D. Giardina, pp. 9–38.

Scientism. Scientifically-based research (SBR). The No Child Left Behind Act and the Reading Excellence Act. The National Research Council's (NRC) "Scientific Research in Education" report (Shavelson & Towne, 2002). Indigenous struggles. Social justice. A radical, progressive democracy. These were the topics within and against which that first Congress struggled, undergirded by a political climate—inaugurated in large measure during the George W. Bush presidency (2001–2009)—filled with Patriot Acts, Faith-Based Initiatives, Homeland Security Administrations, conservative regimes of science and truth, the demonization of public servants and teachers, and unending wars in Iraq and Afghanistan.

Ten years on, the more things have changed, the more they have stayed the same: We still have our (seemingly) unending military engagements in the Middle East. The corporate dictates of the neoliberal university continue to run wild, whether we are talking about tenure and promotion cases, academic freedom, the slashing of research budgets, or the commercialization of knowledge and education (see Giroux, this volume). In the United States, the Republican-controlled House Committee on Science, Space, and Technology wages war on the National Science Foundation (NSF) over the 'value' of what projects the NSF has funded (see Mervis, 2014). Academics are under fire for what they say or do, both in terms of their research agendas and their extramural political speech (see, for example, the case of Steven Salaita). The 'gold standard' of positivism remains intact, yet challenged from all sides.

Qualitative Inquiry—Past, Present, and Future: A Critical Reader sits within this context. More philosophical reflection on the state of the field than how-to handbook, our volume revisits the developments, debates, challenges, and changes that have taken place in qualitative inquiry over the last decade. Before starting on our journey, however, we feel it necessary to revisit the history of the last ten years so as to better understand our *methodologically contested present.*

← ↑ →

The qualitative research community, such that we can speak of it as a community, can best be defined as a wide-ranging collection of loosely affiliated, globally dispersed persons who are working within and against different paradigms and who are attempting to implement a critical interpretive approach that will help them (and others) make sense of the terrifying conditions that define daily life in the second decade of this new century. The open-ended nature of the qualitative research project leads to a perpetual resistance against attempts to impose a single, umbrella-like paradigm over the entire project. There are multiple interpretive projects at play, including the decolonizing methodological project of Indigenous scholars; theories of critical pedagogy; performance (auto)ethnographies; standpoint epistemologies; critical race theory; critical, public, poetic, queer, materialist, feminist, reflexive ethnographies; projects connected to Frankfurt School and the British cultural studies traditions; grounded theorists of several varieties; multiple strands of ethnomethodology; and transnational cultural studies projects. The generic focus of each of these versions of qualitative research involves a politics of the local, and a utopian politics of possibility (see Madison, 2010) that redresses social injustices and imagines a radical democracy that is not yet (Weems, 2002). Which is to say, although constant breaks and ruptures define the field of qualitative research, there is a shifting center to the project: the avowed humanistic and social justice commitment to study the social world from the perspective of the interacting individual. From this principle flow the liberal and radical politics of action that are held by its practitioners.

The International Congress of Qualitative Inquiry was launched in 2005 in an attempt to bring this global community closer together, to offer a venue in which critical scholarship, divergent viewpoints, and political engagement could take place.[2] From 2005 forward, those gathering at the Congress have explored global political, ethical, and methodological challenges to qualitative inquiry. They have resisted calls for the predominance of scientifically-based research (SBR), and contested the over-regulation of human subject research by Institutional Review Boards (IRBs; see Koro-Ljungberg, 2010; Maxwell, this volume). Participants have created spaces for critical action research;

indigenous inquiry discourse; post-qualitative, post-humanist, and materialist-feminist theory; new writing strategies; performance autoethnography; and the use of social media and multimedia methods in art-based inquiries.

Over these last ten years of the Congress, however, one overarching goal has taken precedence: *a focus on the role of critical qualitative research in a historical present when the need for social justice has never been greater.* Each Congress volume that we have edited has privileged a particular facet of that goal, from ethics (2007) and evidence (2008) to advocacy (2012) and global crises (2011).[3] But regardless of any singular topical focus, these nine volumes similarly highlighted the interconnected themes as we come to another punctuation point in the history of qualitative inquiry and qualitative methods in *Qualitative Inquiry—Past, Present, & Future*: philosophy of inquiry; politics of evidence/politics of research; new directions in methodology; and Indigenous and decolonizing interventions.

We are, to put it bluntly, at a pivotal crossroads: We live in a historical present that cries out for emancipatory visions, for visions that inspire transformative inquiries, and for inquiries that can provide the moral authority to move people to struggle and resist oppression.

History, Politics, and Paradigms

To better understand where we are today in our methodologically contested present, to better grasp these current criticisms, it is helpful to revisit the so-called paradigm wars of the 1980s, which resulted in the serious crippling of quantitative research in education. Critical pedagogy, critical theorists, and feminist analyses fostered struggles for power and cultural capital for the poor, non-Whites, women, and the LGBTQ community (Gage, 1989).[4]

Teddlie and Tashakkori's (2003a and b, 2011) history is helpful here. They expand the time frame of the 1980s war. For them, there have been at least three paradigm wars, or periods of conflict: the postpositivist–constructivist war against positivism (1970–1990); the conflict between competing postpositivist, constructivist, and critical theory paradigms (1990–2005); and the current conflict between evidence-based methodologists and the mixed methods, interpretive, and critical theory schools (2005–present). Guba's *Paradigm Dialog* (1990a) signaled an end to the 1980s wars. Postpositivists, constructivists, and critical theorists talked to one another, working through issues connected to ethics, field studies, praxis, criteria, knowledge accumulation, truth, significance, graduate training, values, and politics. By the early 1990s, there was an explosion of published works on qualitative research, and handbooks and new journals appeared. Special interest groups committed to particular paradigms appeared, and some had their own journals.

The second paradigm conflict occurred within the mixed-methods community and involved disputes "between individuals convinced of the 'paradigm purity' of their own position" (Teddlie & Tashakkori, 2003b, p. 7). Purists extended and repeated the argument that quantitative and qualitative methods cannot be combined because of the differences between their underlying paradigm assumptions. On the methodological front, this incompatibility thesis was challenged by those who invoked triangulation as a way of combining multiple methods to study the same phenomenon (Teddlie & Tashakkori, 2003b). Thus was ushered in a new round of arguments and debates over paradigm incompatibility and incommensurability.

A soft, apolitical pragmatic paradigm emerged in the post-1990 period. Suddenly, quantitative and qualitative methods became compatible and researchers could use both in their empirical inquiries (Teddlie & Tashakkori, 2003a). Proponents made appeals to a "what works" pragmatic argument, contending that "no incompatibility between quantitative and qualitative methods exists at either the level of practice or that of epistemology . . . there are thus no good reasons for educational researchers to fear forging ahead with 'what works'" (Howe, 1988, p. 16). Of course, what works is more than an empirical question. It involves the politics of evidence.

This is the space that evidence-based research entered. This is the battleground of war number three, "the current upheaval and argument about 'scientific' research in the scholarly world of education" (Clark & Scheurich, 2008; Scheurich & Clark, 2006, p. 401), which was amplified during the first decade of the 2000s.

Enter Teddlie and Tashakkori's third moment, where mixed methods and evidence-based inquiry meet one another in a soft center. Mills (1959) would say this is a space for *abstracted empiricism*. Inquiry is cut off from politics. Biography and history recede into the background. Technological rationality prevails.

Another Discursive Formation

The field is on the edge of New Paradigm Dialog, a fourth formation existing alongside mixed-methods discourses. This is the space primarily filled by post-qualitative, post-humanist, postmodernist, poststructuralist, critical constructionist, feminist materialists, critical pedagogy, and performance studies (see Jackson & Mazzei, 2012; Lather, 2007; MacLure, 2009; St. Pierre, 2011). These scholars are in a different space altogether. They seldom trouble terms like validity or reliability. Inquiry is put under erasure; theory produces different readings. A disruptive politics of representation is the focus, crafting works that move persons and communities to action.

The pursuit of social justice within a transformative paradigm challenges prevailing forms of inequality, poverty, human oppression, and injustice.[5] This paradigm is firmly rooted in a human rights agenda. It requires an ethical framework that is rights- and social justice-based. It requires an awareness of "the need to redress inequalities by giving precedence … to the voices of the least advantaged groups in society" (Mertens, Holmes, & Harris, 2009, p. 89). It encourages the use of qualitative research for social justice purposes, including making such research accessible for public education, social policy-making, and community transformation.

This is a vision that is open to myriad ways of doing social justice work: social workers handling individual clients compassionately; graduate students serving as language translators for non-English-speaking migrant workers and their children; health researchers collaborating with communities to improve health care delivery systems; qualitative researchers engaging their students in public interest visions of society; Indigenous scholars being trained to work for their own nations using their own values; and teachers fostering the ethical practices of qualitative research through publications and presentations and teaching in both traditional classroom and professional development settings, nationally and internationally (Bloom, 2009, p. 253).

Thus are qualitative inquiry scholars united in the commitment to expose and critique the forms of inequality and discrimination that operate in daily life (Garoian & Gaudelius, 2008). Together, they seek morally informed disciplines and interventions that will help people transcend and overcome the psychological despair fostered by wars, economic disaster, and divisive sexual and cultural politics. As global citizens, we are no longer called to just *interpret* the world, which was the mandate of traditional qualitative inquiry. Today, we are called to *change* the world and to change it in ways that resist injustice while celebrating freedom and full, inclusive, participatory democracy. Such has been the mandate of the Congress; such is the mandate of this volume.

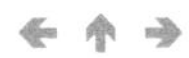

It is here that we find the global community of qualitative researchers midway between two extremes, searching for a new middle and moving in several different directions at the same time. Mixed methodologies and calls for scientifically-based research, on the one hand, and renewed calls for social justice inquiry from the critical social science tradition, on the other, pull from opposite poles. Poststructuralism took away positivism's claim to a God's eye view of the world, that view which said objective observers could turn the world and its happenings into things that could be turned into data (Richardson, 2000, p. 928; St. Pierre, 2011, p. 620). The argument was straightforward (if not radical for the time): things, words, "become data only when theory acknowledges them as data" (St. Pierre, 2011, p. 621). In a single gesture, doubt replaces certainty—no theory, method, discourse, genre, or tradition has "a universal and general claim as the 'right' or privileged form of authoritative knowledge" (Richardson, 2000, p. 928). Indeed, all claims to universal truth "mask particular interests in local, cultural, and political struggles" (Richardson, 2000, p. 928).

Moreover, it is important to remember, as Benozzo, Bell, and Koro-Ljungberg (2013) remind us, that "data" itself is best conceptualized not as something made into being through theory, to then be treated as data, but rather that it might best be thought of as "a wave, a flow, as liquid; ever-changing, inconstant, unreliable, non-interpretable; as a dark forest. Data is already there and here, only partially accessible" (p. 1). It is something that "may not need to be collected but may be lived, sensed, and done" (p. 1). To wit, they implore us to think of data not for "what it produces" or how it is "called into being" but rather for "how it moves and for how it can be lived and sensed by researchers, and how data makes us as people and researchers" (p. 1).[6] What we see, then, as Denzin (2013) posits, is that (something we call) data

> fold into one another, get tangled up in one another. How a thing gets inside the text is shaped by the politics of representation. Language and speech do not mirror experience. They create experience and in the process transform and defer that which is being described. Meanings are always in motion, incomplete, partial, contradictory. There can never be a final, accurate, complete representation of a thing, an utterance, or an action. There are only different representations of different representations. There is no longer any pure presence; description becomes inscription becomes performance. (p. 2)

The evidence- and scientifically-based research (EBR and SBR) communities responded to the critique. Mixed-methods became the new watchword, an old strategy that says data can be both qualitative and quantitative, at once in the same. By keeping a focus on data, and its management, traditional qualitative inquiry texts become complicit in this conversation.[7] As St. Pierre (2013) has argued, too often we see qualitative researchers who "continue to use concepts and practices like bias, objectivity, subjectivity statements, triangulation, audit trails, and interrater reliability that signal they are bound to logical positivism/empiricism, objectivism, and realism" (p. 2), and who likewise reject the performative, the poetic, or interpretive turn.

A Rupture

More is at play, however: there is a rupture that goes beyond mixed methods, evidence, data, and their meanings. The traditional concepts of narrative, meaning, voice, presence, and representation have also been put under erasure, regarded as pernicious leftovers from the twin ruins of postpositivism and humanistic qualitative inquiry (Jackson & Mazzei, 2012, p. vii; St Pierre & Pillow, 2000). Materialist feminist ontologies have inspired a new analytics of data analysis, including defractive readings of data (Jackson & Mazzie, 2012). Post-methodologists, post-humanist, post-empirical, and post-qualitative frameworks call for new models of science, second empiricisms, reimagined social sciences, capacious sciences, sciences of *différance*, a science defined by becoming a double(d) science (Lather, 2007; MacLure, 2011; St. Pierre, 2011, p. 613).

Where do data fit in these new spaces?

Is there any longer even a need for the word?

Why keep the word after you have deconstructed it?

At the same time, in some other wilderness, a radical middle based on social justice and transformational politics engages these competing voices, hoping to make some sense out of everything after having already gotten lost once before (Lather, 2007).[8] It is clear that a great deal is happening. We are beyond the arguments of even ten years ago. Critics are united by commitments to social justice. The arguments for and against data (new or old versions) are debated. New places are sought.

It is time to open up new spaces, time to explore new discourses. We need to find new ways of connecting people and their personal troubles with social justice methodologies. We need to become better accomplished in linking these interventions to those institutional sites where troubles are turned into public issues, and public issues transformed into social policy (Charmaz, 2005; Mills, 1959).

A critical framework modeled after C. Wright Mills (1959), Paulo Freire (2001), bell hooks (2005), and Cornel West (1989, 1991) is central to this project. It privileges practice, politics, action, consequences, performances, discourses, methodologies of the heart, pedagogies of hope, love, care, forgiveness, and healing (Pelias, 2004). It speaks for and with those who are on the margins. As a liberationist philosophy, it is committed to examining the consequences of racism, poverty, and sexism on the lives of interacting individuals (Seigfried, 1996).

It is therefore necessary to confront and work through the criticisms that continue to be directed to qualitative inquiry. Each generation must draw its line in the sand and take a stance toward the past. Each generation must articulate its epistemological, methodological, and ethical stance toward critical inquiry. Each generation must offer its responses to current and past criticisms.

Moving Forward

The agenda for the qualitative inquiry community in the next decade should be defined by the work that interpretive scholars do as they implement the above assumptions. These situations set the stage for qualitative research's transformations in the twenty-first century. As this occurs we anticipate a continued performance turn in qualitative inquiry, with writers performing their texts for others. All of this will likely take place within and against a complex historical field, a global war on terror, a third and fourth methodological movement, the beginning or end of a new moment (Denzin & Lincoln, 2005, p. 3).[9]

So, at the beginning of the second decade of the twenty-first century it is time to move forward. It is time to open up new spaces, time to explore new discourses. We need to find new ways of connecting people and their personal troubles with social justice methodologies. We need to become better accomplished in linking these interventions to those institutional sites where troubles are turned into public issues and public issues transformed into social policy.

A critical framework is central to this project. It privileges practice, politics, action, consequences, performances, discourses, methodologies of the heart, and pedagogies of hope, love, care, forgiveness, and healing. It speaks for and with those who are on the margins (Smith, 2012). As a liberationist philosophy, it is committed to examining the consequences of racism, poverty, and sexism on the lives of interacting individuals.

As part of this agenda, there needs to be a greater openness to alternative paradigm critiques. We need to work through the beliefs that organize our interpretive communities, including our theories of being (ontology), knowing (epistemology), inquiry (methodology), moral conduct (ethics), praxis, politics, truth, voice, and representation (see St. Pierre, 2011, for a critique of these terms). You can't just throw out the word "paradigm" because you don't like it (Lincoln, 2010).

Paradigm proliferation is alive and well, theoretical paradigms are not commensurable—you can't move easily from one to another. Some think quantitative and qualitative methods are not incompatible. Many people in the mixed, multiple, and emergent methods group believe this (Hesse-Biber & Leavy, 2008; Morse & Niehaus, 2009; but see Flick, 2014).

We disagree.

There needs to be a decline in conflict between alternative paradigm proponents. Paths for fruitful dialogue between and across paradigms need to be explored. This means there needs to be a greater openness to and celebration of the proliferation, inter-mingling, and confluence of paradigms and interpretive frameworks (Guba & Lincoln, 2005). Paradigms are beginning to intermingle—for example, participatory action theory and postmodernism, critical theory and critical pedagogy, critical race theory, and performance studies. Paradigm proponents are informing and influencing one another, exposing differences, confluences and controversies.

This is good.

Dominant paradigms *should* be subverted.

Scholars *should* be encouraged to embrace a militant particularism, individual paradigms that embody and reframe inquiry "as a healing process, as a process of being in the service of social justice and social change" (Dillard, 2006, p. 65).

The commensurability and incompatibility theses, as they apply to paradigms and methods, need to be revisited. What is gained and what is lost with these two theses? These two terms address the underlying philosophical foundations of a paradigm, from ontology to axiology, from epistemology to ethics, and from methodology to praxis. If you remove these terms, you lose the philosophical, reflexive cutting-edge that critical inquiry requires.

You can only critique a work from within its paradigm. It makes no sense to apply foundational-positivistic criteria to a poem, or to performance ethnography. In turn, performance criteria should not be applied to a piece of statistical analysis. The two projects rest on different politics of representation. To repeat, *differences in interpretive criteria must be honored.*

It is not easy moving from one interpretive paradigm or space to another; politics, emotions, identities, egos, biographies, reputations, and hard work are involved. New literatures have to be mastered. Old habits have to be let go of; new ways of thinking have to be learned. It can be a risky business moving from one paradigm to another. This movement from one paradigm commitment to another cannot be accomplished overnight. Time and effort will be required, at least as much as one might be willing to invest with a psychotherapist (Guba, 1990b).

The move between and across paradigmatic spaces also operates at the institutional, pedagogical level. Well thought-out, longer than one or two course sequences need to be institutionalized at the undergraduate and graduate student levels. Students need to be taught the languages and critical interpretive skills connected to words like paradigm, ethics, politics, writing, and performance.

Paradigm dominance involves control over graduate curriculums, recruitment, and funding, as well as faculty appointments and tenure. Strong academic departments encourage paradigm diversity. Excellence *within* a paradigm is the operative criterion. Fruitful dialogue is not only a possibility, it is a requirement if a democratic community is to flourish in the academy and within the qualitative inquiry community.

The Chapters

Putting together any kind of critical reader that presumes to speak to/for a field, especially one that is continually in flux and ever-contested, is not a trivial undertaking. That is especially true in this case, where the contents of this reader are drawn from the nine previous Congress volumes that collectively totaled roughly 120 chapters. As such, we necessarily had to make decisions about what to include and, perhaps more problematically, what *not* to include. In surveying the academic climate of the last decade (outlined above), it became clear to us that the four most prominent/important/recurring themes have been:

(I) Philosophy of Inquiry; (II) Politics of Evidence/Politics of Research; (III) Methodological Imperatives; and (IV) Indigenous and Decolonizing Interventions.

Having a firm grounding in the philosophy of inquiry is, for us, a key starting point. Too often, whether in published manuscripts or conference presentations, job talks or colloquia, we have seen a general lack of understanding concerning the philosophy of inquiry and various paradigmatic approaches to research—and what those approaches mean for being, living, asking, and knowing in the social world.[10] For example, as Giardina and Laurendeau elucidate (2013):

> Too often, we see folks speak in the language of 'doing' 'qualitative' research or 'doing' 'quantitative' research as if those are two distinct avenues to 'collecting' 'data' beyond treating such 'data' as 'numerical' or 'nonnumerical' (e.g., using interviews versus surveys conducted on a Likert scale). This dichotomy is fraught with problems, not the least of which is that it betrays a lack of concern with one's own epistemology and ontological grounding; a lack of understanding (or consideration) about the philosophy of science, the philosophy of inquiry. It is not a question of "qualitative" or "quantitative" research "strategies" that we should be concerning ourselves with; it is a question of theory and praxis, of (post-) positivist, humanist, critical theory, postmodernist, and poststructuralist paradigms, and what locating ourselves in (and in some instances, across) one (or more) of those paradigms means for the research act, for the questions we can ask (and whether it is we who should be determining those questions [see, for example, Fisette & Walton, 2014]), the questions we are unable to ask, the questions that are masked, the questions that get erased/privileged/confounded, and, most importantly, for the meanings that are said to be the results of our endeavors. (p. 242)

To that end, the chapters by Kamberelis and Dimitriadis, Christians, Maxwell, and St. Pierre direct attention to the philosophical underpinnings of social science research, presenting the reader with a historically informed and sophisticated set of arguments from which to strengthen his or her understanding of inquiry.

Additionally, as the politics of evidence and the politics of research are inextricably linked in the present moment—a moment in which all research conducted within it is undergirded by the status and consequence of neoliberalism—it is important that readers concern themselves with the debates surrounding such a politicized (and politicizing) space. For within it, knowledge has come to be treated as a commodity, funding councils (such as the National Science Foundation or National Institutes of Health in the United States) are increasingly turning in isolation to supporting 'gold standard,' evidence-based research (but whose evidence?), journals have become increasingly political in their editorial decision making, bureaucratic managerialism has supplanted shared faculty governance, and "universities exist not simply to educate, but also to sell education in a competitive market to customers who in the past were wrongly thought of as just scholars" (Furedi, 2002, pp. 34–35). Written from different disciplinary, geographic, and epistemological positions, the chapters by Janice Morse, Harry Torrance, Antjie Krog, Gloria Ladson-Billings, H. L. (Bud) Goodall, Jr., and Henry Giroux in this second section offer compelling insight into understanding—and ultimately challenging—such a contested landscape.

We have also witnessed new and innovative methodological approaches to research come to the forefront of critical scholarship in the last decade, either as a response to or as an outgrowth of the social, cultural, political, and economic conditions of the last decade. In Section III we thus highlight new developments related to interviewing, research in new/social media spaces, arts-based research, performance studies, and autoethnography. Although numerous different methodologies have highlighted the last decade of Congresses and volumes, we settled on the above approaches as they, for us, push us toward a kind of new performative cultural politics (see Giardina & Denzin, 2011)—toward a critical imagination that is radically democratic, pedagogical, and interventionist—a politics that dialogically inserts itself into the world, provoking conflict, curiosity, criticism, and reflection, and contributes to a public conversation—to a dialogic that puts the very notions of democracy and freedom, citizen, and patriot into play (Carey, 1997, pp. 208, 216). Contributions to this section from Svend Brinkmann, Annette Markham, D. Soyini Madison, Ronald Pelias, Cynthia Dillard, Charles Garoian, and Jean Halley both carve out new methods and, at the same time, enable us to enact (or at least envision) a radical democratic pedagogy (see Denzin, 2009).

The final section of the reader makes clear that we are engaged in a global project, one inflected with power imbalances, diverse epistemologies and ontologies, and innovation. This would include red pedagogy (see Grande, 2004), borderland-Mestizaje feminism (see Saavedra & Nymark, 2008), Kaupapa Māori (Bishop, this volume), and decolonizing (Smith, 2012) methodologies. Such work by Indigenous and decolonizing scholars over the last decade has forced scholars in the Global North to come to terms with the First World/colonial longings embedded within much of Western scholarship. Four of the key scholars in this regard—Linda Tuhiwai Smith, Margaret Kovach, César Cisneros Puebla, and Russell Bishop—contribute chapters to this section, offering a direct challenge to how we understand critical inquiry in the contemporary moment.

In the remainder of this introduction, we present summaries of each chapter in the four sections, as well as touch on the Coda and Epilogue, which point us forward toward the next decade.

Section I begins with George Kamberelis and Greg Dimitriadis ("Chronotopes of Human Science Inquiry"), who open this section by calling for a language of human science inquiry (chronotopes) that stretches across disciplines (education, sociology, anthropology, language studies), epistemologies (positivism, postpositivism, hermeneutics, poststructualism), and methodologies. By isolating four chronotopes—objectivism and representation; reading and interpretation; skepticism, conscientization, and praxis; and power/knowledge and defamiliarization—they underscore the complexity and tensions that currently define the field of qualitative inquiry.

Clifford G. Christians's chapter ("Natural Science and the Ethics of Resistance") follows, and continues in a similar philosophical direction as the previous chapter as he argues that the social sciences must reinvent themselves in qualitative terms after the humanities if they are to realize an ethics and politics of resistance. After first introducing notions of John Stuart Mill's philosophy of social science, value neutrality in the work of Max Weber, and the politics of institutional review boards (IBRs), Christians counters this positivistic frame and works forward to speak to the need for interpretive sufficiency in reinventing power and transforming IRBs with the goal of "enabling the humane transformation of the multiple spheres of community life." This social ethics of resistance, he argues, ultimately works to reintegrate human life with the moral order.

In the next chapter, Joseph A. Maxwell ("A Critical Realist Perspective for Qualitative Research") makes the case that critical realism can make important contributions to the critique of evidence-based research, contributions that are particularly relevant to—and supportive of—qualitative research. Working through arguments outlined by philosophers such as Andrew Abbott and Peter Achinstein, Maxwell argues for a dialogical, postmodern approach to evidence in qualitative research, "one that embraces contrary perspectives such as realism and constructivism, and uses these to gain a better understanding of the phenomena we study."

Elizabeth Adams St. Pierre's chapter ("Refusing Human Being in Humanist Qualitative Inquiry") brings Section I to a close. In it, she calls for the resurgence of postmodernism, a philosophically informed inquiry that will resist calls for scientifically-based forms of research. In so doing, she offers a powerful postmodern critique of conventional humanistic qualitative methodology and argues that it is time for qualitative inquiry to reinvent itself, to put under erasure all that has been accomplished, so that something different can be done—a "rigorous re-imagining of a capacious science that cannot be defined in advance and is never the same again."

Section II begins with Janice M. Morse's chapter ("The Politics of Evidence"), in which she criticizes the evidence-based (or scientifically-based) movement by showing its negative effects in the field of medical research. Morse demonstrates its narrow view of evidence and its myopic vision of health, and the effects such regulation has on research. She then calls for a new ethic of inquiry, what she calls the ultimate ethic—the ability to learn from past mistakes so as to maximize the positive effects of research on human beings.

In Harry Torrance's chapter ("Building Confidence in Qualitative Work: Engaging the Demands of Policy"), he discusses the articulation of evidence and politics in the contemporary moment. Reflecting on the mid-2000s situation in both the United States and the United Kingdom, Torrance begins by reviewing arguments for and against random clinical trials (RCTs) within the broad spectrum of educational research, particularly how they are enmeshed within policy-oriented discursive spaces. From there, he discusses some initial responses of the "qualitative research community," taking care to point out that this is a diverse and disunified arena comprised of numerous scholarly disciplines (for example, anthropology, psychology, social work, and so forth) and differently arrayed national contexts, each with its own applied research and policy settings (education, social work, health studies, and so forth). He goes on to focus specifically on responses within the United Kingdom, particularly the government Cabinet Office's commissioned report by the National Center for Social Research (*Quality in Qualitative Evaluation: A Framework for Assessing Research Evidence*), which, he argues, "comprise[s] a banal and inoperable set of standards which beg all the important questions of conducting and writing up qualitative fieldwork." He follows this examination of the UK context by next turning his attention to similar developments in the United States, such as those conducted under the auspices of the National Science Foundation or by scholarly associations such as the American Educational Researcher Association (AERA). He concludes by offering that we must be willing to engage with policymakers and draw them into the discussion in the pursuit of productive, organic relationships rather than retreating and becoming focused solely on "standards" and "frameworks."

Drawing from her work on the South African Truth and Reconciliation Commission (TRC), Antjie Krog ("In the Name of Human Rights") focuses on the rights of two groups: (1) those living in marginalized areas but who produce virtually on a daily basis intricate knowledge systems of survival, and (2) scholars coming from those marginalized places, but who can only enter the world of acknowledged knowledge in language not their own and within discourses based on foreign and estrange-ing structures. More specifically, Krog shows us the backstage processes of her collaborative work with one particulate individual who testified before the TRC (Mrs. Konile), addressing in the process questions of "academic authority" and voice, of whose voice carries authority to speak, and of the limitations of "disciplines" and "theory." She concludes by imploring us to find ways in which "the marginalized can enter our discourses on their own genres and their own terms so that we can learn to hear them."

Continuing with a focus on marginalized peoples, Gloria Ladson-Billings ("Educational Research in the Public Interest") presents a powerful critique of education policy and contemporary politics that weaves together a narrative of New Orleans (pre- and post-Katrina) with a discussion of its (mis-)educational legacies, poverty, and racial climate. In so doing, she argues that for education research to matter, it must not merely be about data points and effect size and career advancement, but about what kind of real difference such work can make in the lives of real people.

H. L. (Bud) Goodall, Jr., ("I Read the News Today, Oh Boy...: The War on Public Workers") keeps our focus on the political politics of research, presenting us with a stunning rebuke to the assault on public education in the United States (and elsewhere), especially in terms of funding, tenure, and the myth of the current professoriate as the "cultural elite." At the same time, Goodall challenges academics to quit "hiding behind the very traditions that are under attack" and to remember that we are "working-class intellectuals" whose very existence is at stake.

Henry A. Giroux ("Public Intellectuals Against the Neoliberal University") likewise engages with the current intersection of politics and research, as he offers a critical analysis of (North American) higher education under the throes of neoliberalism. He documents the need to reclaim our public institutions from private demands—demands that have turned universities into shopping malls and critical thought into market relations, and have cast civic education and democratic values off to the side. In so doing, he advocates for academics to once again take up the mantel of public intellectualism, rejecting "market-driven pedagogy" in favor of what Edward Said referred to as a "pedagogy of mindfulness," one that combines what Giroux sees as "rigor and clarity, on the one hand, with civic courage and political commitment, on the other."

Section III shifts the discussion of the volume to methodological imperatives of the research act. Svend Brinkmann's chapter ("Interviewing and the Production of the Conversational Self") opens the section, as he addresses the changing formulation of interviewing within a consumer society that is a *de facto* interview society. Viewing all human research as conversational at its core, Brinkmann reveals not only how "our interpersonal social reality is constituted by conversations," but also the self—the "processes of our lives." Pushing back against the growing notion that interviewing is either a passive recording of opinion or an empathetic entrée into someone else's life, he turns to the notion of the epistemic interview (in the vein of Socrates) and its ethical considerations, arguing that such is a most useful approach in the current context.

Keeping with this theme of developing trends in research, Annette Markham ("Remix Cultures, Remix Methods: Reframing Qualitative Inquiry for Social Media Contexts") situates qualitative inquiry in a digital age in which "we are witnessing a startling transformation in the way cultural knowledge is produced and how meaning is negotiated," which includes a "de-privileging of expert knowledge, decentralizing culture production, and unhooking cultural units of information from their origins." We might think of this as YouTube videos that mash together music, words, and video in forms of protest (as we saw in Egypt during the Tahrir Square protests or during the #Ferguson protests in Missouri following the murder of Michael Brown), crowdsourcing, and alternative forms of (noncommercial or noncorporate) journalism. To this end, she examines particular elements of (qualitative) remix that move us toward disrupting traditional ways and means of conducting research in and among digital culture and contexts.

D. Soyini Madison ("Dangerous Ethnography and Utopian Performatives") further grounds the researcher as an active part of the research act, as she illustrates the complex dynamics and contextual politics of researcher positionality, power, privilege, and safety during the conduct of ethnographic research in locales deemed to be quite literally "dangerous" environs. She begins by presenting three vignettes of 'danger,' then 'flips the script' and has us rethink the very idea of danger in the sense of "ourselves as being dangerous," of the researcher acting as an agent of danger in the pursuit of social justice. To this end, she locates the body in performance as the harbinger of danger in the pursuit of utopian performatives.

Related to the focus of the body in research, Ronald J. Pelias ("Performative Writing: The Ethics of Representation in Body and Form") inquires into the ethics of performance, first outlining its definitional complexities before identifying a number of ethical issues in regard to performative writing as a representational form. In so doing, he focuses his gaze most specifically on the embodied, the evocative, the partial, and the material forms. He closes with a resounding performative writing oath for ethical performative writing that embraces the risks associated with such writing in the name of a transformative vision of activism and social justice.

Cynthia B. Dillard ("Learning to Remember the Things We've Learned to Forget: Endarkened Feminisms and the Sacred Nature of Research") next directs our attention to the Global South, and draws on her engagements in Ghana, West Africa, as they relate to questions of race, memory, and identity. Utilizing the idea of the praisesong ("ceremonial and social poems, recited or sung in public at celebrations such as outdoorings or anniversaries or funerals"), Dillard calls on us to consider our very conception of self as it relates to our research practices, our very location *in* our research practices. Thus, her chapter serves as a resounding response to the challenges of living and researching within and against global crises.

Remaining with the arts-based research theme, Charles R. Garoian ("The Exquisite Corpse of Art-based Research") meditates on "educational research that more closely follows the imaginary and improvisational processes and practices of artists, poets, and musicians as compared with inquiry that is commonly associated with the logical-rational approaches in the sciences and social sciences." Engaging with an "Exquisite Corpse process" (or the collective assemblage words and images) for qualitative inquiry, Garoian addresses through five artistic examples how "fragmented research and practice" can enable creative and political agency.

Jean Halley's chapter ("The Death of a Cow") concludes this section, as she offers an autoethnographic account that explores the death of beef cows, and contrasts such deaths with the death of her childhood cat and the sadness in her childhood. She looks at the violence of such deaths, yes, but also in the ways that deaths are a move from one state to another, not only for the dying, but for all those involved in and surrounding death. Through her lyrical, repetitive writing style, she tries to capture the feel, the atmosphere and experience of these changes. Thus is the social history of beef ranching intertwined with both personal and political narratives on the production of life and death.

Section IV directs our attention to interventions with/in Indigenous and decolonizing research. Linda Tuhiwai Smith ("Choosing the Margins: The Role of Research in Indigenous Struggles for Social Justice") opens the section, discussing research in/on Indigenous communities, the assembly of those who have witnessed, have been excluded from, and have survived modernity and imperialism. She further examines the implications for indigenous researchers as they struggle to produce research knowledge that documents social justice, recovers subjugated knowledges, helps create voices of the silenced to speak, and challenges racism, colonialism, and oppression. Such indigenous research activity offers genuine utopian hope for creating and living in a more just and humane social world.

Margaret Kovach's chapter ("Thinking *Through* Theory: Contemplating Indigenous Situated Research and Policy") makes a forceful case that if the "Indigenous voice is not being heard in the research theory that shapes Indigenous policy development, whose voice, then, is being relied upon? How trustworthy is this voice in offering an accounting of Indigenous people's lives?" She turns to policy debates within Indigenous education as a clear example of the theory/research/policy dynamic in action. She concludes by positing how, more often than not, outsider theorizing in research and policy has diminished rather than upheld Indigenous peoples.

César Cisneros Puebla ("Indigenous Researchers and Epistemic Violence") presents us with an impassioned call for a "sociology of our own practices as researchers, as scientists, as persons of flesh and blood." Grounding himself in the modernity of his colonial past as a Latin American scholar, Cisneros Puebla argues that knowing more about ourselves in "historical, geopolitical, and epistemological views" is a major challenge, true, but that knowing more about ourselves is also a matter of "ethics and responsibilities." As such, he delves into discussions concerning core and peripheries in the 'knowledge divide'; specifically, the "historical consequence of the global dynamics of capitalism" that has divided the world into the core and the peripheries—including *researchers*. He then draws from a Mexican example that illustrates this "division of scientific labor in the context of globalized knowledge"; that of so-called "cover-science," or universalizing the local knowledge of 'great authors' of the Global North. Put differently, he critiques the practice of copying, drawing from, or otherwise importing of particular theoretical perspectives or traditions into another context (something, we might say, U.S. scholars did with British cultural studies in the 1990s). He concludes by arguing that "developing autochthonous research methods is decisive to overcome the epistemic...violence," as well as to "enrich our practices as researchers by getting into new ways of experiencing relationships and human interactions."

Russell Bishop's chapter ("Freeing Ourselves: An Indigenous Response to Neo-colonial Dominance in Research, Classrooms, Schools, and Education Systems") concludes this section, as he "demonstrates how theorizing and practice that [have] grown from within Māori epistemologies [have] been applied in a number of settings as counter-narratives to the dominant discourses in New Zealand." He does so by elaborating Kaupapa Māori research examples, such as the "centrality of the process of establishing extending family-like relationships, understood in Māori as *whanaungatanga*," and how such research was then translated to classroom settings in mainstream schools. He then discusses how 'scaling-up' Indigenous-based education reform may hold the promise for "freeing public schools and the education system that supports them from neo-colonial dominance."

Laura L. Ellingson's essay ("Are You Serious? Playing, Performing, and Producing an Academic Life") serves as a coda to the reader, in which she powerfully suggests that researchers need to find room among our seriousness for the "play" of research. She goes on to detail the "passion and pleasure" we might endeavor to locate within our research acts; the "playful immersion" (or deep attention) we might find within our analysis of empirical material; the possibilities heralded by "playing outside the box" (or being creative) with research design; the deploying of the notions of "the trickster" and "playing the fool" (or active performer) to subvert and rethink boundaries; and, methodologically speaking, the assuming of the role of an epistemic player who takes pleasure from multiplicity (that is, one who moves freely among methodological and epistemological possibilities). Ellingson reminds us of the productive place of "play" and how we might use it to our benefit in spite of the rigid and serious boundaries in our professional midst.

As an epilogue of sorts, Michael D. Giardina, Norman K. Denzin, Elizabeth Adams St. Pierre, Svend Brinkmann, Maria del Consuelo Chapela Mendoza, Christopher Poulos, and Marcelo Diversi present a 'coversation' about the past, present, and future of qualitative inquiry, drawing from their diverse locations in the academy to point toward the passions, possibilities, complexities, and contradictions in the current climate of qualitative inquiry.

Coda

We come in many different forms.[11] We are global, we are interpretivists, we are postmodernists, poststructuralists, we are postmaterialists, and critical feminists. We choose lenses that are border, racial–ethnic, hybrid, queer, differently abled, indigenous, margin, center (Lincoln, 2010). We are a global, moral community, a complex network of committed interpretive scholars. It is for this community, stealing a line from Ernest Hemingway (1940), that the bell tolls, for whom this discourse is written. It has been nearly 25 years since Guba (1990b) enumerated emergent themes and agenda items for the international constructivist community. We believe Guba's themes and agenda items can guide us today:

Agenda Items

The Intellectual Agenda

The global community of qualitative inquiry needs annual events where it can deal with the problems and issues that the community confronts at this historical moment. These events should be international, national, regional, and local. They can be held in conjunction with "universities, school systems, health care systems, juvenile justice systems, and the like" (Guba, 1990b, p. 376).

The issues and problems are many and revolve around the following: the implementation of a social justice framework in an increasingly hostile environment; dialogue, conflict, and controversy surrounding interpretive frameworks, paradigms, and their epistemologies and methodologies; the articulation of a transdisciplinary, empowerment ethical mode; an agreed upon set of interpretive, poetic, political, and artistic criteria, which can be applied to any form of critical qualitative inquiry.

The Advocacy Agenda

The community needs to develop "systematic contacts with political figures, the media …, the professional press and with practitioners such as teachers, health workers, social workers, [and] government functionaries" (Guba, 1990b, p. 376). Advocacy includes the following: (a) showing how qualitative work addresses issues of social policy; (b) critiquing federally mandated ethical guidelines for human subject research; and (c) critiquing outdated, positivist modes of science and research.

The Operational Agenda

Qualitative researchers are encouraged to engage in self-learning, and self-criticism, to re-socialize themselves. Their goals should include building productive relationships with professional associations, journals, policy makers, and funders (Guba, 1990b). Representatives from many different professional associations—the American Educational Research Association, the American Sociological Association, the American Anthropological Association, and so on—need to be brought together.

To these we add an additional item.

The Ethical Agenda

The qualitative inquiry community needs an empowerment code of ethics that cross-cuts disciplines, honors Indigenous voices, implements the values of love, care, compassion, community, spirituality, praxis, and social justice.

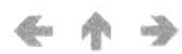

A common ground can be found, a global meeting place. We all want social justice. Many of us want to influence social policy. All of us—positivists, postpositivists, post-structuralists, post-humanists, feminists, queer theorists, social workers, nurses, sociologists, educators, and anthropologists—share this common commitment, in some form or another.

Turning against one another, criticizing one another's writing style or language, or debunking another's paradigm will not move any of us any closer to this goal. We are all bricoleurs, trained to use whatever resource or method is at hand to accomplish a socially worthwhile goal. If we work back from the consequences of our actions to these goals and intentions, then there is no cause for alarm. The meaning of an interpretation lies in its ability to make life better for a person, or a group of persons. We can live side-by-side under a big tent, postpositivists and interpreters, if, as pragmatists in the William James (1909) tradition, we abide by this simple pragmatic maxim. In this way, we can begin to implement a truly global social justice agenda.

We have a job to do; let's get to it.

Notes

1 Denzin is at the University of Illinois; Giardina is now at Florida State University.

2 The Congress has grown in numbers from roughly 500 attendees that first year to more than 1,300 in year ten—with delegates representing upwards of 50 countries.

3 The previous nine titles are: *Qualitative Inquiry and the Conservative Challenge* (2006); *Ethical Futures in Qualitative Research* (2007); *Qualitative Inquiry and the Politics of Evidence* (2008); *Qualitative Inquiry and Social Justice* (2009); *Qualitative Inquiry and Human Rights* (2010); *Qualitative Inquiry and Global Crises* (2011); *Qualitative Research and the Politics of Advocacy* (2012); *Global Dimensions of Qualitative Research* (2013); and *Qualitative Research Outside the Academy* (2014). A tenth volume, *Qualitative Research and the Politics of Research*, is forthcoming in 2015.

4 This section is drawn directly from Denzin (2014).

5 This section draws from Denzin (2010, pp. 101–103).

6 In a related piece in which she frames data as a "vital illusion," Koro-Ljungberg (2013) similarly makes the case that "Data is a proxy or anti-substance, a real that never really is because it is always a reproduction of something that escapes itself as being constructed" (p. 1). She continues:

> Data's meaning is only illustrative; data has no meaning since it has all possible meanings. Data is deprived of its meaning by its own escape. There is no more real data, just reproductions and probabilities of data since data may only signify ontological absence from itself. Instead, data could be conceptualized as an image of the believed real, imagined signifier, or manufactured sign of experience—a vital illusion.... By assigning meanings to objects and signifiers, data is produced, consumed, admired, collected, validated, interpreted, constructed, and destroyed, *but data is not necessarily ontologically related to the Real.* (p. 2, emphasis ours)

7 Complicit, too, are those who call for the use of computer-assisted qualitative data analysis software (CAQDAS; see Davidson & di Gregorio, 2011, p. 627).

8 This is not the radical mixed-methods middle outlined by Onwuegbuzie (2012).

9 Mixed methods research is Teddlie and Tashakkori's third movement or moment. The first movement is quantitative research, and the second is qualitative inquiry. The third movement offers a middle ground that mediates quantitative and qualitative disputes (see Teddlie & Tashakkori, 2003a, p. x; 2003b, pp. 4–9).

10 This should not be surprising, for far too increasingly students are not exposed to the philosophical debates concerning inquiry, research paradigms, and so forth in any real depth at the graduate level.

11 This section is drawn directly from Denzin (2014)

References

Benozza, A., Bell, H., & Koro-Ljungberg, M. (2013). Moving between nuisance, secrets, and splinters as data. *Cultural Studies⇔Critical Methodologies, 13*(4), 309–315.

Bloom. L. (2009). Introduction: Global perspectives on poverty and social justice. *International Journal of Qualitative Studies in Education, 22*(3), 253–261.

Carey, J. (1997). "A republic, if you can keep it": Liberty and public life in the age of Glasnost. In E. Munson & C. Warren (Eds.), *James Carey: A critical reader* (pp. 207–227). Minneapolis: University of Minnesota Press.

Charmaz, K. (2005). Scrutinizing standards: Convergent questions in medical practice and qualitative inquiry. *Symbolic Interaction, 28*(2), 281–289.

Clark, M. C., & Scheurich, J. J. (2008). Editorial: The state of qualitative research in the early twenty-first century—Take 2. *International Journal of Qualitative Studies in Education, 21*, 313.

Davidson, J., & di Gregorio, S. (2011). Qualitative research and technology in the midst of a revolution. In N. K. Denzin & Y. S. Lincoln (Eds.). *The SAGE handbook of qualitative research* (pp. 627– 643), 4/e. Thousand Oaks, CA: Sage.

Denzin, N. K. (2004). *The qualitative manifesto: A call to arms.* Walnut Creek, CA: Left Coast Press, Inc.

Denzin, N. K. (2009). Critical pedagogy and democratic life, or, a radical democratic pedagogy. *Cultural Studies⇔Critical Methodologies, 9*(3), 379–397.

Denzin, N. K. (2013). The death of data. *Cultural Studies ⇔ Critical Methodologies, 13*(4), 353–356.

Denzin, N. K. (2014). Reading the challenges of a global community and the sociological imagination. *Qualitative Inquiry, 20*(9), 1122–1127.

Denzin, N. K., & Lincoln, Y. S. (2005) Introduction: The discipline and practice of qualitative research. In N. K. Denzin & Y. S. Lincoln (Eds.), *The SAGE handbook of qualitative research* (pp. 1–32), 3/e. Thousand Oaks, CA: Sage.

Dillard, C. B. (2006). When the music changes, so should the dance: Cultural and spiritual considerations in paradigm "proliferation." *International Journal of Qualitative Studies in Education, 19*, 59–76.

Fisette, J., & Walton, T. (2014). 'If you really knew me' ... I am empowered through action. *Sport, Education, and Society, 19*(2), 131–152.

Flick, U. (2014). Challenges for qualitative inquiry as a global endeavor: Introduction to the special issue. *Qualitative Inquiry, 20*(9), 1059–1063.

Freire, P. (2001). *Pedagogy of the oppressed: With an introduction by Donaldo Macedo* (30th anniversary ed.). New York: Continuum.

Furedi, F. (2002). The bureaucratization of the British university. In D. Hayes & R. Wynward (Eds.), *The McDonaldization of higher education* (pp. 33–42). Westport, CT: Bergin & Garvey.

Gage, N. L. (1989). The paradigm wars and their aftermath: A "historical sketch" of research and teaching since 1989. *Educational Researcher, 18*(7), 4–10.

Garoian, C. R., & Gaudelius, Y. M. (2008). *Spectacle pedagogy: Art, politics and visual culture.* Albany, NY: SUNY Press.

Giardina, M. D., & Denzin, N. K. (2011). Acts of activism⇔Politics of possibility: Toward a new performative cultural politics. *Cultural Studies⇔Critical Methodologies, 11*(4), 319–327.

Giardina, M. D., & Laurendeau, J. (2013). Truth untold? Evidence, knowledge, and research practice(s). *Sociology of Sport Journal, 30*(3), 237–255.

Giroux, H. A. (2009). Academic labor in dark times. *CounterPunch.* Retrieved December 5, 2014, from www.counterpunch.org/2009/03/11/academic-labor-in-dark-times/

Grande, S. (2004). *Red pedagogy: Native American social and political thought.* Lanham, MD: Rowman & Littlefield.

Guba, E. (Ed.) (1990a).(Ed.), *The paradigm dialog.* Thousand Oaks, CA: Sage.

Guba, E. (1990b). Carrying on the dialog. In E. Guba (Ed.), *The paradigm dialog* (pp. 368–378). Thousand Oaks, CA: Sage..

Guba, E., & Lincoln, Y. S. (2005). Paradigmatic controversies, and emerging confluences. In N. Denzin & Y. Lincoln (Eds.), *Handbook of qualitative research* (3rd ed., pp. 191–216). Thousand Oaks, CA: Sage.

Hemingway, E. (1940). *For whom the bell tolls.* New York: Charles Scribner's Sons.

Hesse-Biber, S. N., & Leavy, P. (2008). Introduction: Pushing on the methodological boundaries—The growing need for emergent methods within and across the disciplines. In S. N. Hess-Biber & P. Leavy (Eds.), *Handbook of emergent methods* (pp. 1–15). New York: Guilford Press.

hooks, b. (2005). *Soul sister: Women, friendship, and fulfillment.* Boston: South End Press.

Howe, K. R. (1988). Against the quantitative-qualitative incompatibility theses, or, dogmas die hard. *Educational Researcher, 17*(8), 10–16.

Jackson, A. Y., & Mazzei, L. A. (2009). *Voice in qualitative inquiry: Challenging conventional, interpretive, and critical conceptions in qualitative research.* London: Routledge.

Jackson, A. Y., & Mazzei, L. A. (2012). *Thinking with theory in qualitative research: Viewing data across multiple perspectives.* London: Routledge.

James, W. (1909). *The meaning of truth.* New York: Longmans.

Koro-Ljungberg, M. (2010). Validity, responsibility and aporia. *Qualitative Inquiry, 16*(8), 603–610.

Koro-Ljungberg, M. (2013). "Data" as vital illusion. *Cultural Studies ⇔ Critical Methodologies, 13*(4), 274–278.

Lather, P. (2007). *Getting lost: Feminist efforts toward a double(d) science*. Albany, NY: SUNY Press.

Lincoln, Y. S. (2010). "What a long, strange trip it's been . . .": 25 Years of qualitative and new paradigm research. *Qualitative Inquiry, 16*, 3–9.

MacLure, M. (2009). Broken voices, dirty words: On the productive insufficiency of voice. In A. Y. Jackson & L. A. Mazzei (Eds.), *Voice in qualitative inquiry: Challenging conventional, interpretive, and critical conceptions in qualitative research* (pp. 97–114). London: Routledge.

MacLure, M. (2011). Qualitative inquiry: Where are the ruins? *Qualitative Inquiry, 17*(10), 997–1005.

Madison, S. D. (2010). *Acts as activism: Human Rights as radical performance*. New York: Cambridge University Press.

Maxwell, J. A. (2004). Reemergent scientism, postmodernism, and dialogue across differences. *Qualitative Inquiry, 10*(1), 35–41.

Mertens, D. M., Holmes, H. M., & Harris, R. L. (2009). Transformative research and ethics. In D. M. Mertens & P. E. Ginsberg (Eds.), *The handbook of social research ethics* (pp. 85–101). Thousand Oaks, CA: Sage.

Mervis, J. (2014, October 2). Battle between NSF and House science committee escalates: How did it get this bad? *Science*. Retrieved December 5, 2014, from news.sciencemag.org/policy/2014/10/battle-between-nsf-and-house-science-committee-escalates-how-did-it-get-bad

Mills, C. W. (1959). *The sociological imagination*. New York: Oxford University Press.

Morse, J. M., & Niehaus, L. (2009). *Mixed method design: Principles and procedures*. Walnut Creek, CA: Left Coast Press, Inc.

Onwuegbuzie, A. I. (2012). Introduction: Putting the MIXED back into quantitative and qualitative research in educational research and beyond: Moving toward the radical middle. *International Journal of Multiple Research Approaches, 6*(3), 192–219.

Pelias, R. J. (2004). *A methodology of the heart*. Walnut Creek, CA: AltaMira Press.

Richardson, L. (2000). Writing: A method of inquiry. In N. K. Denzin & Y. S. Lincoln (Eds.), *The handbook of qualitative research* (pp._923–948), 2/e. Thousand Oaks: Sage.

Saavedra, C., & Nymark, E. D. (2008). Borderland-mestizaje feminism: The new tribalism. In N. K. Denzin, Y. S. Lincoln, & L. T. Smith (Eds.),

The SAGE handbook of critical and Indigenous methodologies (pp. 255–276). Thousand Oaks, CA: Sage.

Scheurich, J. J., & Clark, M. C. (2006). Qualitative studies in education at the beginning of the twenty-first century. *International Journal of Qualitative Studies in Education, 19*, 401.

Seigfried, C. H. (1996). *Pragmatism and feminism*. Chicago: University of Chicago Press.

Shavelson, R. J., & Towne, L. (Eds.). *Scientific research in education*. Washington, DC: National Academy Press.

Smith, L. T. (2012). *Decolonizing methodologies: Research and Indigenous peoples*, 2/e. London: Zed Books.

St. Pierre, E. A. (2011). Post qualitative research: The critique and the coming after. In N. K. Denzin & Y. S. Lincoln (Eds.), *The SAGE handbook of qualitative research* (pp. 611–626), 4/e. Thousand Oaks, CA: Sage.

St. Pierre, E. A. (2013). The appearance of data. *Cultural Studies ⇔ Critical Methodologies, 13*(4), 223–227.

St. Pierre, E. A., & Pillow, W. (Eds.). (2000). *Working the ruins: Feminist poststructural methods in education*. New York: Routledge.

Stronach, I., Garratt, D., Pearce, C., & Piper, H. (2007). Reflexivity, the picturing of selves, the forging of method. *Qualitative Inquiry, 13*(2), 179–203.

Teddlie, C., & Tashakkori, A. (2003a). Preface. In A. Tashakkori & C. Teddlie (Eds.), *Handbook of mixed-methods in social and behavioral research* (pp. ix–xv). Thousand Oaks, CA: Sage

Teddlie, C., & Tashakkori, A. (2003b). Major issues and controversies in the use of mixed methods in the social and behavioral sciences. In A. Tashakkori & C. Teddlie (Eds.), *Handbook of mixed-methods in social and behavioral research* (pp. 3–50). Thousand Oaks, CA: Sage.

Teddlie, C., & Tashakkori, A. (2011). Mixed methods research. In N. K. Denzin & Y. S. Lincoln (Eds.), *Handbook of qualitative research* (4th ed., pp. 285–299). Thousand Oaks, CA: Sage.

Weems, M. (2002). *I speak from the wound in my mouth*. New York: Peter Lang.

West, C. (1989). *The American evasion of philosophy: A genealogy of pragmatism*. Madison: University of Wisconsin Press.

West, C. (1991). Theory, pragmatisms and politics. In J. Arac & B. Johnson (Eds.), *Consequences of theory* (pp. 22–38). Baltimore, MD: Johns Hopkins University Press.

Section 1

Philosophy of Inquiry

Chapter 2

Chronotopes of Human Science Inquiry

George Kamberelis
Greg Dimitriadis

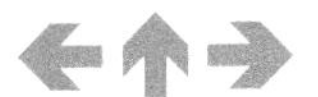

In this chapter, we hope to add to a growing "complicated conversation" (Pinar, 2004) about qualitative research methods. We argue for a language that can work across and through multiple approaches in sophisticated and nuanced ways, in ways that can open a more nuanced discussion that might enable truly inter- and multimethodological approaches. Specifically, we offer an account of what we see to be the prevalent *chronotopes* of inquiry that ground and inform most qualitative research (and the social sciences generally). Our task is akin to the one undertaken by Birdwhistell (1977) in response to his students' queries about whether Margaret Mead and Gregory Bateson had a methodology. These queries led Birdwhistell to argue that theory-method complexes, which he termed "logics-of-inquiry," guide all research.

Our task is also similar to Strike's (1974) construct of "expressive potential." Strike argued that all research endeavors are governed by an expressive potential that delimits the objects worthy of investigation, the research questions that may be asked, the units of analysis that are relevant, the analyses that may be conducted, the claims that may be made about the objects of

Originally published in *Qualitative Inquiry and the Conservative Challenge*, edited by Norman K. Denzin and Michael D. Giardina, pp.3–30. © 2006 Left Coast Press, Inc., Walnut Creek, CA. Republished in *Qualitative Inquiry—Past, Present, and Future: A Critical Reader*, edited by Norman K. Denzin and Michael D. Giardina, pp. 41–68 Left Coast Press, Inc. All rights reserved.

investigation, and the forms of explanation that may be invoked. We argue here for a new language that can be used to talk across a range of disciplinary and methodological approaches, from ethnography to genealogy and rhizomatics. In working toward such a language, we highlight both the possibilities and dangers of this moment of meta-disciplinary coalescence. Informed by this, we close by offering a new metaphor for the qualitative researcher—that of the genealogist.

Why Chronotopes?

Although similar to "logics-of-inquiry" or "expressive potentials," the construct of chronotopes of inquiry also extends these constructs in important ways. To the best of our knowledge, Bakhtin (1981) borrowed the term "chronotope," which literally means "time-space," from Einstein and applied it to the study of language and literature For Bakhtin, chronotopes do not simply link particular times and spaces with specific cultural events. Instead, they delineate or construct sedimentations of concrete, motivated social situations or figured worlds (Holland et al., 1998) replete with typified plots, themes, agents, forms of agency, scenes, objects, affective dispositions, kinds of intentionality, ideologies, value orientations, and so on. In this regard, chronotopes are like "x-rays of the forces at work in the culture system from which they spring" (Bakhtin, 1981, pp. 425–426).

Chronotopes are normalizing frames that render the world as "just the way things are" by celebrating the prosaic regularities that make any given world, day after day, recognizable and predictable for the people who live in it (Morson & Emerson, 1990, p. 87). They connote specific ways to understand context and the actions, agents, events, and practices that constitute those contexts. Bakhtin was clear about the fact that chronotopes are not a priori structures but durable structuring structures (e.g., Bourdieu, 1990; Giddens, 1979) constituted within concrete histories of human activity across time and space. Among the ways in which he illustrated this idea was to show how the public square in ancient Greece or the family at the height of the Roman Empire were constitutively related to specific modes of rhetorical and literary activity common to those time-spaces.

Chronotopes are a lot like what cultural studies scholars (e.g., Grossberg, 1992; Hall, 1992; Hebdidge, 1979; Willis, 1977) refer to as cultural formations—historically formed/informed and socially distributed modes of engagement with particular sets of practices for particular reasons. Chronotopes describe the lines of force that locate, distribute, and connect specific sets of practices, effects, goals, and groups of actors. Such articulations not only involve selections and configurations from among the available practices, but also a distribution of the chronotopes themselves within and across social time and space. To understand and describe a chronotope requires a reconstruction of its context—the dispersed yet structured field of objects, practices, agents, and so on by which the specific articulation reproduces itself across time and space. Chronotopic assertions are thus "strategems" of genealogy. All chronotopes have their own "common cultural sense," "sensibilities," "tastes," "logics," and so on. These dimensions of being become embodied in the people who work within a chronotope such that they become part of the chronotope itself. What seems natural, proper, and obvious to individuals becomes aligned with what is the "common cultural sense" within the chronotope. For our purposes, then, *chronotopes of qualitative inquiry index durable historical realities that constitute what is common, natural, and expected by collectives of social scientists who conduct particular kinds of qualitative research.*

Although other scholars might argue for slightly fewer or slightly more, we focus on four primary chronotopes of inquiry currently operating in powerful and pervasive ways within the contemporary scene of educational research, especially in relation to literacy studies. We settled on the following "names" for the chronotopes that we believe most commonly ground qualitative inquiry within education and literacy studies:

1. Objectivism and Representation
2. Reading and Interpretation
3. Skepticism, Conscientization, and Praxis
4. Power/Knowledge and Defamiliarization

All four chronotopes engage with the Enlightenment project, but in different ways—some more resonantly and some more dissonantly. Each chronotope embodies a different set of assumptions about the world, knowledge, the human subject, language, and meaning. Each also embodies or indexes a particular set of approaches/methods for framing and conducting research. Finally, in different ways and to different degrees, each has exerted considerable power in sustaining and reproducing particular logics of inquiry within our field and within the larger world of the social sciences. We propose this loosely coupled taxonomy simply as a heuristic for understanding some of the different ways in which qualitative inquiry is typically framed and how different frameworks predispose researchers to embrace different epistemologies, theories, approaches, and strategies.

Chronotope I: Objectivism and Representation

Perhaps the roots of this chronotope extend back to early critiques of "correspondence theories of truth" and a "logics of verification" that inhabited representational approaches to research in anthropology and philosophy (e.g., Clifford & Marcus, 1986; Rorty, 1979). "Correspondence theories of truth" posit the possibility of directly and unproblematically mapping symbolic representations onto the facts in the world in a one-to-one fashion. Approaches driven by "correspondence theories of truth" derive from Descartes's dualism of mind and body and have become all but synonymous with the scientific method. This dualism renders the individual human subject as radically separate from the external world but able to know this world through reflection and thought. A variety of methods and research tools have been developed within the chronotope of objectivism and representation. These methods and tools are predicated on the inviolability of the mind-body binary. Language is construed as a neutral medium for accurately *representing* observed relations in the external world.

A considerable amount of the qualitative research that is conducted in the field of language and literacy, for example, fits comfortably within the chronotope of objectivism and representation. E. D. Hirsch's (1987) work on cultural literacy is one example. Within a cultural literacy framework, it is assumed that there is a neutral canon of key cultural knowledge that all students should know. It is also assumed that this body of knowledge exists outside of the individual subject and can be learned, usually through direct instruction and study. This neutral body of knowledge is transmitted to individual subjects through the neutral medium of Standard English. Finally, Hirsch asserts that if students lack a particular and prescribed set of cultural knowledge, they will be unable to read and write adequately and to function productively in society. The cultural knowledge that Hirsch has in mind is presumed to be "common culture," not elite culture, even though it derives primarily from canonical works within a white, European American, middle- to upper-class heterosexist tradition.

Knowledge here is considered to be entirely separate from power relations or any other dimensions of context. A radical separation of subject and object is assumed. Language and literacy practices are assumed to be neutral vehicles for representing equally neutral facts. The real world and talking or writing about the real world are held radically separate. The idea that language and literacy might be able to shape and constitute thought, practice, or circulation of power is eclipsed. Such a construal renders language and literacy practices as little more than conduits or vehicles for preexistent thoughts or conditions, and it occludes the idea that such practices have ontological substance and constitutive power themselves. Questions about whether our relations with and within the world are at least partially constituted by language and literacy practices become unimportant. Little, if any, conceptual room is allocated for political praxis or social change through language and literacy practices because fact and value are believed to be independent of each other. Instead, language and literacy practices are evaluated according to their relative *effectiveness* in representing a priori cognitive or communicative entities or events. Positing effectiveness as a primary (or sole) evaluative criterion galvanizes the tendency to view language and literacy as little more than simple conduits for communicating established perspectives or existing sets of conditions, and it eclipses processes of imagining the constitutive roles that these practices might play in the construction of knowledges, identities, and fields of social practice.

Accepting the separation of subject and object or language and world as "given" or "natural" positions the field of language and literacy studies as a second-order field of inquiry that is de facto subservient to more legitimate fields and dependent on their theories and methods for its existence. It is not surprising, then, that many of the constructs and methods deployed within research on language and literacy conducted within the chronotope of objectivism and representation derive from other disciplines such as psychology (e.g., schema, motivation), sociology (e.g., symbolic interactionism, conversation analysis), anthropology (e.g., speech event, participant observation) or literary studies (e.g., reader response, genre studies). By drawing heavily on conceptual frameworks developed in other fields (especially psychology), research agendas often focus not on actual language and literacy practices but on internal or hidden variables such as readers' motivations (e.g., Turner, 1995) or writers' intentions (e.g., Flower & Hayes, 1981). When language and literacy research are located within the chronotope of objectivism and representation, one wonders exactly what language and literacy practices are involved and where they can be found. Are the reasons for practices always to be found outside of the practices themselves—in some hidden or deep structures or an Oz behind the curtain? Is nothing important evident in the surface of things? As we move through the discussions of all four chronotopes, we will show how actual, observable practices have become increasingly important as legitimate resources for explaining the nature and functions of language and literacy activities. And their increasing legitimation as both data and interpretive/explanatory resources has presented serious challenges to canonical ways of thinking about qualitative research practice.

Chronotope II: Reading and Interpretation

Not all approaches to research conducted within a modernist framework adhere to positivist epistemologies and their attendant assumptions. One framework that is modernist but not positivist is what we call the chronotope of reading and interpretation. Grounded in social constructionist epistemologies, this chronotope is not predicated on a complete rejection of Enlightenment perspectives on knowledge, rationality, and truth, but it does rearticulate these perspectives to render knowledge, truth, and rationality as relative (or perspectival) rather than absolute. Such a move rescues these constructs from the hegemonic clutches of scientism and instrumental reasoning without jettisoning these perspectives altogether. Knowledge, reason, and truth are no longer conceived as the representational mirroring (through language and other semiotic media) of an already existing world. Instead, knowledge, reason, and truth are believed to be constructed through the symbolic acts of human beings in relation to the world and to others (e.g., Heidegger, 1962; Rorty, 1979). Concomitantly, science is no longer about verification within a correspondence theory of truth but about human interaction, communication, dialogue, and reasoned argument.

Modernism, then, embraces not only scientistic modes of reason grounded in objectivist epistemologies but also modes of reason that are linguistically (or semiotically) mediated and grounded in the experience of "being-in-the-world." As we noted earlier, chronotopes are fluid, leaky, and flexible, and it is possible to have both objectivist-modernist articulations as well as interpretive-modernist ones. From this perspective, the existence of a real world external to human subjects is assumed, but faith in the timeless, universal nature of the world-knowledge relation and thus the possibility of generating representations that map that world in absolute or foundational terms is rejected.

This shift from "brute facts" to semiotically mediated facts is far from trivial. Among other things, it marks the need to replace a correspondence theory of truth with a consensus theory of truth, which implies a human discourse community as the arbiter of knowledge and truth claims. Gadamer's (1972) work is instructive here. Gadamer argued that truth does not emerge through the application of technical tools or methods but within and through embodied engagement within a "horizon" of experience within a human community. He went even further to claim that truth will always elude capture by technical methods because knowledge is always semiotically and dialogically constructed. Truth is never an act of reproduction but always an act of production within the limited horizon of a community's texts and meanings. Because knowledge (and thus truth) always emerges out of the embodied, rich, and messy process of being-in-the-world, it is always perspectival and conditional.

Within the chronotope of reading and interpretation, the subject-object dualism of the Enlightenment project is also assumed, but subject and object are placed in dialogic tension. This tension is a hallmark of philosophical hermeneutics, which is the foundation (i.e., antifoundation) on which the chronotope of reading and interpretation was built. The term "hermeneutics" derives from the Greek word hermeneuein with its obvious linkages to Hermes, the fleet-footed messenger of the gods. This derivation would suggest, then, that the origins of the chronotope of reading and interpretation lie in early Greek thought. Most philosophers of science and social theorists, however, usually place the beginnings of the chronotope reading and interpretation in nineteenth-century German philosophy, especially the work of Schleiermacher and Dilthey.

Although the term *verstehen* is often used as a generic term for interpretive social science, Dilthey (1976/1900) has been credited with developing a specific verstehen approach to understanding. This approach basically refers to the process of understanding from another subject's point of view. The verstehen approach, according to Dilthey, is achieved through the psychological reenactment or imaginative reconstruction of the experiences of others. In other words, it is intersubjectivity achieved basically through empathy. The extreme psychologism of Dilthey's position has been challenged and tempered by other philosophers including Husserl, Heidegger, and Gadamer.

Most contemporary uses of the term "hermeneutics" refer to the general process of coming to understand a phenomenon of interest (e.g., text, experience, social activity) or constructing an interpretation of such a phenomenon without placing such a heavy burden on intersubjectivity through empathy. Instead, hermeneutic or interpretive inquires are predicated on understanding meanings and practices in relation to the situations in which they occur. Such modes of inquiry draw on the notion of the "hermeneutic circle" as a unique and powerful strategy for understanding and knowledge building. Using this strategy, understanding the "part" (a text, an act, a person) always involves also understanding the whole (the context, the activity setting, the life history) and vice versa.

Heavily influenced by this notion of the hermeneutic circle, qualitative inquiry conducted within the chronotope of reading and interpretation does not aim to generate foundational knowledge claims. Instead, it aims to refine and deepen our sense of what it means to understand other people and their social practices (including language and literacy practices) within relevant contexts of interaction and communication. Put in philosophical terms, these forms of inquiry link the Enlightenment or modernist project of discovering knowledge with a genuine interest in understanding and enriching the "life worlds" (Habermas, 1987) or "lived experience" of others (i.e., our research participants). Researchers operating within a chronotope of reading and interpretation espouse a linguistically mediated view of existence and knowledge wherein both are constituted (and not just represented) in and through human language practices. They study language practices such as conversation, storytelling, disciplinary writing, and the like in order to reveal and understand the contexts and ontologies that they index.

Although the historical roots of the chronotope of reading and interpretation may be traced to nineteenth-century German philosophy, it has grown exponentially during the past two decades. Interestingly, and a bit ironically, this trend was not particularly visible in the major language and literacy journals until just a few years ago, even though it has been quite visible in journals from allied disciplines (e.g., *Anthropology and Education Quarterly*, *International Journal of Qualitative Studies in Education*). It has also been quite visible for some time within dissertations, presentations at professional literacy conferences, and books. The fact that research conducted within the chronotope of reading and interpretation was resisted in our mainstream journals and had to be smuggled into our field through less mainstream venues is testimony to the powerful, pervasive, and long-lasting grip that the chronotope of objectivism and representation has had and still has on qualitative inquiry in our field. Nevertheless, the chronotope of reading and interpretation has managed finally to become a force to be reckoned with in research on language and literacy.

Among the earliest and most durable instances of literacy research representing this force grew out of the ethnography of communication (EOC) tradition, with its focus on the relations among language, community, and identity. Shirley Brice Heath's (1983) now classic *Ways with Words* is one of the best exemplars of this tradition.

In outlining the research strategies she used to conduct the research for her book, Heath (1982) virtually recreated earlier descriptions of the hermeneutic circle, arguing that her research involved "the collection of artifacts of literacy, descriptions of contexts of uses, and their spatial and temporal distribution within the life of members of the community" (p. 47). She went on to claim that she studied how people used literacy artifacts, the activities and events within which the artifacts were used, whether links were made between symbolic representations and their real-world equivalents, how artifacts were presented to children, and what children then did with them (p. 47). Clearly, she came to understand parts in relation to wholes and vice versa.

A central question that motivated Heath's research was "what were the effects of preschool, home and community environments on the learning of those language structures which were needed in classrooms and job settings?" (1982, p. 2). Heath explored and documented language and literacy practices common in the homes of families in three different communities in the Piedmont Carolinas: a working-class black community (Trackton), a working-class white community (Roadville), and an integrated middle-class community (Maintown). Based on findings from ten years of research, Heath argued convincingly for how the knowledges and "ways with words" of people living in these different communities were historically and socially constructed in very different ways. In Heath's words, "the place of language in the cultural life of each social group is interdependent with the habits and values of behaving shared among members of that group" (p. 11). For example, the kinds of interactions that parents and children from the three communities engaged in while reading storybooks were linked to different ways of living, eating, sleeping, worshipping, using space, and spending time. These interactions were also linked to different notions of play, parenting, truth, and morality.

More generally, Heath explained that "for the children of Trackton and Roadville ... and for the majority of the mill workers and students in the Piedmont schools the ways [of the people of Maintown] are far from natural and they seem strange indeed" (1982, p. 262). Importantly, these differences resulted in different consequences for children's success in school. Finally, Heath traced constitutive relations between the identities of people in these communities and their language and literacy practices. In this regard, Heath worked with teachers in the local schools—all of whom were from Maintown—to understand the "ways with words" of the children they taught and to adapt their classroom practices to be more culturally relevant. This process induced changes in the identities, knowledges, and language practices of teachers and students alike.

Central to the work of Heath and other researchers working from within the chronotope of reading and interpretation is the fundamental notion that language practices constitute both individual and community identities. All of these studies presuppose the central assumption that it is not biology or geography or universal structure that constitutes identity and community but the discursive construction of shared meanings and practices. In Heath's work, for example, the predispositions toward books and reading held by the children and parents of Roadville or Trackton have no a priori existence but are continually produced and reproduced through the specific language and literacy practices common to the respective communities. As important as these practices are, however, Heath (and others located within the chronotope of reading and interpretation) never addresses questions about the larger social, political, and economic forces that make specific language and literacy practices visible and available in the first place. These questions are more central to the chronotopes we discuss later in the chapter.

The chronotope of reading and interpretation is embedded within a social constructionist epistemology and deploys hermeneutics as its most common theory-approach complex. From within this chronotope, language is theorized not as a vehicle for representing an already existent world but as the most powerful means available to human beings for constructing what is "really real" (Geertz, 1973) and fundamentally meaningful about that world. This chronotope holds onto the modernist notion of the individual rational subject but views this individual as fundamentally grounded in and constructed within the language and literacy practices of the speech and discourse communities in which he or she participates.

From within the chronotope of reading and interpretation, scholars also reject the idea that science is fundamentally about prediction and control, technical-instrumental rationality, and the gradual accumulation of all knowledge. Instead, researchers operating within this chronotope are committed to reflexively participating in the "language games" (Wittgenstein, 1958) of hermeneutics and the communities that they study with a desire and a willingness to enter into the conversations they find there. From this perspective, ongoing dialogue between researchers and research participants is a primary requirement of knowledge production and understanding.

Chronotope III: Skepticism, Conscientization, and Praxis

Although the chronotope of reading and interpretation constituted the very foundation of early qualitative research, it came under attack for failing to deal adequately with the power-laden political contexts in which presumably "open dialogue" occurs and "genuine understanding" is constructed. In other words, classical interpretivism rooted in hermeneutics did not address the ways in which dialogue can readily become complicit with the hegemonic structures of power in which it is always embedded. Historically, for example, many ethnographers have also been missionaries or military personnel whose "dialogue" with natives was motivated largely by religious and colonial interests masquerading as paternalistic (or maternalistic) benevolence. This social fact is true even into the middle of the twentieth century, when ethnographers shifted their gaze from "exotic" natives in distant places to equally "exotic" natives in American inner cities (e.g., Blacks, Asians, Jews, etc.). Accusations about the absence of attention paid to ideology and domination within the chronotope of reading and interpretation promoted the development of more critical forms of interpretivism within the Enlightenment or modernist project. We refer to these forms under the rubric of a chronotope of skepticism, conscientization, and praxis.

The roots of a chronotope of skepticism, conscientization, and praxis can be traced to linkages between the hermeneutic tradition and various strands of critical social theory within the tradition of neo-Marxism during the middle of the twentieth century. The name for the chronotope itself is a play on the term "hermeneutics of suspicion," which was introduced by Paul Ricoeur (1970) to refer to modes of interpretation that are radically skeptical about whatever is presumed to be the truth. Building on Ricoeur's basic insights, John B. Thompson (1990) constructed a systematic theory-method complex, which he called depth hermeneutics. Echoing the classic line attributed to Karl Marx, Ricoeur and Thompson argued that ideologies often "operate behind people's backs," which makes it impossible to escape completely the bonds of "false consciousness." Gadamer (1972) had something similar in mind when he claimed that, more than our judgments, our interests or our prejudices constitute who we are. Built largely on the neo-Marxist concerns with ideology and ideology critique, the goal of a critical or depth hermeneutics is to deconstruct or unmask the "reality" or "truth" of prejudicial understanding and to reveal the contingency, relativity, and historicity of consciousness, other people, and the world. Finally, we included Freire's (1970) term "conscientization" in the name of this chronotope to underscore its *praxis* orientation. For Freire, conscientization refers to critical reflection and its articulation with social action to enact individual and collective emancipation.

Like the chronotope of reading and interpretation, the chronotope of skepticism, conscientization, and praxis is grounded in social constructionist epistemologies. Unlike the chronotope of reading and interpretation, the chronotope of skepticism, conscientization, and praxis embraces the challenge of interrogating how ideology functions to "naturalize" and privilege some forms of knowledge and being-in-the-world over others. It also embodies an imperative for democratic social change. Operating within this chronotope, researchers assume that surface-level meanings and actions hide deep structural conflicts, contradictions, and falsities that function to maintain the status quo.

The neo-Marxist foundations of Chronotope III

To better understand the chronotope of skepticism, conscientization, and praxis warrants a detour into neo-Marxism. Certain neo-Marxists, including Antonio Gramsci (1971), George Lukács (1971), and Louis Althusser (1971), challenged the economic determinism of traditional Marxism, arguing that power derives not so much from base economic conditions but from cultural ideologies, which are only informed by economic/political configurations (e.g., feudalism, capitalism, socialism).

Another group of neo-Marxist thinkers known as the Frankfurt School theorists concerned themselves with understanding what they believed to be a set of constitutive relations among capitalism, epistemology, and politics. Although steeped in modernism, many Frankfurt School theorists were downright suspicious about the Enlightenment vision of an increasingly free and more democratic society through technical-instrumental rationality (i.e., science). In the words of Horkheimer and Adorno (1988), "in the most general sense of progressive thought, the Enlightenment has always aimed at liberating men from fear and establishing their authority. Yet the fully enlightened earth radiates disastrous triumph" (p. 3). The radical skepticism of the Frankfurt School did not so much mark a break with the Enlightenment or modernism project as an extension of it, which included a radical critique of the technical-instrumental rationality that had become so central to the project. Frankfurt School theorists were fundamentally concerned with interrogating why the presumed social progress of the project had resulted in "the fallen nature of modern man" (Horkheimer & Adorno, 1988, p. xiv), and the goal of their work was to rescue and reanimate "the hopes of the past" (p. xv).

Frankfurt School theorists did not attempt to disrupt the subject-object dichotomy central to Enlightenment and modernist work, however. Indeed, they struggled to preserve the idea that individuals are both rational and free but wanted to demonstrate how these inalienable characteristics had become distorted and corrupted by what Adorno (1973, p. 5) called "identity logic." Identity logic, according to Adorno, is radically subjectivistic and embodies the desperate human need to eliminate the distance between subject and object. It is rooted in the hubristic desire to know "things-in-themselves," to experience first hand what is indexed by the notion of a "correspondence theory of truth." The propensity for mastery and control, which is implicit in Adorno's identity logic and which was central to the Enlightenment project's notion of human freedom (and freedom from suffering), was viewed by Adorno and other neo-Marxists as the primary cause of the Enlightenment's demise and the disintegration of a logic of verification within the logical positivist tradition. Although Adorno often "affirm[ed] the wildest utopian dreams of the Enlightenment project" (Bernstein, 1992, p. 43), he thought that equating human reason and technical-instrumental rationality would negate the possibility of a critique of ideology and critical self-reflexivity. In this regard, he saw lived experience and material reality as far richer and more complex than could ever be captured by human thought and language. To imagine otherwise, he believed, was wrongheaded and arrogant. Worse than this, he argued that such arrogance eclipsed people's capacity for reflexivity and self-reflexivity in human thought and action.

The work of Frankfurt School scholar, Jürgen Habermas, perhaps went the furthest in laminating an emancipatory logic onto the basic modernist project. In his theory of communicative action, Habermas (1984, 1987) offered a critique of modernism, which shifted the locus of human agency from the Cartesian ego to the possibilities of dialogue inherent in language itself. Importantly, this shift entailed a concomitant shift in the locus of agency from the individual to the social. Finally, he rejected the technical-instrumental rationality of the Enlightenment without rejecting rationality itself, an issue we take up below.

Habermas's (1984, 1987) theory of communicative action is both a theory of rationality and a theory of society. In this regard, he viewed rationality as a social, dialogic process with both political and ethical valences. According to this view, rationality is not a property of the transcendental ego or individual subject. Instead, it is produced within "ideal speech situations" wherein people engage in communicative acts that are free, unconstrained, dialogic, and therefore undistorted. Ideal speech situations are defined or constituted by four "validity claims." Whatever speakers say must be

(a) meaningful, (b) true, (c) justified, and (d) sincere. Truth is the goal or promise of this model, and it is defined in terms of agreement or consensus achieved through critical dialogue and debate. Rational consensus is determined on the basis of who offers the better argument with the most adequate evidence and warrants. Reasoned argumentation is thus the ultimate court of appeal.

Habermas's insistence on the importance of the ideal speech situation was rooted in his ethical and political commitments. Because he believed that the colonizing forces of capitalism were rooted in technical-instrumental rationality, he rejected this form of rationality and posited two alternatives: (a) practical rationality and (b) emancipatory rationality. Practical rationality (or Habermas's version of praxis) is the means by which people reach mutual understandings through unfettered dialogue. Emancipatory rationality is a mode of thinking/being that allows people to escape the lures of hegemony and oppression through self-reflection. By acknowledging the workings of these three forms of rationality in social life, Habermas was able to account for how language is a constitutive force *both* in generating shared understandings (and thus truth) *and* in the exercise of power and domination. Social movements such as second-wave feminism, the civil rights movement, and the ecology movement are good examples of how Habermas's rational, emancipatory, de/recolonization project have been concretely realized in history. In our own field, one might argue that "whole language" pedagogies, Gravesian versions of the "writing process" pedagogies, and many incarnations of the "critical literacy" pedagogies are all grounded in Habermas's practical and emancipatory forms of rationality, as well as how these pedagogies have been assaulted by hegemonic regimes rooted in and legitimated by technical-instrumental rationality.

The praxis turn

The general interest in practical reason or praxis has a long history in philosophy. Aristotle (e.g., Nichomachean Ethics, Book VI) contrasted poesis with praxis, arguing that poesis involves instrumental action that results in *making* or *producing* things whereas praxis involves action that results in acting or doing things with and for others that promote moral goodness and "the good life." Thus, praxis always has to do with what people *do* in relation to each other to enhance their respective lives. Aristotle also believed that, through these acts, people also promote the democratic goals of the state.

More generally, the term "praxis" has often been used to refer to the general process of linking theory and practice, knowledge and action to enhance the possibilities of *communitas* and to make the world a better place to live in for all people. For the most part, knowledge has remained the privileged term in this binary but practical knowledge and not knowledge for its own sake has been emphasized. Since the so-called crisis of representation in anthropology (e.g., Marcus & Fisher, 1986), praxis has often been used to refer to the practical and dialogic/reciprocal relationships that researchers may forge with research participants. Within these relationships, researchers have often imposed mandates on themselves to work with research participants to help them improve the conditions of their lives (e.g., Lather, 1991, 1997). Less common, but at least as important, is a political sense of praxis such as that developed by Gramsci (1971). This sense of praxis unites theory and practice in such a way that neither is subservient to the other. Researchers and research participants enter into reciprocal relationships wherein the common work experience has to be as much a venue for both intellectuals and workers to advance their points of view and interests. Reciprocal relationships must lead to the development of common goals, and these goals must in some ways express the transformative possibilities of a dialogic community.

Chronotope IV: Power/Knowledge and Defamiliarization

When most people think about "critical" qualitative research, they presume that it is always framed within postmodern and/or poststructural epistemologies and theories. Although we argued against this generalization in the previous section, critical qualitative research has been increasingly grounded in postmodern and poststructural perspectives. Because power/knowledge and defamiliarization are constructs that are central to these perspectives, we have used them to characterize the next chronotope we discuss. Partly because of its almost exclusive alignment with postmodernism and poststructuralism rather than modernism and structuralism, this chronotope is partially discontinuous with the chronotope of skepticism, conscientization, and praxis.

Power/knowledge and games of truth

Perhaps the hallmark of postmodern and poststructural critical theorists is the extent to which they debunked modernist notions of knowledge, arguing that knowledge is always related to power. For example, they rejected Habermas's (1984, 1987) dialogic/consensus model of knowledge made possible by the inherent potential of language to afford an "ideal speech situation." Contra Habermas, Baudrillard (1983), Foucault (1977), Lyotard (1984), and others warned that consensus is a hopeless vestige of modernism that actually elicits complicity with totalizing regimes of knowledge and truth, and they set out to demonstrate the ways in which knowledge and power are co-constitutive. Foucault's (1975, 1977, 1990) genealogies of madness/the asylum, criminality/the prison, and the discourses of sexuality, for example, showed how what is considered true or false is dependent on specific "games of truth" or "regimes of power" upon which the possibilities of making any and all knowledge claims depend. Different games of truth afford and allow different knowledge claims. For example, Foucault (1990) raised several doubts about the presumed "repressive hypothesis" of modern society beginning with the Victorian age:

> First doubt: Is sexual repression truly an established historical fact? ... Second doubt: Do the workings of power, and in particular those mechanisms that are brought into play in societies such as ours, really belong primarily to the category of repression? ... Third and final doubt: Did the critical discourse that addresses itself to repression come to act as a roadblock to a power mechanism that had operated unchallenged up to that point, or is it not in fact part of the same historical network as the thing it denounces (and doubtless misrepresents) in calling it "repression"? [p. 10]

Foucault went on to claim that these doubts about the repressive hypothesis "are aimed less at showing it to be mistaken than at putting it back within a general economy of discourses on sex in modern societies since the seventeenth century" (1990, p. 10). And he argued that this relocation ushers in new (and more important) questions about sexuality such as "Why has sexuality been so widely discussed, and what has been said about it? What were the effects of power generated by what was said? What are the links between these discourses, these effects of power, and the pleasures that were invested by them? What knowledge (*savoir*) was formed as a result of this linkage?" (p. 10).

The human subject

Besides reconceptualizing knowledge in relation to power, postmodern/poststructural critical theorists went much further than modernist critical theorists in decentering Enlightenment notions about the human subject and displacing the locus of rationality from the mind of this subject. For example, although Habermas (1984, 1987) rejected the idea of the Cartesian subject and argued for viewing rationality not as a possession of the individual subject but as a dialogic social process rooted in the potential for an "ideal speech situation" inherent in language, he still viewed subjectivity as coherent and progressive.

For postmodern/poststructural critical theorists, the subject is neither autonomous nor coherent nor teleological in nature. Instead, the subject is constructed within various "discursive systems" or "discourses" that normalize what it means to be a subject in the first place (Foucault, 1977, 1990). These discourses are not linguistic and textual alone but involve habituated and largely unconscious ways of thinking, talking, feeling, acting, and being. Discourses are practical "grids of specification" (Foucault, 1972, 1977, 1996) for classifying, categorizing, and diagramming the human subject in relation to the social. Discourses are forms of power that both literally and metaphorically inscribe/produce the individual and the collective social body. Indeed, the residue of such production processes litters our vocabulary: "the culturally literate citizen," "the naturally literate child," "the educated gentleman," "the child author," "the reader of romance," "the functional illiterate," and "the academically prepared student." These classifications are almost always also classed, raced, and gendered.

Language

Although we have already touched on the views of language and discourse central to the chronotope of power/knowledge and defamiliarization, we want to return to this topic and to address it more explicitly. The roots of understanding language and discourse within this framework seem to lie in postmodern notions of deconstruction. Importantly, however, like Habermas's communicative ethics, deconstruction never entirely escaped from the inherent dualism of transcendental philosophy or the foundational status of subjective experience. Again, Foucault offered some insights that allow us to address/redress these problems. So, we will outline the contours of deconstruction and then show how Foucault identified and responded to some of their inherent weaknesses.

Deconstruction decentered traditional notions of the relationsbetween signs and their referents (e.g., Saussure's signifiers and signifieds). Derrida (1976), for example, made the provocative claim that there is nothing outside of language (or semiotics more broadly conceived). Extending the "negative dialectics" of Adorno, he argued that we can never make the relation between the sign and its referent identical. In uncompromising terms, this claim brought into high relief the possibility that that the referents of all signs and symbols, including those of natural language, are not objects in the world but other signs and symbols. Unmediated knowledge of the referents in themselves is a radical impossibility.

No particular signifier (sign) can ever be regarded as referring to any particular signified (referent). Baudrillard (1983) extended this idea further with his construct of the "simulacrum." According to this construct, the sign is actually more real that the reality it represents. The real forever recapitulates the imagined. Postmodernity, Baudrillard argued, is "hyperreal." We do not live in reality but "hyperreality" where everything is simulation and objects seduce subjects rather than subjects rationally choosing objects. What he meant here is that the boundary between the real and the imaginary has been dissolved. Reality is no longer a court of appeal for experience and knowledge. The "more real than real" has become existence itself. In an age of "hyperreality," signs exert more power and influence over people than material reality, and reality itself is experienced as mysterious and illusionary to a large extent.

Defamiliarization

The construct of defamiliarization becomes important for exploring the tactics at the heart of conjunctural analysis, and for understanding the ways in which Chronotope IV reflects a sharp break from the other chronotopes, especially with regard to the nature and process of research, and the stances of researchers toward the "objects" of their research. In his efforts to imagine an ethnography for the late twentieth and early twenty-first centuries, Clifford (1988) talked about a "hermeneutics of vulnerability," which foregrounds the ruptures of fieldwork, the multiple and contradictory positionings of researchers and research participants, the imperfect control of the ethnographer, and the utility of self-reflexivity.

In one sense, self-reflexivity involves making transparent the rhetorical and poetic work of the ethnographer in representing the object of her or his study. In another perhaps more important sense, self-reflexivity refers to the efforts of researchers and research participants to engage in acts of defamiliarization in relation to each other. In this regard, Probyn (1993) discussed how fieldwork always seems to result in being "uneasy in one's skin" and how this experience often engenders a virtual transformation of the identities of both researchers and research participants even as they are paradoxically engaged in the practice of consolidating them. This is important theoretically, because it allows for the possibility of constructing a mutual ground between researchers and research participants even while recognizing that the ground is unstable and fragile. Self-reflexivity as defamiliarization is also important because it encourages reflection on ethnography as the practice of both knowledge gathering and self-transformation through self-reflection and mutual reflection with the other. Importantly, these acts of defamiliarization can help people recognize the fragmentary, historically situated, partial, and unfinished nature of their "selves" and promote processes of self-construction/reconstruction in relation to new discourses and others.

Summary and Conclusions

The taxonomy we have used to organize our argument is not meant to be read as a taxonomy in the classic Aristotelean sense. Instead, it should be used as a heuristic device that helps move us down the road in our thinking about the complex and nuanced ways in which particular epistemes, epistemologies, theories, and methods have coalesced in emergent ways to become "regimes of truth" that inform inquiry practices in powerful and pervasive ways. Importantly, we did not find these regimes of truth lying around in the basement of a philosophy department; we produced them. They are neither "real" in any universal sense nor are they mutually exclusive. Together, however, they constitute a useful continuum for thinking about how different articulations or assemblages of subjectivity, rationality, language, knowledge, and truth emerged historically, became durable chronotopes, and continue to affect in very powerful ways how qualitative inquiry is imagined and practiced within literacy studies, education, and the social sciences. Imagined as points positioned on a continuum, the chronotope of objectivism and representation embodies many traditional Enlightenment logics such as Descartes's rational subject and a correspondence theory of truth, whereas the chronotope of power/knowledge and defamiliarization probably goes the furthest in disrupting these particular logics and replacing them with alternatives.

Translating these ideas to research practice, perhaps what is most important is to generate as good a fit as possible between research questions or objects of interest and where to locate oneself on this continuum of chronotopes. This requires deep reflection on the relations among various epistemologies, theories, approaches, and strategies. In some ways, each chronotope is uniquely valuable for pursuing some research projects more than others. But this is a bit of an overstatement. Seldom is a researcher ever really located within a single chronotope. Additionally, depending on their values and goals, two different researchers might choose to locate ostensibly the same research project within different chronotopes. For example, although Heath's famous *Ways with Words* (1983)—the classic ethnography of reading across three communities in the Piedmont Carolinas—located itself quite firmly in Chronotope II, one could imagine locating similar work within Chronotopes III or IV. Indeed, certain critiques of Heath's work have suggested that this might have been a good idea—that it should be less descriptive and more critical. Similarly, Luke's

(1992) poststructual work on discipline and reading in Australian elementary schools could readily have been conducted within Chronotope II. Indeed, many more "neutral" interpretive accounts of read-alouds and story discussions have been written.

So where does this all leave us and our fellow qualitative researchers today? How might our philosophical and historical reflections inform the ways in which we imagine and enact research practices as we move through the twenty-first century? Many metaphors have recently been proposed to describe the possible futures of qualitative inquiry. Each is predicated on particular ontological and epistemological assumptions, and each calls attention to the complexities and difficulties of conducting research a globalized, fast-capitalist, media-saturated world. We conclude with brief descriptions of a subset of these metaphors.

Locating themselves primarily within Chronotope IV, Denzin and Lincoln (1994) famously call for qualitative researchers to be "bricoleurs," mixing and matching the multiple logics and tools of qualitative inquiry in pragmatic and strategic ways to "get the job done," whatever one imagines that job to be. The goal of research, according to this metaphor, is to produce "a complex, dense, reflexive collage-like creation that represents the researcher's images, understandings, and interpretations of the world or phenomenon under analysis" (p. 3).

Located more in Chronotopes I and II, Hammersly (1999) responded to this metaphorically informed call with another one rooted in more cautionary, pragmatic, neomodernist impulses. Briefly, he argues that qualitative researchers should imagine themselves not as bricoleurs but as "boatbuilders." This metaphor derives from what is known as Neurath's boat, named after the German sociologist Otto Neurath, who compared the work of scientists with the work of sailors who must often rebuild their ships at sea, never able to start from scratch and always aware that their reconstructions must result in a coherent whole that floats. Hammersly goes on to argue that producing collage and pentimento can never be a basis for good boat building and that the impulse toward "bricolage" threatens to "sink" the qualitative inquiry ship. "A central message that ought to be taken from Neurath's metaphor," Hammersly claims, "is that because we are always faced with the task of rebuilding our craft at sea, everything cannot be questioned at once" (p. 581). He argues further that "those who want to be poets or political activists, or both, should not pretend that they can simultaneously be social researchers" (p. 583). Unabashedly modernist, Hammersly urges that we "develop a coherent sense of where we are going and of how we need to rebuild our vessel to sail in the right direction" (p. 579), which, among other things, will require thoroughgoing knowledge of where we have been.

A third metaphor, and the one that motivated many of our arguments in this chapter, is the "genealogist." Thinking genealogically forces us to see disciplines as the ongoing work of invested actors, not as paradigms we must uncritically occupy. Traditionally, researchers have been encouraged to see research traditions and methods as immutable, with parameters that are defined a priori. Genealogists have no given lineages, but different histories at their disposal.

Using these histories, they attempt to understand how any "subject" (e.g., a person, a social formation, a social movement, an institution) has been constituted out of particular intersections of forces and systems of forces by mapping the complex, contingent, and often contradictory ways in which these forces and systems of force came together to produce the formation in the precise way that that it did and not some other way. From the perspective of genealogy,

> [h]istory becomes "effective" to the degree that it introduces discontinuity into our very being—as it divides our emotions, dramatizes our instincts, multiplies our body and sets it against itself. "Effective" history deprives the self of the reassuring stability of life and nature, and it will not permit itself to be transported by a voiceless obstinacy toward a millennial ending. It will uproot its traditional foundations and relentlessly disrupt its pretended continuity. This is because knowledge is not made for understanding; it is made for cutting. [Foucault, 1981, p. 88]

Guided by this sense that knowledge is "for cutting," we choose methodological directions strategically but with full knowledge that there no "safe spaces," no alibis for our decisions. Although genealogists call into question naive realism and the authority of experience, they also try to deploy such constructs in thoughtful and partial ways. Deleuze and Guattari (1987), for example, do not claim to rid the world of binaries but to create new ones that are more productive for achieving democratic ideals. Genealogists realize that they need to appropriate extant epistemologies theories, approaches, and strategies to do their work, but they are aware that there are no "pure" choices, no guarantees about what these appropriations will produce or how they will produce it. To understand such outcomes requires intense retrospective analysis, constantly looking back and trying to understand how our accounts were constructed in the ways they were and not in other ways.

In closing, we want to underscore that we have presented these three metaphors because we believe that all of them (as well as others we might have discussed) are powerful and productive for thinking about the central topic of this book—the logics of qualitative inquiry—past, present, and future. These metaphors index tensions that have always existed in the field of qualitative inquiry and will probably always exist. Together, they map the many imperatives and impulses that we, as qualitative researchers, must struggle with in our daily work, especially with respect to locating ourselves strategically within and across chronotopes and creating epistemology-theory-approach-strategy assemblages that are both principled and pragmatic.

References

Adorno, T. (1973). *Negative dialectics* (E. B. Ashton, Trans.). New York: Continuum.

Althusser, L. (1971). *Lenin and philosophy*. New York: Monthly Review Press.

Bakhtin, M. M. (1981). *The dialogic imagination* (C. Emerson & M. Holquist, Trans.). Austin: University of Texas Press.

Baudrillard, J. (1983). *Simulations*. New York: Semiotext(e).

Bernstein, R. (1992). The new constellation: The ethical/political horizons of modernity/postmodernity. Cambridge, MA: MIT Press.

Birdwhistell, R. L. (1970). *Kinesics and context: Essays on body motion communication*. Philadelphia: University of Pennsylvania Press.

Bourdieu, P. (1990). *The logic of practice* (R. Nice, Trans.). Stanford, CA: Stanford University Press.

Clifford, J. (1988). *The predicament of culture: Twentieth-century ethnography, literature, and art.* Cambridge, MA: Harvard University Press.

Clifford, J., & Marcus, G. (Eds.). (1986). *Writing culture: The poetics and politics of ethnography.* Berkeley: University of California Press.

Deleuze, G., & Guattari, F. (1987). *A thousand plateaus: Capitalism and schizophrenia* (B. Massumi, Trans.). Minneapolis: University of Minnesota Press.

Denzin, N. K., & Lincoln, Y. S. (Eds.). (1994). *Handbook of qualitative research.* Thousand Oaks, CA: Sage.

Derrida, J. (1976). *Of grammatology* (G. Spivak, Trans.). Baltimore: Johns Hopkins University Press.

Dilthey, W. L. (1976/1900). *Selected writings.* Cambridge, UK: Cambridge University Press.

Flower, L., & Hayes, J. (1981). A cognitive process theory of writing. *College Communication and Composition, 32*, 365–387.

Foucault, M. (1972). *The archaeology of knowledge* (A. M. Sheridan Smith, Trans). New York: Pantheon Books.

Foucault, M. (1975). *The birth of the clinic. An archaeology of medical perception* (A. Sheridan, Trans.). New York: Vintage.

Foucault, M. (1977). *Discipline and punish: The birth of the prison* (A. Sheridan, Trans.). New York: Vintage Books.

Foucault, M. (1990). *The history of sexuality: An introduction* (Vol. 1) (R. Hurley, Trans.). New York: Vintage. (Original work published in 1978.)

Foucault, M. (1996). History, discourse and discontinuity. In S. Lotringer (Ed.), *Foucault live (Interviews, 1961–1984)* (pp. 33–50). New York: Semiotext(e). (Original essay published in 1972.)

Freire, P. (1970). *Pedagogy of the oppressed.* New York: Continuum.

Gadamer, H. G. (1972). *Knowledge and human interests* (J. J. Shapiro, Trans.). Boston: Beacon.

Geertz, C. (1973). *The interpretation of cultures: Selected essays.* New York: Basic Books.

Giddens, A. (1979). *Central problems in social theory.* Berkeley: University of California Press.

Gramsci, A. (1971). *Selections from the prison notebooks of Antonio Gramsci* (Q. Hoare & G. N. Smith, Eds. and Trans.). New York: International.

Grossberg, L. (1992). *We gotta get out of this place: Popular conservatism and postmodern culture.* New York: Routledge.

Habermas, J. (1984). *The theory of communicative action: Reason and the rationalization of society* (Vol. 1) (T. McCarthey, Trans.). Boston: Beacon.

Habermas, J. (1987). The *theory of communicative action: Lifeworld and system* (Vol. 2) (T. McCarthy, Trans.). Boston: Beacon.

Hall, S. (1992). Cultural studies and its theoretical legacies. In L. Grossberg, C. Nelson, & P. Treichler (Eds.), *Cultural studies* (pp. 277–294). New York: Routledge.

Hammersly, M. (1999). Not bricolage but boatbuilding. *Journal of Contemporary ethnography, 28*(5), 574–585.

Heath, S. B. (1982). Ethnography in education: Defining the essentials. In P. Gilmore & A. A. Glatthorn (Eds.), *Children in and out of school: Ethnography and education* (pp. 33–55). Washington, DC: Center for Applied Linguistics.

Heath, S. B. (1983). *Ways with words: Language, life, and work in communities and classrooms*. Cambridge, UK: Cambridge University Press.

Hebdige, R. (1979). *Subculture: The meaning of style*. London: Routledge.

Heidegger, M. (1962). *Being and time* (R. MacQuarrie, Trans.). New York: Harper & Rowe.

Hirsch, E. D. (1987). *Cultural literacy*. Boston: Houghton Mifflin.

Holland, D., Lachiotte, W., Skinner, D., & Cain, C. (1998). *Identity and agency in cultural worlds*. Cambridge, MA: Harvard University Press.

Horkheimer, M., & Adorno, T. (1988). *The dialectic of enlightenment* (J. Cummings, Trans.). New York: Continuum.

Lather, P. (1991). *Getting smart: Feminist research and pedagogy with/in the postmodern*. New York: Routledge.

Lather, P. (1997). Drawing the lines at angels: Working the ruins of feminist ethnography. *Qualitative Studies in Education, 10*(3), 285–304.

Lukács, G. (1971). *History of class consciousness: Studies in Marxist dialectics* (R. Livingstone, Trans.). Cambridge, MA: MIT Press.

Luke, A. (1992). The body literate: Discourse and inscription in early literacy training. *Linguistics and Education, 4*(1), 107–129.

Lyotard, F. (1984). *The postmodern condition: A report on knowledge* (G. Bennington & B. Massumi, Trans.). Minneapolis: University of Minnesota Press.

Marcus, G., & Fischer, M. (1986). *Anthropology as cultural critique: An experimental moment in the human sciences*. Chicago: University of Chicago Press.

Morson, G., & Emerson, C. (1990). *Mikhail Bakhtin: Creation of a prosaics*. Stanford, CA: Stanford University Press.

Pinar, W. (2004). *What is curriculum theory?* Hillsdale, NJ: Lawrence Erlbaum.

Probyn, E. (1993). *Sexing the self: Gendered positions in cultural studies*. London and New York: Routledge.

Ricoeur, P. (1970). *Freud and philosophy: An essay on interpretation*. New Haven, CT: Yale University Press.

Rorty, R. (1979). *Philosophy and the mirror of nature*. Princeton, NJ: Princeton University Press.

Strike, K. (1974). On the expressive potential of behaviorist language. *American Educational Research Journal, 11*(2), 103–120.

Thompson, J. B. (1990). The methodology of interpretation. In J. B. Thompson (Ed.), *Ideology and modern culture* (pp. 272–327). Stanford, CA: Stanford University Press.

Turner, J. C. (1995). The influence of classroom contexts on young children's motivation for literacy. *Reading Research Quarterly, 30*, 410–441.

Willis, P. (1977). *Learning to labor: How working class kids get working class jobs*. New York: Columbia University Press.

Wittgenstein, L. (1958). *Philosophical investigations* (G. E. M. Anscombe, Trans.). Oxford, UK: Basil Blackwell.

Chapter 3

Neutral Science and the Ethics of Resistance

Clifford G. Christians

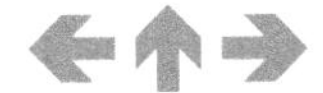

The subject-object dichotomy dominated the Enlightenment mind.[1] Isaac Newton's *Principia Mathematica* (1687) described the world as a lifeless machine built on uniform natural causes in a closed system, and Newton inspired the eighteenth century as much as anyone. Descartes (1596–1690) presumed clear and distinct ideas, objective and neutral, apart from anything subjective. The physical universe became the only legitimate domain of knowledge. On the positive side, it unlocked an excitement to explore and rule the natural world that formerly had controlled them. In fact, Descartes limited his interests to precise mechanistic knowledge because he wished that "we should make ourselves masters and possessors of nature" ([1637] 1916, pt. VI). Natural science played a key role in setting people free. Achievements in mathematics, physics, and astronomy provided unmistakable evidence that by applying reason to nature and to human beings in fairly obvious ways, people could live progressively happier lives. Crime and insanity, for example, no longer needed repressive theological explanations, but instead were deemed capable of mundane empirical solutions. Science

Originally published in *Ethical Futures in Qualitative Inquiry*, edited by Norman K. Denzin and Michael D. Giardina, pp.47–66. © 2007 Left Coast Press, Inc., Walnut Creek, CA. Republished in *Qualitative Inquiry—Past, Present, and Future: A Critical Reader*, edited by Norman K. Denzin and Michael D. Giardina, pp. 69–87. Left Coast Press, Inc. All rights reserved.

gained a stranglehold on truth, with its ideology of hard data versus subjective values.

It is a hallmark of modernity that the character of the social sciences revolves around the theory and methodology of the natural sciences. As the social sciences and the liberal state emerged and overlapped historically, Enlightenment thinkers in eighteenth-century Europe advocated the techniques of experimental reasoning to support the state and citizenry. The basic institutions of society were designed to ensure "neutrality between different conceptions of the good" (Root, 1993, p. 12; cf. pp. 14–15).[2] Objects and events situated in space-time were considered to contain all the facts there are. Value-free experimentalism in Enlightenment terms has defined the theory and practice of mainstream social science until today. Only a reintegration of research practice and the moral order provides an alternative paradigm. For an ethics and politics of resistance, the social sciences must reinvent themselves in qualitative terms after the humanities.

Value-Neutral Experimentalism

Mill's Philosophy of Social Science

For John Stuart Mill, neutrality is necessary to promote autonomy. Planning our lives according to our own ideas and purposes is sine qua non for autonomous beings in his *On Liberty* ([1859] 1978): "The free development of individuality is one of the principal ingredients of human happiness, and quite the chief ingredient of individual and social progress" (p. 50; see also Copleston, 1966, p. 303, n. 32). This neutrality, based on the supremacy of individual autonomy, is the foundational principle in his *Utilitarianism* (Mill, [1861] 1957), and in *A System of Logic* (Mill, [1843] 1893) as well. In addition to bringing classical utilitarianism to its maximum development and establishing with Locke the liberal state, Mill delineated the foundations of inductive inquiry as social scientific method. In terms of the principles of empiricism, he perfected the inductive techniques of Francis Bacon as a problem-solving methodology to replace Aristotelian deductive logic.

According to Mill, syllogisms contribute nothing new to human knowledge. If we conclude that because "all men are mortal" the

Duke of Wellington is mortal by virtue of his manhood, then the conclusion does not advance the premise (see Mill, [1843] 1893, II, 3, 2, p. 140). The crucial issue is not reordering the conceptual world but discriminating genuine knowledge from superstition. In the pursuit of truth, generalizing and synthesizing are necessary to advance inductively from the known to the unknown. Mill seeks to establish this function of logic as inference from the known, rather than certifying the rules for formal consistency in reasoning (Mill, [1843] 1893, bk. 3). Scientific certitude can be approximated when induction is followed rigorously, with propositions empirically derived and the material of all our knowledge provided by experience.[3] For the physical sciences, he establishes four modes of experimental inquiry: agreement, disagreement, residues, and the principle of concomitant variations (Mill, [1843] 1893, III, 8, pp. 278–288). He considers them the only possible methods of proof for experimentation, as long as one presumes the realist position that nature is structured by uniformities.[4]

In Book 6 of *A System of Logic*, "On the Logic of the Moral Sciences," Mill ([1843] 1893) develops an inductive experimentalism as the scientific method for studying "the various phenomena which constitute social life" (VI, 6, 1, p. 606). Although he conceived of social science as explaining human behavior in terms of causal laws, he warned against the fatalism of full predictability. "Social laws are hypothetical, and statistically-based generalizations by their very nature admit of exceptions" (Copleston, 1966, p. 101; see also Mill, [1843] 1893, VI, 5, 1, p. 596). Empirically confirmed instrumental knowledge about human behavior has greater predictive power when it deals with collective masses than when we are dealing with individual agents.

Mill's positivism is obvious throughout his work on experimental inquiry.[5] Based on the work of Auguste Comte, he defined matter as the "permanent possibility of sensation" (Mill, 1865b, p. 198) and believed that nothing else can be said about metaphysical substances.[6] With Hume and Comte, Mill insisted that metaphysical substances are not real and only the facts of sense phenomena exist. There are no essences or ultimate reality behind sensations, therefore Mill (1865a, 1865b) and Comte ([1848] 1910) argued that social scientists should limit themselves to particular data as a factual source out of which experimentally valid laws can be derived. For both, this is the only kind of knowledge that yields practical benefits (Mill, 1865b, p. 242); in fact, society's salvation is contingent on such scientific knowledge (p. 241).[7]

Mill's philosophy of social science is built on a dualism of means and ends. Citizens and politicians are responsible for articulating ends in a free society and science is responsible for the know-how to achieve them. Science is amoral, speaking to questions of means but with no wherewithal or authority to dictate ends. Methods in the social sciences must be disinterested regarding substance and content, and rigorously limited to the risks and benefits of possible courses of action. Research cannot be judged right or wrong, only true or false. "Science is political only in its applications" (Root, 1993, p. 213). Given his democratic liberalism, Mill advocates neutrality "out of concern for the autonomy of the individuals or groups" social science seeks to serve. It should "treat them as thinking, willing, active beings who bear responsibility for their choices and are free to choose" their own conception of the good life by majority rule (Root, 1993, p. 19).

Value Neutrality in Max Weber

When twenty-first-century mainstream social scientists contend that ethics is not their business, they typically invoke Weber's essays written between 1904 and 1917. Given Weber's importance methodologically and theoretically for sociology and economics, his distinction between political judgments and scientific neutrality is given canonical status.

Weber distinguishes value freedom from value relevance. He recognizes that in the discovery phase, "personal, cultural, moral, or political values cannot be eliminated; ... what social scientists choose to investigate ... they choose on the basis of the values" that they expect their research to advance (Root, 1993, p. 33). But he insists that social science be value free in the presentation phase. Findings ought not to express any judgments of a moral or political character. Professors should hang up their values along with their coats as they enter their lecture halls.

"An attitude of moral indifference," Weber ([1904] 1949b) writes, "has no connection with scientific objectivity" (p. 60). His meaning is clear from the value-freedom/value-relevance distinction. For the social sciences to be purposeful and rational, they must serve the "values of relevance."

> The problems of the social sciences are selected by the value relevance of the phenomena treated. ...The expression "relevance to values" refers simply to the philosophical interpretation of that specifically scientific "interest" which determines the selection of a given subject matter and problems of empirical analysis. [Weber, (1917) 1949a, pp. 21–22]

Whereas the natural sciences, in Weber's ([1904] 1949b, p. 72) view, seek general laws that govern all empirical phenomena, the social sciences study those realities that our values consider significant. Whereas the natural world itself indicates what reality to investigate, the infinite possibilities of the social world are ordered in terms of "the cultural values with which we approach reality" ([1904] 1949b, p. 78). However, even though value relevance directs the social sciences, as with the natural sciences, Weber considers the former value free. The subject matter in natural science makes value judgments unnecessary, and social scientists by a conscious decision can exclude judgments of "desirability or undesirability" from their publications and lectures ([1904] 1949b, p. 52). "What is really at issue is the intrinsically simple demand that the investigator and teacher should keep unconditionally separate the establishment of empirical facts ... and his own political evaluations" (Weber, [1917] 1949a, p. 11).

Weber's practical argument for value freedom and his apparent limitation of it to the reporting phase have made his version of value neutrality attractive to twenty-first-century social science. He is not a positivist such as Comte or a thoroughgoing empiricist in the tradition of Mill. He disavowed the positivists' overwrought disjunction between discovery and justification, and he developed no systematic epistemology comparable to Mill's. Nevertheless, Weber's value neutrality reflects the Enlightenment's subject-object dichotomy in a fundamentally similar fashion. In the process of maintaining his distinction between value relevance and value freedom, he separates facts from values and means from ends. He appeals to empirical evidence and logical reasoning rooted in human rationality. "The validity of a practical imperative as a norm," he writes, "and the truth-value of an empirical proposition are absolutely heterogeneous in character" (Weber, [1904] 1949b, p. 52). "A systematically correct scientific proof in the social sciences" may not be completely attainable, but that is most likely "due to faulty data" not because it is conceptually impossible ([1904] 1949b, p. 58).[8] For Weber, as with Mill, empirical science deals with questions of means, and his warning against inculcating political and moral values presumes a means-ends dichotomy (see Weber, [1917] 1949a, pp. 18–19, [1904] 1949b, p. 52).

As Michael Root (1993) concludes, "John Stuart Mill's call for neutrality in the social sciences is based on his belief" that the language of science "takes cognizance of a phenomenon and endeavors to discover its laws" (p. 205). Max Weber likewise "takes it for granted that there can be a language of science—a collection of truths—that excludes all value-judgments, rules, or directions for conduct" (Root, 2003, p. 205). In both cases, scientific knowledge exists for its own sake as morally neutral. For both, neutrality is desirable "because questions of value are not rationally resolvable" and neutrality in the social sciences is presumed to contribute "to political and personal autonomy" (Root, 1993, p. 229). In Weber's argument for value relevance in social science, he did not contradict the larger Enlightenment ideal of scientific neutrality between competing conceptions of the good.

Institutional Review Boards

In an academic world of value-free social science, codes of ethics for professional and academic associations are the conventional format for moral principles. By the 1980s, each of the major scholarly associations had adopted its own code for directing an inductive science of means toward majoritarian ends. And institutional review boards (IRBs) likewise embody the same agenda of instrumentalist, neutral social science. In terms of the IRBs' scope, assumptions, and procedures, data that are internally and externally valid are the coin of the realm, experimentally and morally. Scientific research is presumed to benefit society by uncovering facts about the human condition. The guidelines entailed by IRB policy themselves establish the ends by which the scientific study of society is evaluated as moral.

In 1978, the U.S. National Commission for the Protection of Human Subjects in Biomedical and Behavioral Research was established. As a result, three principles, published in what became known as the Belmont Report, were developed as the moral standards for research involving human subjects: respect for persons, beneficence, and justice.

1. The section on respect for persons reiterates the codes' demands that subjects enter the research voluntarily and with adequate information about the experiment's procedures and possible consequences. On a deeper level, respect for persons incorporates two basic ethical tenets: "First, that individuals should be treated as autonomous agents, and second, that persons with diminished autonomy [the immature and incapacitated] are entitled to protection" (University of Illinois, 2006, n.p.).

2. Under the principle of beneficence, researchers are enjoined to secure the well-being of their subjects. Beneficent actions are understood in a double sense as avoiding harm altogether, and if risks are involved for achieving substantial benefits, minimizing as much harm as possible:

> In the case of particular projects, investigators and members of their institutions are obliged to give forethought to the maximization of benefits and the reduction of risks that might occur from the research investigation. In the case of scientific research in general, members of the larger society are obliged to recognize the longer term benefits and risks that may result from the improvement of knowledge and from the development of novel medical, psychotherapeutic, and social procedures. [University of Illinois, 2006, n.p.]

3. The principle of justice insists on fair distribution of both the benefits and burdens of research. An injustice occurs when some groups (e.g., welfare recipients, the institutionalized, or particular ethnic minorities) are overused as research subjects because of easy manipulation or their availability. And when research supported by public funds leads to "therapeutic devices and procedures, justice demands that these not provide advantages only to those who can afford them" (University of Illinois, 2006, n.p.).

These principles reiterate the basic themes of value-neutral experimentalism—individual autonomy, maximum benefits with minimal risks, and ethical ends exterior to scientific means. The authority of IRBs was enhanced in 1989 when Congress passed the National Institutes of Health Revitalization Act and formed the Commission on Research Integrity. The emphasis at that point was on the invention, fudging, and distortion of data. Falsification, fabrication, and plagiarism continue as federal categories of misconduct, with a new report in 1996 adding warnings against unauthorized use of confidential information, omission of important data, and interference (that is, physical damage to the materials of others).

With IRBs, the legacy of Mill, Comte, and Weber comes into its own. Value-neutral science is accountable to ethical standards through rational procedures controlled by value-neutral academic institutions in the service of an impartial government. Consistent with the way anonymous bureaucratic regimes become refined and streamlined toward greater efficiency, the regulations rooted in scientific and medical experiments now extend to humanistic inquiry. Protecting subjects from physical harm in laboratories has grown to encompass human behavior, history, and ethnography in natural settings. In Jonathon Church's metaphor, "a biomedical paradigm is used like some threshing machine with ethnographic research the resulting chaff" (2002, p. 2). Whereas Title 45/Part 46 of the Code of Federal Regulations (45 CFR 46) designed protocols for research funded by seventeen federal agencies, at present most universities have multiple project agreements that consign all research to a campus IRB under the terms of 45 CFR 46.

While this bureaucratic expansion has gone on unremittingly, most IRBs have not changed the composition of their membership. Medical and behavioral scientists under the aegis of value-free neutrality continue to dominate. And the changes in procedures have generally stayed within the biomedical model also. Expedited review under the Common Rule, for social research with no risk of physical or psychological harm, depends on enlightened IRB chairs and organizational flexibility. Informed consent, mandatory before medical experiments, is simply incongruent with interpretive research not on human subjects but with other human beings. Despite technical improvements, "[i]ntellectual curiosity remains actively discouraged by the IRB. Research projects must ask only surface questions and must not deviate from a path approved by a remote group of people. ... Often the review process seems to be more about gamesmanship than anything else. A better formula for stultifying research could not be imagined" (Blanchard, 2002, p. 11).

In its conceptual structure, IRB policy is designed to produce the best ratio of costs to benefits. IRBs ostensibly protect the subjects who fall under the protocols they approve. However, given the interlocking utilitarian functions of social science, the academy, and the state that Mill identified and promoted, IRBs in reality protect their own institutions rather than subject populations in society at large (see Vanderpool, 1996, chaps. 2–6).[9]

The Current Crisis

Underneath the pros and cons of administering a responsible social science, the structural deficiencies in its epistemology have become transparent (Jennings, 1983, pp. 4–7). A positivistic philosophy of social inquiry insists on neutrality regarding definitions of the good, and this worldview has been generally discredited. The Enlightenment model, setting the subject at odds with the objective world, is bankrupt. Reworking professional codes of ethics so they are more explicit and less hortatory will make no fundamental difference. Requiring ethics workshops for graduate students and faculty is of marginal significance. Strengthening government policy is desirable but not transformative. Refining the IRB process and exhorting IRBs to account for the pluralistic nature of academic research are insufficient.

Certainly, levels of success and failure are open to dispute even within the social science disciplines themselves. More unsettling for the empiricist mainstream than disappointing performance is the recognition that neutrality is not pluralistic but imperialistic. Reflecting on past experience, disinterested research under presumed conditions of value freedom is increasingly seen as de facto reinscribing the agenda in its own terms. Empiricism is procedurally committed to equal reckoning, regardless of how research subjects may constitute the substantive ends of life. But experimentalism is not a neutral meeting ground for all ideas; rather, it is a "fighting creed" that imposes its own ideas on others while uncritically assuming the very "superiority that powers this imposition." In Foucault's (1979, pp. 170–195) more decisive terms, social science is a regime of power that helps maintain social order by normalizing subjects into categories designed by political authorities (see Root, 1993, chap.7). A liberalism of equality is not neutral but represents only one range of ideals, and is itself incompatible with other goods.

This noncontextual, nonsituational model that assumes "a morally neutral, objective observer will get the facts right" ignores "the situatedness of power relations associated with gender, sexual orientation, class, ethnicity, race, and nationality." It is hierarchical (scientist-subject) and biased toward patriarchy. "It glosses the ways in which the observer-ethnographer is implicated and embedded in the 'ruling apparatus' of the society and the culture." Scientists "carry the mantle" of university-based authority as they venture out into "local community to do research" (Denzin, 1997, p. 272; see also Ryan, 1995, pp. 144–145). There is no sustained questioning of expertise itself in democratic societies that belong in principle to citizens who do not share this specialized knowledge (see Euben, 1981, p. 120).

A Social Science Ethics of Resistance

Over the past decade, a social ethics of resistance has made a radical break with rationalist presumption of Western canonical ethics. Rather than searching for neutral principles to which all parties can appeal, ethics is understood to rest on a complex view of moral judgments as integrating various perspectives into an organic whole—everyday experience, beliefs about the good, and feelings of approval and shame. This is a philosophical approach that situates the moral domain within the general purposes of human life that people share contextually and across cultural, racial, and historical boundaries. Ideally, it engenders a new occupational role and normative core for social science research.

Within a social ethics of resistance, the mission of social and cultural research is interpretive sufficiency. In contrast to an experimentalism of instrumental efficiency, this paradigm seeks to open up the human world in all its dynamic dimensions. The thick notion of sufficiency supplants the thinness of the technical, exterior, and statistically precise received view. Rather than reducing social issues to financial and administrative problems, social science research helps people come to terms with their everyday experiences themselves.

Interpretive sufficiency means taking seriously lives that are loaded with multiple interpretations and grounded in cultural complexity (Denzin, 1989, pp. 77, 81). How the moral order works itself out in community formation is the issue, not first of all what researchers or funding agencies consider virtuous. The challenge for those writing culture is not to limit their moral perspectives to their own generic and neutral principles, but to engage the same moral space as the people they study. In this perspective, research strategies are not assessed, first of all in terms of "experimental robustness," but for their "vitality and vigor in illuminating how we can create human flourishing" (Lincoln & Denzin, 2000, p. 1062).

Reinventing Power

Thus, a basic norm for interpretive research is enabling the humane transformation of the multiple spheres of community life. To accomplish that revolution, Paulo Freire speaks of the need to reinvent the meaning of power:

> For me the principal, real transformation, the radical transformation of society in this part of the century demands not getting power from those who have it today, or merely to make some reforms, some changes in it. ... The question, from my point of view, is not just to take power but to reinvent it. That is, to create a different kind of power, to deny the need power has as if it were metaphysics, bureaucratized, anti-democratic. [quoted in Evans, Evans, & Kennedy, 1987, p. 229]

Certainly oppressive power blocs and monopolies—economic, technological, and political—need the scrutiny of researchers and their collaborators. Given Freire's political-institutional bearing, power for him is a central notion in social analysis. But, in concert with him, qualitative research refuses to deal with power in cognitive terms only. The issue is how people can empower themselves instead.

The dominant understanding of power is grounded in non-mutuality; it is interventionist power, exercised competitively and seeking control. In Freire's alternative, power is relational, characterized by mutuality rather than sovereignty. Power from this perspective is reciprocity between two subjects, a relationship not of domination, but of intimacy and vulnerability—power akin to that of Alcoholics Anonymous, in which surrender to the community enables the individual to gain mastery. As understood so clearly in the indigenous Kaupapa Māori approach to research, "the researcher is led by the members of the community and does not presume to be a leader, or to have any power that he or she can relinquish" (Denzin, 2003, p. 243).

Dialogue is the key element in an emancipatory strategy that liberates rather than imprisons us in manipulation or antagonistic relationships. Although the control version of power considers mutuality weakness, the empowerment mode maximizes our humanity and thereby banishes powerlessness. In the research process, power is unmasked and engaged through solidarity as a researched-researcher team. There is certainly no monologic "assumption that the researcher is giving the group power" (Denzin, 2003, p. 243). Rather than play semantic games with power, researchers themselves are willing to march against the barricades.

In Freire's (1973) terms, the goal is conscientization, that is, a critical consciousness that directs the ongoing flow of praxis and reflection in everyday life. In a culture of silence, the oppressor's language and way of being are fatalistically accepted without contradiction. But a critical consciousness enables us to exercise the uniquely human capacity of "speaking a true word" (Freire, 1970b, p. 75). Under conditions of sociopolitical control, "the vanquished are dispossessed of their word, their expressiveness, their culture" (1970b, p. 134). What is nonnegotiable in Freire's theory of power is participation of the oppressed in directing cultural formation. If an important social issue needs resolution, the most vulnerable will have to lead the way.[10] Through conscientization the oppressed gain their own voice and collaborate in transforming their culture (Freire, 1970a, pp. 212–213). Therefore, research is not the transmission of specialized data but, in style and content, a catalyst for critical consciousness. Without what Freire

(1970b, p. 47) calls "a critical comprehension of reality" (that is, the oppressed "grasping with their minds the truth of their reality"), there is only acquiescence in the status quo.

The resistance of the empowered is more productive at the interstices—at the fissures in social institutions where authentic action is possible. Effective resistance is nurtured in the backyards, the open spaces, voluntary associations, among neighborhoods, schools, and interactive settings of mutual struggle without elites. Because only nonviolence is morally acceptable for sociopolitical change, there is no other option except an educational one—having people's movements gain their own voice and nurturing a critical conscience through dialogic means. People-based development from below is not merely an end in itself, but a fundamental condition of social transformation.

Transforming the IRB

Interpretive sufficiency as a philosophy of social science fundamentally transforms the IRB system in form and content. As with IRBs, it emphasizes relentless accuracy, but understands it as the researcher's authentic resonance with the context and the subject's self-reflection as a moral agent. In an Indigenous Māori approach to knowledge, for example, "concrete experience is the criterion of meaning and truth," and researchers are "led by the members of the community to discover them" (Denzin, 2003, p. 243). However, because the research-subject relation is reciprocal, the IRBs' invasion of privacy, informed consent, and deception are nonissues. In an ethics of resistance, conceptions of the good are shared by the research subjects, and researchers collaborate in bringing these definitions into their own. "Participants have a co-equal say in how research should be conducted, what should be studied, which methods should be used, which findings are valid and acceptable, how the findings are to be implemented, and how the consequences of such actions are to be assessed" (Denzin, 2003, p. 257).

Interpretive sufficiency transcends the current regulatory system governing research on human subjects. Therefore, it recommends a policy of strict territorialism for the IRB regime. Given its roots historically in biomedicine, and with the explosion in both genetic research and privately funded biomedical research,

45 CFR 46 should be confined to medical, biological, and clinic studies and the positivist and postpositivist social science that is epistemologically identical to them. Research methodologies that have broken down the walls between subjects and researchers ought to be excluded from IRB oversight. As Denzin observes:

> Performance autoethnography, for example falls outside this [IRB] model, as do many forms of participatory action research, reflexive ethnography, and qualitative research involving testimonies, life stories, life-history inquiry, personal narrative inquiry, performance autobiography, conversation analysis, and ethnodrama. In all of these cases, subjects and researchers develop collaborative, public, pedagogical relationships. [2003, p. 249]

Because participation is voluntary, subjects do not need "to sign forms indicating that their consent is 'informed.'" Confidentiality is not an issue, "for there is nothing to hide or protect. Participants are not subjected to pre-approved procedures, but 'acting together, researchers and subjects work to produce change in the world'" (Denzin, 2003, pp. 249–250).

Given their different understanding of human inquiry, the review of their research protocols ought to be given to peers in academic departments or units familiar with these methodologies. The Oral History Association (OHA), for example, was excluded from IRB policy on September 22, 2003, in a letter from the Office for Human Research Protection (OHRP): "Oral history interviewing activities, in general, are not designed to contribute to generalizable knowledge and, therefore, do not involve research a defined by Department of Health and Human Services (HHS) regulations at 45 CFR 46.102d."

The OHA had argued that the regulations inscribed in the Common Rule were inconsistent with oral history methodology and inhibited critical inquiry. The IRB regulatory system is "based on a definition of research far removed from historical practice. Moreover, historians are acutely aware of the ethical dimensions of [their] work and have well-developed professional standards governing oral history interviewing" (Shopes, 2000. p. 8; cf. Shopes and Ritchie, 2004). Against the background of the American Historical Association's "Standards of Professional

Conduct" adopted on January 6, 2005, the OHA has codified a set of principles and responsibilities for guiding its own work in lieu of submitting research protocols for IRB review. Ambiguities in interpretation remain, given historical research and interviews designed for generalizable knowledge. Three years after the ruling by the OHRP, studies indicated that most university IRBs had not yet formally implemented the oral history exclusion (Townsend, 2006).[11] Despite the limited gains, and even though the IRBs' canon of rationalist knowledge is not contradicted, OHA's exclusion represents an important challenge to the "mission creep" of IRB bureaucracy (Gunsalus et al., 2005).

Conclusion

As Guba and Lincoln (1994) argue, the issues in social science ultimately must be engaged at the worldview level. "Questions of method are secondary to questions of paradigm, which we define as the basic belief system or worldview that guides the investigator, not only in choices of method but in ontologically and epistemologically fundamental ways" (Guba & Lincoln, 1994, p. 105). The conventional view, with its extrinsic ethics, gives us a truncated and unsophisticated paradigm that needs to be conceptually transformed. This historical overview of theory and practice points to the need for an entirely new model of research ethics in which human action and conceptions of the good are interactive.

When rooted in a positivist worldview, explanations of social life are considered incompatible with the renderings offered by the participants themselves. In problematics, lingual form, and content, research production presumes greater mastery and clearer illumination than the nonexperts who are the targeted beneficiaries. Protecting and promoting individual autonomy have been the philosophical rationale for value neutrality since its origins in Mill. But the incoherence in that view of social science is now transparent. By limiting the active involvement of rational beings or judging their self-understanding to be false, empiricist models contradict the ideal of rational beings who "choose between competing conceptions of the good" and make choices "deserving of respect." The verification standards of an instrumentalist system "take away what neutrality aims to protect: a community of free and equal rational beings legislating their own principles of conduct" (Root, 1993, p. 198). A social ethics of resistance escapes this contradiction by reintegrating human life with the moral order.

Notes

1 For a more detailed essay on value-free experimentalism, though with a different orientation, see Christians (2005, pp. 130–164).

2 Michael Root (1993) is unique among philosophers of the social sciences in linking social science to the ideals and practices of the liberal state on the grounds that both institutions "attempt to be neutral between competing conceptions of the good" (p. xv). Root's interpretations of Mill and Weber are crucial to my own formulation. As will be seen, neutrality is the common linkage among IRB conceptions of science, the university structure, and the state apparatus.

3 Although committed to what he called "the logic of the moral sciences" in delineating the canons or methods for induction, Mill shared with natural science a belief in the uniformity of nature and the presumption that all phenomena are subject to cause-and-effect relationships. His five principles of induction reflect a Newtonian cosmology.

4 In his *A System of Logic*, Mill ([1843] 1893) combines the principles of French positivism (as developed by Auguste Comte) and British empiricism into a single system.

5 For an elaboration of the complexities in positivism—including reference to its Millian connections—see Lincoln and Guba (1985, pp. 19–28).

6 Mill's realism is most explicitly developed in his *Examination of Sir William Hamilton's Philosophy* (1865b). Our belief in a common external world, in his view, is rooted in the fact that our sensations of physical reality "belong as much to other human or sentient beings as to ourselves" (p. 196; see also Copleston, 1966, p. 306, n. 97).

7 Mill (1969) specifically credits to Comte his use of the inverse deductive or historical method: "This was an idea entirely new to me when I found it in Comte; and but for him I might not soon (if ever) have arrived at it" (p. 126). Mill explicitly follows Comte in distinguishing social statics and social dynamics. He published two essays on Comte's influence in the *Westminster Review*, which were reprinted as *Auguste Comte and Positivism* (Mill, 1865a; see also Mill, 1969, p. 165).

8 The rationale for the Social Science Research Council (SSRC) in 1923 is multilayered, but in its attempt to link academic expertise with policy research, and in its preference for rigorous social scientific methodology, the SSRC reflects and implements Weber.

9 For a sociological and epistemological critique of IRBs, see Denzin (2003, pp. 248–257).

10 Because of his fundamental commitment to dialogue, empowering for Freire avoids the weaknesses of monologic concepts of empowerment in which researchers are seen to free up the weak and unfortunate (summarized by Denzin [2003, pp. 242–245] citing Bishop, 1998). Although Freire represents a radical perspective, he does not claim "as more radical theorists" do that "only they and their theories can lead" the researched into freedom (Denzin, 2003, p. 246, citing Bishop, 1998).

11 This specific evidence regarding OHA in 2006 is consistent with Denzin and Lincoln's conclusion regarding twenty years of debate over IRBs: "Institutional review boards appear, at least on some campuses, to be less, rather than more, sensitive to new epistemological concerns in the field, and more, rather than less, sensitive to newer forms of inquiry, including action research and participatory action research" (2001, p. xlv).

References

Bishop, R. (1998). Freeing ourselves from neo-colonial domination in research: A Māori approach to creating knowledge. *International Journal of Qualitative Studies in Education*, *11*(2), 199–219.

Christians, C. G. (2005). Ethics and politics in qualitative research. In N. K. Denzin & Y. Lincoln (Eds.), *The Sage handbook of qualitative research*, 3rd ed. (pp. 139–164). Thousand Oaks, CA: Sage.

Church, J. T. (2002). Should all disciplines be subject to the common rule? Panel, U. S. Department of Health and Human Services. Available online at http://www.aaup.org/publications/Academe/02mj/02mjftr.htm. Accessed December 17, 2006.

Comte, A. (1910). *A general view of positivism* (J. H. Bridges, Trans.). London: Routledge. (Original work published 1848; subsequently published as the first volume of *Positive philosophy*, 2 vols. [H. Martineau, Trans.]. London: Trübner, 1853.)

Copleston, F. (1966). *A history of philosophy*, vol. 8. Garden City, NY: Doubleday.

Denzin, N. K. (1989). *Interpretive biography*. Newbury Park, CA: Sage.

Denzin, N. K. (1997). *Interpretive ethnography: Ethnographic practices for the 21st century*. Thousand Oaks, CA: Sage.

Denzin, N. K. (2003). *Performance ethnography: Critical pedagogy and the politics of culture*. Thousand, Oaks, CA: Sage.

Denzin, N. K., & Lincoln, Y. S. (2001). *The American tradition of qualitative research*, vol. 1. Thousand Oaks, CA: Sage.

Descartes, R. (1916). *Discourse on method* (J. Veitch, Trans.). London: J. M. Dent & Sons, Ltd. (Original work published 1637.)

Euben, J. P. (1981). Philosophy and the professions. *Democracy, 2*(2), 112–127.

Evans, A. F., Evans, R. A., & Kennedy, W. B. (1987). *Pedagogies for the non-poor.* Maryknoll, NY: Orbis.

Foucault, M. (1979). *Discipline and punish: The birth of the prison* (A. Sheridan, Trans.). New York: Random House.

Freire, P. (1970a). *Education as the practice of freedom: Cultural action for freedom.* Cambridge, MA: Harvard Educational Review/Center for the Study of Development.

Freire, P. (1970b). *Pedagogy of the oppressed.* New York: Seabury.

Guba, E. G., & Lincoln, Y. S. (1994). Competing paradigms in qualitative research. In N. K. Denzin & Y. S. Lincoln (Eds.), *Handbook of qualitative research* (pp. 105–117). Thousand Oaks, CA: Sage.

Gunsalus, C. K., Bruner, E. M., Burbules, N. C., Dash, L., Finkin, Goldberg, J. P, Greenough, W. T., Miller, G. A., Pratt, M. G., Iriye, M., & Aronson, D. (2005). Improving the system for protecting human subjects: Counteracting IRB "mission creep." Available online at http://www.law.uiuc.edu/conferences/whitepaper/papers/SSRN-id902995.pdf. Accessed February 15, 2007.

Lincoln, Y. S., & Denzin, N. K. (2000). The seventh moment: Out of the past. In N. K. Denzin & Y. S. Lincoln (Eds.), *Handbook of Qualitative Research*, 2nd ed. (pp. 1047–1065). Thousand Oaks, CA: Sage.

Lincoln, Y. S., & Guba, E. G. (1985). *Naturalistic inquiry.* Beverly Hills, CA: Sage.

Mill, J. S. ([1865a] 1907). *Auguste Comte and positivism.* London: Kegan Paul, Trench, Trubner & Co.

Mill, J. S. (1865b). *Examination of Sir William Hamilton's philosophy and of the principal philosophical questions discussed in his writings.* London: Longman, Green, Roberts & Green.

Mill, J. S. (1893). *A system of logic, ratiocinative and inductive: Being a connected view of the principles of evidence and the methods of scientific investigation*, 8th ed. New York: Harper & Brothers. (Original work published 1843.)

Mill, J. S. (1957). *Utilitarianism.* Indianapolis: Bobbs-Merrill. (Original work published 1861.)

Mill, J. S. (1969). *Autobiography.* Boston: Houghton Mifflin. (Original work published posthumously 1873.)

Mill, J. S. (1978). *On liberty.* Indianapolis: Hackett. (Original work published 1859.)

Root, M. (1993). *Philosophy of social science: The methods, ideals, and politics of social inquiry*. Oxford: Blackwell.

Ryan, K. E. (1995). Evaluation ethics and issues of social justice: Contributions from female moral thinking. In N. K. Denzin (Ed.), *Studies in symbolic interaction: A research annual*, vol. 19 (pp. 143–151). Greenwich, CT: JAI.

Shopes, L. (2000). Institutional review boards have a chilling effect on oral history. *Perspectives online*. Available online at http://www.theaha.org/perspectives/issues/2000/0009/0009vie1.cfm. Accessed December 17, 2006.

Shopes, L., & Ritchie, D. (2004). Exclusion of oral history from IRB review: An update. *Perspectives online*. Available online at http://www.historians.org/Perspectives/Issues/2004/0403new1.cfm. Accessed December 17, 2006.

Townsend, R. B. (2006). Oral history and review boards: Little gain and more pain. *American historical association perspectives*. Available online at http://www.historians.org/perspectives/issues/2006. Accessed December 17, 2006.

University of Illinois at Urbana-Champaign, Institutional Review Board. (2006). Part II: Fundamental guidelines. A. Ethical principles. In *Investigator handbook: For the protection of human subjects in research*. Available online at http://www.irb.uiuc.edu. Accessed December 17, 2006.

Vanderpool, H. Y. (Ed.). (1996). *The ethics of research involving human subjects: Facing the 21st century*. Frederick, MD: University Publishing Group.

Weber, M. (1949a). The meaning of ethical neutrality in sociology and economics. In E. A. Shils & H. A. Finch (Eds. & Trans.), *The methodology of the social sciences* (pp. 1–47). New York: Free Press. (Original work published 1917.)

Weber, M. (1949b). Objectivity in social science and social policy. In E. A. Shils & H. A. Finch (Eds. & Trans.), *The methodology of the social sciences* (pp. 50–112). New York: Free Press. (Original work published 1904.)

Chapter 4

Evidence

A Critical Realist Perspective for Qualitative Research

Joseph A. Maxwell

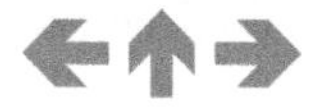

The topic of evidence is so central for research and scholarship that it is extraordinary how little direct attention it has received.

—Chandler, Davidson, & Harootunian, 1994, p. 1

The concept of evidence, largely neglected by researchers in the social sciences for many years, has recently become a hotly contested one, largely because of the rise of movements for "evidence-based" practice and policy (Denzin & Giardina, 2008; Pawson, 2006).[1] Much of the critique of the evidence-based movement by qualitative researchers has been based on a social constructivist or postmodern epistemology that challenges the basic concept of "evidence." This has also been true of the larger debate over evidence in the social sciences, and has "threatened to reduce the role of evidence, facts, and proof to the point of nonexistence" (Chandler, Davidson, & Harootunian, 1994, p. 5).

However, there have also been significant challenges to this movement, and to the push for "science-based" research in general,

Originally published in *Qualitative Inquiry and Social Justice*, edited by Norman K. Denzin and Michael D. Giardina, pp.108–122. Republished in *Qualitative Inquiry—Past, Present, and Future: A Critical Reader*, edited by Norman K. Denzin and Michael D. Giardina, pp. 88–102. Left Coast Press, Inc.

from a realist perspective (Hammersley, 1992b; Maxwell, 2004a; Pawson, 2006). In this chapter, I argue that critical realism[2] can make important contributions to the critique of evidence-based research, contributions that are particularly relevant to, and supportive of, qualitative research. However, although I think that critical realism is a significant and valuable voice in that critique, I'm not arguing that critical realism is the single, correct philosophical stance for qualitative research. In fact, I'm skeptical that there is such a thing as a "correct" philosophical stance for qualitative research.

My thinking about this approach has been influenced by the work of the sociologist Andrew Abbott (2001, 2004), who has argued for what he calls a "fractal" view of the grand debates over epistemological and methodological issues in the social sciences. (The basic idea of a fractal is self-similarity at different scales or levels.) His view is that if we take any of a large number of debates between polar positions, such as positivism versus interpretivism, analysis versus narrative, realism versus constructivism, and so on, these issues can play out at many different levels, even within communities of scholars that have adopted one or the other of these positions at a broader level. Thus, within the community of sociologists of science, which is generally seen as constructivist in orientation, there are internal debates that play out in terms of realist or constructivist "moves" by particular scholars within that community.

Abbott claims that philosophical paradigms, rather than constituting grand overarching frameworks that inform and control the theories and practices of particular disciplines and subfields, instead function as heuristics, conceptual tools that can be applied in an endless number of specific situations to break out of theoretical blocks and generate new questions and theories. He even suggests that this is the way these grand paradigmatic positions originated: as useful heuristics that later became abstracted and formalized into high-level philosophical systems.

One of the many examples that Abbott provides is Daniel Chambliss's (1989) ethnographic study of competitive swimming. Chambliss argued that there is no such thing as "talent" as an explanation of high performance; it is a social construction that romanticizes and mystifies what he called "the mundanity of excellence." This is a constructivist move in the debate over sports performance. He supported this claim with detailed evidence from observations of, and interviews with, swimmers, showing that high performance is simply the result of dozens of small skills, learned or stumbled on, that are repeatedly practiced and synthesized into a coherent whole. However, an essential part of this argument was a realist move, identifying the actual skills and practices that led to excellence.

Abbott argues that the heuristic uses of such polar positions as realism and constructivism are not aimed at demolishing or debunking the opposition. Instead, their function is to open up the debate, to provoke discussion, and increase understanding, revealing new ways of making sense of the things we study. This perspective has a great deal in common with postmodernism, which rejects "totalizing metanarratives" and emphasizes diversity and irreconcilability (Bernstein, 1992).

From this perspective, philosophical positions look less like the traditional view of paradigms, and more like tools in a toolkit. "Logical consistency" is the wrong standard to apply to a toolkit. You don't care if the tools are all consistent with some axiomatic principle; you care if, among them, they enable you to do the job, to create something that can meet your needs or accomplish your goals. In the same way, consistency is the wrong standard to apply to an individual's or a community's ontological and epistemological views. These views, seen as heuristics, are resources for getting your work done.

The essential characteristic of critical realism (discussed below) is that it combines ontological realism with epistemological constructivism in a productive, if apparently inconsistent, "constellation" (Bernstein, 1992) of positions. Smith and Deemer (2000) argue that this combination is contradictory, and therefore a fatal flaw in critical realism. From Abbott's perspective, this is not a valid criticism, any more than arguing that an automobile having both a battery and a gasoline engine is contradictory. The question is not whether they are logically consistent, but whether they are compatible in their actual functioning. I argue (Maxwell, 2008) that ontological realism and epistemological constructivism are not only compatible, but, like the battery and gasoline engine in a hybrid car, are more effective than a consistent position.

Realism

Schwandt (2007, p. 256) defines realism in a broad sense as "the doctrine that there are real objects that exist independently of our knowledge of their existence," and argues that "most of us probably behave as garden-variety empirical realists—that is, we act as if the objects in the world (things, events, structures, people, meanings, etc.) exist as independent in some way from our experience with them." However, there are many varieties of realism, ranging from naive or direct realism—the view that we directly perceive things as they actually are—to more sophisticated positions that recognize that our concepts and theories necessarily mediate our perceptions of reality.

Many of the latter positions adopt an ontological realism, but an epistemological constructivism, asserting that there is not, even in principle, a "God's eye view" that is independent of any particular perspective or stance. I will refer to these positions as forms of "critical" realism. Lakoff states that such versions of realism assume "that 'the world is the way it is,' while acknowledging that there can be more than one scientifically correct way of understanding reality in terms of conceptual schemes with different objects and categories of objects" (1987, p. 265). Such positions can be seen as postmodern in the sense that they reject the idea that there must be a single correct account or interpretation of a complex reality.

I have argued elsewhere (Maxwell, 2004a, 2004c, 2008) that these positions are both compatible with, and can make a number of valuable contributions to, qualitative research. In particular, they reject the Humean, regularity concept of causation that has dominated both quantitative research and the evidence-based movement and adopt a process-oriented view of causality; they emphasize the importance of context and particular understanding, rather than focusing entirely on general conclusions and laws; and they accept the reality of mental phenomena and the necessity of incorporating these in our understanding and explanation of human action.

In what follows, I present how I see these positions contributing to our understanding of evidence and how they can provide a concept of evidence that is both useful for qualitative researchers and can defend qualitative research from the criticisms of advocates of a narrowly conceived evidence- or science-based approach to social research.

Evidence

Schwandt (2007, p. 98) defines evidence as "information that bears on determining the validity (truth, falsity, accuracy, etc.) of a claim or what an inquirer provides, in part, to warrant a claim." From a different perspective, Chandler, Davidson, and Harootunian, discussing Collingwood's view of evidence in history, likewise argue that "question and evidence are therefore 'correlative' in the sense that facts can only become evidence in response to some particular question" (1994, p. 1).

Schwandt's definition and Collingwood's argument point to the inextricable connections between evidence, claim, and validity. A key property of evidence is that it does not exist in abstraction but only in relation to some claim (theory, hypothesis, interpretation, etc.). There is no such thing as evidence in general; evidence is always evidence *relative to* some particular claim, account, or theory. Evidence is thus in the same position as validity—it can't be assessed in context-independent ways, but only in relation to the particular question and purpose to which it is applied.

In particular, evidence can't be evaluated solely in terms of the methods used to obtain it. Any attempt to establish a context-free hierarchy of kinds of evidence based entirely on the methods used to create that evidence, as proponents of evidence-based approaches typically do, is inevitably flawed. Although this emphasis on the context-dependence of evidence and conclusions is a key feature of critical realist approaches, it is shared by a much broader community of scholars. Phillips states what seems to be a widely held view in the philosophy of science: "In general it must be recognized that there are no procedures that will regularly (or always) yield either sound data or true conclusions" (1987, p. 21).

Shadish, Cook, and Campbell, in what is currently the definitive work on experimental and quasi-experimental research, are quite explicit on this point with respect to validity, and thus for evidence: "Validity is a property of inferences. It is not a property of designs or methods, for the same designs may contribute to more or less valid inferences under different circumstances. ... No method guarantees the validity of an inference" (2002, p. 34). Brinberg and McGrath make the same point: "Validity is not a commodity that can be purchased with techniques. ... Rather, validity is like integrity, character, and quality, to be assessed relative to purposes and circumstances" (1985, p. 13)

The philosopher Peter Achinstein, who has probably done the most to systematically critique and reformulate the traditional philosophical view of evidence (2001, 2005), makes the related point that evidence isn't a single thing, but several; there is no essential property that all uses of "evidence" possess (2001, p. 15). This position is strikingly similar to the philosopher Nancy Cartwright's concept of causal pluralism. Cartwright has provided a detailed argument for the view that what causes are and what they do depends on the particular situation in which they are employed. I would similarly argue for evidential pluralism. To borrow Cartwright's phrasing, what evidence is and what it does varies from case to case, and "there is no single interesting characterizing feature of [evidence]; hence no off-the-shelf or one-size-fits-all method for [identifying] it, no 'gold standard' for judging [evidence]" (Cartwright, 2007, p. 2).

In particular, there is a key difference between the uses of evidence in quantitative and qualitative research, or more specifically between what Mohr (1982) called "variance theory" and "process theory." Variance theory deals with variables and the relationship between them, and the main use of evidence is to show that a particular relationship exists between different variables, whether these are constructs measured using a test or survey, or manipulated in an experiment. Process theory, in contrast, is mainly concerned with events and processes, rather than variables, and the main use of evidence (and the primary strength of qualitative research) is to support claims about these events and processes—to get inside the "black box" of variance theory and to argue for what is actually happening in specific cases.

By "what is happening," I (and critical realists in general) include participants' meanings, intentions, beliefs, and perspectives, which are essential parts of these events and processes (Maxwell, 2004a). Evidence for claims about meanings and perspectives, which fall under the general category of "interpretive" claims, require quite different sorts of evidence than claims about behavior, let alone claims about the relationships between variables. Thus, the kinds of claims, and the nature and evaluation of the evidence for these claims, are very different in qualitative research than those in quantitative research, and evidential standards appropriate for quantitative and experimental research can't legitimately be applied to qualitative research.

Achinstein draws a number of other conclusions from this claim-dependence and context-dependence of evidence. First, whether some fact is evidence for a particular claim depends on how the fact is obtained or generated (Achinstein, 2001, p. 8). This does not conflict with the previous point that evidence can't be assessed strictly in terms of the methods used to obtain it. It simply asserts that how the evidence was obtained is often relevant to the support it lends to a particular claim, because the methods used may create certain validity threats that threaten the claim.

Second, the significance of evidence depends on the context of *other* evidence and hypotheses relevant to the claim being supported. A particular piece of data might by itself be evidence for a claim, but not when considered in combination with other evidence. In addition, the degree of support that a particular piece of evidence provides for a particular claim depends on the plausibility of (and evidence for) *alternative* claims regarding the phenomena in question (Achinstein, 2001, pp. 7–10). Achinstein provides several examples from different sciences in which a finding that was once believed to be convincing evidence for a particular claim was no longer thought to be so when new evidence was developed or alternative explanations were proposed. Thus, part of the context that evidence for a particular claim depends on for its assessment is the context of alternative possible theories and explanations for the phenomenon in question.

Achinstein addresses this issue by referring to what he calls the "epistemic situation" in which the use of particular data to support a claim is located (2001, pp. 20–21). This situation consists of what the researcher knew and believed at the time, and what this person was *not* in a position to know or believe. For Achinstein, any justification for saying that a claim is supported by a particular body of evidence is relative to this epistemic situation, rather than being a context-independent truth, and "since justification is relativized to an epistemic situation, so is the concept of evidence based on it."[3] Researchers often agree on the data relative to some claim, but disagree on whether these constitute evidence for the claim. Evidence is therefore an interpretation of the data or observations, and "evidence" is an essentially contested concept.

Third, the previous point entails that whether a fact or observation is evidence for some claim is an empirical question, not a logical one (Achinstein, 2001, p. 9). The evidence can only be assessed in the context of the particular claim that the evidence is asserted to support, the way the evidence was generated, and the epistemic situation in which these claims are made. This context is not given a priori but needs to be empirically discovered. Achinstein argues that one of the main reasons that actual researchers have paid so little attention to philosophical work on evidence is that this work usually presumes that the link between claim and evidence is strictly logical, semantic, or mathematical, something that can be established by calculation rather than empirical investigation.

Finally, Achinstein argues that for a fact to be evidence for some claim, simply because the fact increases the probability that the claim is true isn't enough; there must be some *explanatory connection* between the fact and the claim (2001, p. 145ff.). This is an essential component of realist approaches to explanation in general—that a valid explanation does not simply support the view *that* x causes y, but must address *how* it does so (Manicas, 2006; Salmon, 1998; Sayer, 1992, 2000). This lack of attention to the *process* by which a causal influence takes place is a major flaw in most evidence-based approaches (Maxwell, 2004a, 2008).

A recent study by Leibovici (2001) illustrates this point. Liebovici conducted a double blind, randomized clinical trial of the effectiveness of intercessory prayer on a number of outcomes for hospital patients. To avoid problems of patient consent, reactivity, and patient attrition, the author selected a sample of hospital records of 3,393 adult patients—every patient who had been diagnosed with a bloodstream infection between 1990 and 1996. These records were randomly divided into an intervention group and a control group, and a short prayer was said for the well-being and recovery of the intervention group as a whole. (This intervention took place four to ten years after the patient had left the hospital.) Examination of the records showed that the patients in the intervention group had had a mean length of stay in the hospital and duration of fever shorter than those in the control group ($p<.01$ and $p<.04$, respectively). Mortality was also lower in the intervention group, but this difference was not statistically significant.

Even if there are doubts that the study was rigorously conducted, the main threat to the credibility of this study's results as evidence for the author's conclusion—that intercessory prayer was effective in reducing the morbidity and mortality of the patients—is that no plausible mechanism can be provided for the causal conclusion. The author addresses this problem head-on: "No mechanism known today can account for the effects of remote, retroactive intercessory prayer said for a group of patients with a bloodstream infection" (Leibovici, 2001, p. 1451). He argues that this case is similar to that of James Lind, who, in 1753, found that lemons and limes cured scurvy without having any knowledge of Vitamin C, let alone an understanding of the mechanism by which this can prevent and cure scurvy.

The difference between these two cases is that for limes and scurvy, even in 1753, the idea that something in limes could cure scurvy was not implausible and could serve as a plausible explanatory connection between the evidence and the claim. For retroactive intercessory prayer, an explanatory connection is difficult to imagine, except in an "epistemic situation" in which the power of God to do anything, even on the basis of a perfunctory prayer said for an entire category of people, is an accepted mechanism.

Achinstein does not directly address the evidence-based approaches that have made evidence a critically important issue for social researchers and evaluators, as opposed to philosophers. However, his reformulations of the concept of evidence challenge many of the premises of these approaches. Evidence is not a context-free entity that can unproblematically be aggregated to generate conclusions about "what works"; what counts as evidence varies from case to case and depends not only on the methods used, but the epistemic situation; and the use of evidence is dependent on the process by which the program or intervention is theorized to affect the outcome, not simply to whether it does so.

The methodologist and evaluation researcher Ray Pawson (2006) has applied a realist perspective to the evidence-based policy movement, specifically to the central idea of "systematic review" promoted by this movement, particularly by the Cochrane Collaborative (in medicine) and the Campbell Collaborative (in program evaluation). The purpose of such reviews is to produce conclusions about what works based on the "best evidence" culled from available studies.

The failures of this approach that Pawson identifies and systematically criticizes, and the strengths of the realist alternative that he proposes, are too numerous to fully present here, and I will focus on only the most important and intrinsic of these for the use of evidence in research. In particular, I will not address the critique that the very idea that policy should be evidence-based or "research-based" is problematic (Hammersley, 2005; Pawson, 2006).

First, practitioners of the evidence-based approach largely ignore the *process* by which programs or interventions influence the outcomes of interest. Consistent with the Humean, regularity view of causation that they accept, the review focuses on finding evidence on *whether* the intervention influenced the outcome, not *how* it did so—what Shadish, Cook, and Campbell (2002, p. 9) call "causal description" rather than "causal explanation." Instead of trying to understand the mechanisms and processes by which a program has its effects, it attempts to identify causal generalizations, "main effects" across studies and situations.

Second, in seeking these causal generalizations, such reviews systematically neglect the importance of context in understanding why a program may or may not have particular outcomes. For realists, context is intrinsically involved with process in influencing outcomes, and evidence about the effect of the specific context is essential for assessing the likely results of a program or intervention. Causality is thus fundamentally particular rather than general, and an adequate understanding how causes operate requires evidence about the contextual influences operating in the specific case.

Pawson summarizes these two points as follows:

> The nature of causality in social programmes is such that any synthesis of evidence on whether they work will need to investigate how they work. This requires unearthing information on mechanisms, contexts, and outcomes. The central quest is to understand the conditions of programme efficacy and this will involve the synthesis in investigating for whom, in what circumstances, and in what respects a family of programmes work. (2006, p. 25)

It is ironic that these are issues for which qualitative research can make a significant contribution (Maxwell, 2004a). However, the theory of causation on which the evidence-based movement relies, and the bias toward quantitative and experimental methods that this produces, has largely excluded qualitative evidence from the research syntheses that the movement generates.

In part because of this bias, qualitative researchers have long been either defensive about their use of evidence, or dismissive of the entire concept of evidence. I argue that there is no good reason for either of these reactions. A realist reformulation of the concept of evidence can provide a strong justification for the value of the evidence generated by qualitative research, and qualitative researchers have their own ways of obtaining and using such evidence that are just as legitimate for their purposes as quantitative researchers' are for theirs (Maxwell, 2004c).

Finally, I want to say something about the relationship between ethics and evidence. I would argue that evidence and ethics are separate issues, and that there is sometimes a tradeoff between them. It may be impossible, in any particular study, to maximize both of these. As Hammersley (1992a) has argued about critical theory, it is an illusion to believe that there must be a solution in which all "progressive" goals are compatible and can be optimally achieved.

An example of this tradeoff is Stanley Milgram's experimental studies[4] on obedience to authority (1974), in which he recruited participants to participate in a purported study of reinforcement and learning. This study was clearly unethical in that it subjected participants to potentially psychologically damaging experiences without informing them of the nature of the study or of these risks, but that doesn't discredit the evidence that his study produced to support the view that most people will readily inflict severe pain on others when told to do so by someone seen as an authority. Milgram, in fact, argues that some participants in the study claimed that their lives were transformed by the experience, leading them to be much more concerned about ethical ideals and the need to resist unjust authority.

In conclusion, I am arguing for a dialogical (Greene, 2007), postmodern approach to evidence in qualitative research, one that embraces contrary perspectives such as realism and constructivism and uses these to gain a better understanding of the phenomena we study. This approach can help us make better use of the concept of evidence and help us challenge misguided appropriations of this concept.

Notes

1 An additional work that directly and insightfully addresses many of the issues discussed in this paper, but which was published too recently to be included in the text of the chapter, is Donaldson, Christie, & Mark (2009).

2 The phrase "critical realism" was coined by Roy Bhaskar to refer to his influential version of realism as a philosophy of social science (Archer et al., 1998; Bhaskar, 1978, 1989). However, there are many other systematically developed positions that combine ontological realism with a more constructivist epistemology, by both philosophers (Haack, 2003; Manicas, 2006; Putnam, 1990, 1999) and social scientists (Lakoff, 1987; Lakoff & Johnson, 1999; Pawson, 2006; Pawson & Tilley, 1997; Sayer, 1992, 1999; Shweder, 1991), including qualitative researchers (Hammersley, 1992b; Huberman & Miles, 1985; Maxwell, 1992, 1999, 2004a, 2004b, 2004c, 2008). Although these positions differ on many specific points of philosophy and method, I will refer to all of them, broadly, as "critical realist."

3 Achinstein claims that the dependence of evidence on the epistemic situation still leaves this an objective rather than a subjective definition of "evidence" (2001, p. 21), because the epistemic situation is defined not entirely by what the person believes, but on what the person *is in a position* to know or believe, which can be objectively assessed. However, it is certainly a *context-dependent* definition of what counts as evidence, and includes the person's beliefs as part of that context. In addition, as noted above, Achinstein recognizes that evidence is not a single thing, but a variety of things, one of

which he calls "subjective evidence," which *is* based on the subjective beliefs of some person at some time (2001, p. 23). I therefore see Achinstein's position as at least a major step away from objectivism toward a constructivist epistemology. Achinstein is clearly an ontological realist in treating hypotheses and theories as referring to a real world, rather than as simply useful constructions (2001, p. 145 ff., 263–265).

4 Despite the title, these studies combined quantitative/experimental and qualitative methods. Milgram provided detailed case studies of how particular individuals responded to the experimental situation and interviewed participants following the experimental procedure to understand their perception of the situation and why they responded as they did (Maxwell & Loomis, 2003).

References

Abbott, A. (2001). *Chaos of disciplines.* Chicago: University of Chicago Press.

Abbott, A. (2004). *Methods of discovery: Heuristics for the social sciences.* New York: W. W. Norton.

Achinstein, P. (2001). *The book of evidence.* Oxford: Oxford University Press.

Achinstein, P. (Ed.). (2005). *Scientific evidence: Philosophical theories and applications.* Baltimore: Johns Hopkins University Press

Archer, M., Bhaskar, R., Collier, A. Lawson, T., & Norrie, A. (1998). *Critical realism: Essential readings.* London: Routledge.

Bernstein, R. (1992). *The new constellation: The ethical-political horizons of modernity-postmodernity.* Cambridge MA: MIT Press.

Bhaskar, R. (1978). *A realist theory of science*, 2nd ed. Brighton, UK: Harvester.

Bhaskar, R. (1989). *Reclaiming reality: A critical introduction to contemporary philosophy.* London: Verso.

Brinberg, D. & McGrath, J. E. (1985). *Validity and the research process.* Newbury Park, CA: Sage .

Cartwright, N. (2007). *Hunting causes and using them: Approaches in philosophy and economics.* Cambridge: Cambridge University Press.

Chambliss, D. (1989). The mundanity of excellence: An ethnographic report on stratification and Olympic swimmers. *Sociological Theory*, 7, 70–86.

Chandler, J., Davidson, A., & Harootunian, H. (1994). *Questions of evidence: Proof, practice, and persuasion across the disciplines.* Chicago: University of Chicago Press.

Denzin, N. K. & Giardina, M. D. (2008). *Qualitative inquiry and the politics of evidence.* Walnut Creek, CA: Left Coast Press, Inc.

Donaldson, S. I., Christie, C. A., & Mark, M. M. (2009). *What counts as credible evidence in applied research and evaluation practice?* Thousand Oaks, CA: Sage.

Greene, J. (2007. *Mixed methods in social inquiry.* New York: Wiley.

Haack, S. (2003). *Defending science—within reason.* Amherst, NY: Prometheus Press.

Hammersley, M. (1992a). Critical theory as a model for ethnography. In M. Hammersley (Ed.), *What's wrong with ethnography? Methodological explorations*, pp. 96–125. London: Routledge.

Hammersley, M. (1992b). Ethnography and realism. In M. Hammersley (Ed.), *What's wrong with ethnography? Methodological explorations*, pp. 43–56. London: Routledge.

Hammersley, M. (2005). The myth of research-based practice: The critical case of educational inquiry. *International Journal of Social Research Methodology, 8*(4), 317–330.

Huberman, A. M. & Miles, M. B. (1985). Assessing local causality in qualitative research. In D. N. Berg & K. K. Smith (Eds.), *Exploring clinical methods for social research*, pp. 351–382. Beverly Hills, CA: Sage.

Lakoff, G. (1987). *Women, fire, and dangerous things: What categories reveal about the mind.* Chicago: University of Chicago Press.

Lakoff, G. & Johnson, M. (1999). *Philosophy in the flesh: The embodied mind and its challenge to Western thought.* New York: Basic Books.

Leibovici, L. (2001). Effects of remote, retroactive, intercessory prayer on outcomes in patients with bloodstream infection: Randomised controlled trial. *British Medical Journal, 323*, 1450–1451.

Manicas, P. T. (2006). *A realist philosophy of social science: Explanation and understanding.* Cambridge: Cambridge University Press.

Maxwell, J. A. (1992). Understanding and validity in qualitative research. *Harvard Educational Review, 62*, 279–300.

Maxwell, J. A. (1999). A realist/postmodern concept of culture. In E. L. Cerroni-Long (Ed.), *Anthropological theory in North America*, pp. 143–173. Westport, CT: Bergin & Garvey.

Maxwell, J. A. (2004a). Causal explanation, qualitative research, and scientific inquiry in education. *Educational Researcher, 33*(2), 3–11.

Maxwell, J. A. (2004b). Re-emergent scientism, postmodernism, and dialogue across differences. *Qualitative Inquiry, 10*, 35–41.

Maxwell, J. A. (2004c). Using qualitative methods for causal explanation. *Field Methods, 16*, 243–264.

Maxwell, J. A. (2008). The value of a realist understanding of causality for qualitative research. In N. K. Denzin & M. D. Giardina (Eds.), *Qualitative inquiry and the politics of evidence*, pp. 163–181. Walnut Creek, CA: Left Coast Press, Inc.

Maxwell, J. A. & Loomis, D. (2003). Mixed methods design: An alternative approach. In A. Tashakkori & C. Teddlie (Eds.), *Handbook of mixed methods in social and behavioral research*, pp. 241–271. Thousand Oaks, CA: Sage.

Milgram, S. (1974). *Obedience to authority: An experimental view.* New York: Harper and Row.

Mohr, L. B. (1982). *Explaining organizational behavior.* San Francisco: Jossey-Bass.

Pawson, R. (2006). *Evidence-based policy: A realist perspective.* London: Sage.

Pawson, R. & Tilley, N. (1997). *Realistic evaluation.* London: Sage.

Phillips, D. C. (1987). Validity in qualitative research: Why the worry about warrant will not wane. *Education and Urban Society*, 20, 9–24.

Putnam, H. (1990). *Realism with a human face*, edited by James Conant. Cambridge: Harvard University Press.

Putnam, H. (1999). *The threefold cord: Mind, body, and world.* New York: Columbia University Press.

Salmon, W. C. (1998). *Causality and explanation.* New York: Oxford University Press.

Sayer, A. (1992). *Method in social science: A realist approach*, 2nd ed. London: Routledge.

Sayer, A. (2000). *Realism and social science.* London: Sage.

Schwandt, T. A. (2007). *Qualitative inquiry: A dictionary of terms*, 3rd ed. Thousand Oaks, CA: Sage.

Shadish, W. R., Cook, T. D., & Campbell, D. T. (2002). *Experimental and quasi-experimental designs for generalized causal inference.* Boston: Houghton Mifflin.

Shweder, R. A. (1991). *Thinking through cultures: Expeditions in cultural psychology.* Cambridge, MA: Harvard University Press.

Smith, J. K. & Deemer, D. K. (2000). The problem with criteria in the age of relativism. In N. K. Denzin & Y. S. Lincoln (Eds.), *The handbook of qualitative research*, 2nd ed., pp. 877–922. Thousand Oaks, CA: Sage.

Chapter 5

Refusing Human Being in Humanist Qualitative Inquiry

Elizabeth Adams St. Pierre

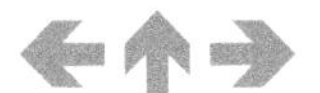

What I call "conventional humanist qualitative inquiry" is grounded in the human being of humanism—the individual, person, or self who has an identity. I have discussed that description in detail elsewhere (St. Pierre, 2000) and will not repeat it here. We generally say that the modern subject began with Descartes's ([1637] 1993) statement we remember well, "I think, therefore I am" (p. 18), and that human was elaborated differently by others, including Locke ([1690] 1924), who is generally referred to as the first of the British empiricists as well as the founder of liberalism. Locke disputed Descartes, describing a "self," an "individual," with a personal identity (sameness over time) based on consciousness whose mind is, at the beginning, a blank slate with no innate ideas.

The descriptions of human being these two Enlightenment thinkers invented, as well as variations introduced by others (e.g., Hegel's unitary, reflexive self-identical subject), pervade the social and natural sciences. In general, they assume an epistemological, knowing, rational, conscious, a priori, grammatical doer who

Originally published in *Qualitative Inquiry and Global Crises*, edited by Norman K. Denzin and Michael D. Giardina, pp. 40–55. Republished in *Qualitative Inquiry—Past, Present, and Future: A Critical Reader*, edited by Norman K. Denzin and Michael D. Giardina, pp. 103–118.

exists ahead of the deed. That is, they believe in the truth of grammatical categories, for example, that, in Descartes's sentence there actually exists a subject "I" that precedes the verb "think." But those particular descriptions of human being and the philosophy of the subject elaborated from them have always been contested, especially in the last century, when the horrors of World War II proved humans' capacity for evil and inhumane behavior.

Post-war French thought identified the "growing instability of the subject in the writings of Koyéve, Hyppolite and Sartre" (Butler, 1987, p. 185) until proclamations declared the death of that human being who no longer seemed either self-evident or desirable. As Peters and Marshall (1993) explained, some took the radical position that that "construct is merely a philosophical and cultural mystification which sought to persuade people that they 'had' … this unique personal identity" (p. 21). In other words, we began to realize that all those descriptions of human being we'd been led to believe were true and real were merely *descriptions*. We'd become trapped in believing in "permanence, identity, and substantiality" (Finke, 1993, p. 15), trapped in old "habits of saying 'I' and 'we'" (Rajchman, 2000, p. 97). We realized we could now think and live human being differently. Foucault ([1981] 1997a) explained as follows:

> There were two possible paths that led beyond this philosophy of the subject. The first of these was the theory of objective knowledge as an analysis of systems of meaning, as semiology. This was the path of logical positivism. The second was that of a certain school of linguistics, psychoanalysis, and anthropology—all grouped under the rubric of Structuralism. (p. 176)

I would argue that conventional humanist qualitative inquiry took up both paths Foucault identified above—logical positivism and structuralism—as well as theories and practices that emerged from the interpretive and critical turns in the social sciences. But the concept repeated with minor variation in all those social science approaches is the human being of humanism.

The Individual in Humanist Qualitative Inquiry

We generally think of qualitative inquiry as interpretive, but the logical positivism and structuralism Foucault identified are quite evident in qualitative inquiry. The stubborn persistence of positivism is evident, for example, when researchers cling to an objectivist epistemology by using terms like "bias" and "triangulation," believe that knowledge *accumulates* and has *gaps* that *findings* can fill, believe in the clarity and transparency of language, and treat data (words in interview transcripts and field notes) as *brute data* and then code them out of context. Structural tendencies are normalist and rationalist and evident when, for example: (1) Researchers cling to linearity in concepts like research "process," "development," and "systematicity"; (2) they create structured wholes with underlying systems of regularities and inner meaning (e.g., humans who have an essential, authentic, inner voice); and (3) they force what might be always already disordered, contingent, and/or arbitrary into supposedly ordered, coherent, rational structures of meaning (e.g., organizing data into *themes* and *patterns* and *linear narratives*).

But qualitative inquiry early on resisted positivist and structuralist approaches and leaned toward interpretivism with its focus on the relation among "what is studied, the means of investigation, and the ends informing the investigator" (Rabinow & Sullivan, 1979, p. 13). Researchers' aim in interpretive research is to try to understand the meaning ordinary people (the person, the individual) make of their lives, to do fieldwork in natural settings where participants live, to elicit their descriptions of everyday lived experience in their own language, and then to reproduce as accurately as possible that meaning and experience in detailed descriptions in the research report. In that work, however, meaning-making and experience too often go untroubled and are assumed to be natural, real, authentic, simply the "way it is." For that reason, interpretive social science is critiqued for too much description and not enough theoretical analysis. Nonetheless, rich, thick description (especially of the individual, of participants) is a hallmark of much qualitative inquiry, even in supposedly critical research, which one would expect to critique the naturalness of oppression in identity.

Social justice agendas popular in qualitative inquiry are also mostly grounded in an essentialist liberal humanist individual, but in this research the focus is on the intentionality, innate agency, and free will of participants. In this work, an emancipatory model of agency claims that individuals can lift themselves out of oppression and alienation—once their consciousness is raised—no matter the circumstances, though it is debatable, for example, whether it is a kindness to tell children who live on the wrong side of all the identity categories—for example, race, class, gender, sexuality—that they can be whoever they want to be. In such circumstances, free will can become a heavy burden. Such romanticized, individualist approaches to liberation—guaranteed as they are by America's founding documents, themselves inspired by Enlightenment humanism—require and restore the humanist individual in both researchers who as liberators can hear and understand stories of oppression—the enlightened, privileged saviors who can recognize and act on injustice when they see it—and in participants—the oppressed who are required to "speak for themselves," to name their oppression.

In the first instance, however, we have learned the hard lesson that those we identify as oppressed may not agree with our diagnosis and may prefer that impositional emancipators leave them alone. In the second, as Spivak (1988, 1999), for example, argued some time ago, the oppressed individual, the subaltern, cannot speak for herself—she is not "authentic" or natural but rather the product of the very ideological, cultural, historical, and hegemonic conditions that oppress her. Neither her identity nor her voice is self-evident. Her speech, her voice, is not originary, primary, fundamental, true, or brute but only speech, and the experience it describes is the normalized and regulated product of her positioning and subjection. Social justice work in qualitative inquiry grounded in the liberal individual of humanism, then, may well secure rather than upend an essentialist, oppressed identity, which seems at odds with the goal of transformation.

An example of the refusal to interrogate the essentialist, humanist individual occurs when qualitative researchers celebrate and empathize with their participants by "letting the data speak for themselves" (professing to present transparent, primary truth as if the researcher's selection of the data is not itself a mediation, an interpretation, an analysis) and/or simply "tell stories" of experience that maintain the naturalness of the oppression and do not provide needed critique. These practices, found in interpretive approaches also, assume there is a deep truth about the human that can be brought to light, expressed in language, and known. As Scott (1991) argued, however, experience (stories, narratives) doesn't exist outside naturalized, established meaning; it cannot serve as uncontestable, reliable evidence; and it cannot serve as the origin or ground of our knowing. Experience is, rather, that which we must explain. Data cannot speak for themselves, and stories can simply endlessly repeat oppression. Even though experience matters a great deal, the work of the researcher is not to revel in the swamps of experience for too long but to investigate the discursive and material conditions that constrain what can be said and lived.

The privileging of uninterpreted experience, stories, narratives, and so forth in much conventional humanist qualitative inquiry not only points to the humanist individual but also to an overreliance on the empirical (Science), as if what we sense (hear, see, etc.) can legitimate what we know—but this is a tenet of logical positivism that rejects metaphysics. It is dangerous to believe in what we hear and see without theorizing what enables us to sense as we do (Philosophy). Of course, we're aware that such reliance can be dangerous—that's why in qualitative research we use concepts like "triangulation" and "member checks" as correctives. Nonetheless, the empiricism we practice assumes a founding, sensing, meaning-making individual separate from what it senses, and that assumption enables troubling binary oppositions: subject/object, mind/body, man/nature, self/other, human/not human, and so on.

In addition, privileging and celebrating experiences, stories, and practices exhibits nostalgia for the *real,* the *true,* the *authentic*—what we imagine is a foundational, immaculate, pure origin outside being itself to which we long to return. But that truth and that real are chimeras, fictions, and *neither can ever be outside human being* but can only ever be human being—the contingent, chaotic, impoverished limit of our imaginations and practices. We do organize and reorganize human being during different historical periods in different cultures using theories and practices laden with politics, power relations, values, and desire—not necessarily evil or mistaken, but surely in need of interrogation. The point is that the description of human being we live now is not the same as past descriptions nor must it continue in the future.

In sum, a particular description of human being is at the center of what I call "conventional humanist qualitative inquiry," whether it employs positivist, interpretive, critical, or other approaches in the social sciences; and that description, that assumption, that belief, enables descriptions of other linked concepts—e.g., truth, reality, experience, freedom—that form a "grid of intelligibility" (Foucault, [1976] 1978, p. 93) that organizes and structures a certain way of understanding the world. To rethink that understanding, we must rethink and disperse that central figure, human being.

Post Human Being: Subjectivity and Agency

Our task, then, is to problematize the individual, the self, the human being of humanism rather than to perpetuate it; "to cultivate an attention to the conditions under which things become evident ... and therefore seemingly fixed, necessary, and unchangeable" (Rabinow, 1997, p. xix) and to attend to the "historical constitution of various forms of the subject" (Foucault, [1984] 1997b, p. 291). We must move away from the philosophy of the subject offered by humanism and understand the modern subject as a "historical and cultural reality—which means something that can eventually change" (p. 177). It can be quite startling to realize that humanism's human is not real but only a description, to understand that we've learned to recognize human being in a particular way, and that we could, in the same way, recognize ourselves differently.

As I mentioned earlier, by the end of World War II, it seemed imperative to rethink the humanist description of human being that had come to such a terrible fruition, and various scholars in the humanities and social sciences who were later labeled "postmodern" and/or "poststructural" began to deconstruct that subject by questioning the notion that it could be centered and "present" to itself (Derrida), to track its descent and emergence using genealogical analyses (Foucault), and to question its ontological status

(Deleuze and Guattari). In effect, they followed Foucault's (1982) advice that "maybe the target nowadays is not to discover what we are but *to refuse what we are*—we have to promote new forms of subjectivity through the refusal of this kind of individuality" (p. 216; emphasis added).

This refusal was evidenced, for example, by avoiding concepts linked to humanism's human being, concepts like "I," "me," "myself," "individual," and "identity." A different concept that had been in use for some time, "subject," a deliberately ambiguous term, seemed useful in that it attempts to capture the ongoing construction of human being—the always already partial, fragmented, in-process nature of human being that is, at the same time, both subject to the disciplinary and normalizing aspects of power relations, discursive formations, and practices *and* able to resist subjection. Related concepts such as "subjectivity" and "subject position" began to be used. Subject position refers to fairly well-defined and recognized culturally constructed categories within which people live, categories that assume certain attitudes, beliefs, and practices (and thus experiences) that one must take up to perform that position acceptably—mother, husband, teenager, homosexual, professor, feminist, and so on. Subject positions can conflict as, for example, when one is, at once, a son chided by an elderly parent and a university professor preparing for a doctoral seminar.

Subjectivity implies the ongoing construction of human being, human being in flux, in process—at every moment being disciplined, regulated, normalized, produced, and, at the same time, resisting, shifting, changing, producing. But the concept subjectivity is often bandied about as if it is a synonym for identity and so is often pluralized—subjectivities—which implies there are unique wholes that can indeed be pluralized. Subjectivity, however, *implies* multiplicity, which can't be located or fixed in identity. It's not that we have multiple subjectivities; *we are subjects*—that's all we need to say (and, after Deleuze and Guattari, we don't need to say *we*).

An example of confusing subjectivity with identity, especially in qualitative inquiry, is the use of a "subjectivity statement," a document the researcher is supposed to write before he begins a study in which he's expected to describe his history, his positionality, his assumptions, his values, his investments in the project, and so on—he's expected to come clean, tell all, confess, reveal his true, inner self. Before he begins fieldwork, he must identify himself: "Here I am; this is who I am, where I came from, what I think, what I believe. I am a white, middle-class, well-educated, heterosexual female who grew up in a large farming family in Iowa. I ... I ... I. ..." This work is about identification. I suspect this kind of text, the subjectivity statement, came from Peshkin's (1988) article in which, perhaps gesturing toward the poststructural, he claimed to identify several of his own "subjectivities," though I would argue he meant something like "roles," a concept from sociology, as in "the roles I play in my research project." I believe the subjectivity statement is really an identity statement grounded in the humanist description of human being.

One problem with this kind of identity work is that researchers too often assume that once they've acknowledged their commitments at the beginning of a study, they're home free. Another is "reflection,"[1] the basis of the subjectivity statement, which alerts us to at least two other problems. The first is the notion that there is, indeed, a stable, conscious identity upon which to reflect. The second is that reflection can serve as a corrective and, thus, help guarantee the validity of a study. The idea is that if we reflect enough, especially in the subjectivity statement before we begin the study, we can *know who we are* and thus know when we're being "biased" or "subjective." All this is not to say that reflection is not useful, but that it is embedded in a particular description of human being and related concepts (validity/truth, objectivity).

Importantly, in all this, we see the notion that there is a researcher who exists ahead of the research—which is out there somewhere—a self-contained individual who moves right through the process from beginning to end, whole, intact, and unencumbered, already identified and secured in the subjectivity statement.

A question that inevitably comes up when discussing subjectivity is agency, choice, free will, freedom. If we no longer believe that an individual is born with innate agency, where lies freedom? Keenan (1997) argued that freedom is possible "only when the subject is not taken for granted" (p. 66), only when the subject is *not* given in advance. Butler (1995) doubted that agency is possible for an a priori subject, when identity is secured in advance of living, because the essentialist, humanist individual "always and already knows its transcendental ground, and speaks only and always from that ground. To be so grounded is nearly to be buried: it is to refuse alterity, to reject contestation, to decline that risk of self-transformation perpetually posed by democratic life" (pp. 131–132).

Butler's point is that an essentialist individual cannot be free, cannot change or be transformed because its foundational, organizing essence must stay the same throughout time and across all occasions of living. At the core, that individual can only ever be "I." That we believe this idea to be true is illustrated by the common statement, "This is the way I am. Take it or leave it." That statement can be made only in a discursive and material formation that assumes an essentialist human being who cannot change, who is, in fact, stuck, shut down.

But Butler (1990) argued that freedom lies in our ability *not to repeat ourselves,* in the possibility of practicing "*subversive repetition*" (p. 42) or "*subversive citation*" (Butler, 1995, p. 135; emphases added). If the subject is not given in advance, then it must be constructed within everyday living, within linguistic, cultural, and material formations and practices organized within power relations, values, and so on. "To be constituted by language is to be produced within a given network of power/discourse which is open to resignification, redeployment, subversive citation from within, and interruption and inadvertent convergences with other such networks. 'Agency' is to be found precisely at such junctures where discourse is renewed" (Butler, 1995, p. 135).

Butler's point is that freedom, agency, and choice are possible even though not innate. Freedom does not exist prior to living but becomes available through cultural practices, both existing and invented, in the course of everyday living. What is important is that we can employ those practices of freedom and choose not to repeat ourselves—to be identical. But if we choose not to repeat practices that identify us to others, if we refuse what we are as

Foucault advised, if we repeat ourselves differently too often, it can be disturbing for others who might say something like, "You haven't been yourself lately. What happened?" as if there's something wrong. And, of course, if we are too different, we may be labeled "abnormal," "insane," "disordered," and so on. But those who have lived long lives and know nothing about poststructuralism often acknowledge that they're not the same person they were when they were 20 or 30 or 60. In numerous relations over time and space, they have indeed produced themselves and been produced differently. They may choose to take up and inhabit subject positions (son, father) that are recognizable, often for the comfort of others, but they know they are not the same.

I believe that a different ethics comes into play with the dismantling of the essentialist human of humanism because one *can* choose not to repeat, perhaps not as much as we'd like because we are always being subjected even as we resist that subjection, but, nonetheless, we can be different. For that reason, we can no longer get off the hook by saying, "This is just the way I am." We have to learn a new responsibility both for how we produce ourselves as subjects and how, in relations, we produce others, how we subject them. It seems to me that this ethics, which is enabled by a different description of human being, was the desire of the post–World War II scholars, as well as everyday people, who were horrified by the practices of humanism's individual who could imagine and put into play the Holocaust, the atomic bomb, and the genocide and horrors that humans continue to repeat in the name of humanity.

Butler's powerful idea of agency through subversive repetition and Foucault's through the refusal of what we are (i.e., how we've been subjected and subject ourselves) are very useful in rethinking possibilities for human being. And Deleuze and Guattari ([1980] 1987) added much to that work by offering, in their normative ontology, a variety of interlocking concepts to move away from the "I," including "haecceity," "rhizome," and "assemblage." But it's not just Philosophy that enables different human being, it's also Science. Quantum physics' theory of entanglement, in my thinking, works hand-in-hand with haecceity and assemblage because both imply different conceptions of space/time in which the human and nonhuman are not simply separate entities tangled or assembled but are so imbricated that they never were and never can be separate. Barad (2007) explained entanglement in quantum theory as follows:

> To be entangled is not simply to be intertwined with another, as in the joining of separate entities, but to lack an independent, self-contained existence. Existence is not an individual affair. Individuals do not preexist their interactions; rather, individuals emerge through and as part of their entangled intra-relating. Which is not to say that emergence happens once and for all, as an event or as a process that takes place according to some external measure of space and of time, but rather that time and space, like matter and meaning, come into existence, are iteratively reconfigured through each intra-action, thereby making it impossible to differentiate in any absolute sense between creation and renewal, beginning and returning, continuity and discontinuity, here and there, past and future. (p. ix)

Quantum physics also disrupts humanism's notions of space and time in which space is a container for stable, bounded, "authentic" places where individuals live and move through the same time together (e.g., in a culture) and can be observed and studied. Space and time in modernity are separate, but in quantum physics space-time is dynamic, fractured, porous, paradoxical, and nonindividual, with sets of space-time relations existing simultaneously, rhizomatically, and overlapping, interfering with each other. When people begin to think of human being as entanglement, haecceity, assemblage, rhizome, "something happens to them that they can only get a grip on again by letting go of their ability to say 'I'" (Blanchot, as cited in Deleuze & Guattari, [1980] 1987, p. 265).

Implications for Qualitative Inquiry

And there's the rub. Once the "I" fails, qualitative inquiry, dependent as it is on humanism's description of human being, fails as well. Its deeply phenenomenological approach, which "gives priority to the observing subject, which attributes a constituent role to an act, which places its own point of view at the origin of all historicity—which, in short leads to a transcendental consciousness" (Foucault, [1966] 1970, p. xiv)—no longer works. The observing subject is, of course, also the knowing, speaking, inquiring subject of qualitative inquiry. The description of the qualitative researcher is, as our texts tell us, one who collects data using interviews and observations, methods of data collection grounded in "being there" (Geertz, 1988), in *presence*, Derrida's ([1966] 1970) bane.

Qualitative researchers use those two face-to-face methods to go deep, to interview repeatedly in order to get closer and closer to the center, the core of participants' being. They are also advised to observe repeatedly for lengthy periods of time to get closer to the core, the real meaning, of practice, of experience, of life. In fact, we are taught that repeated interviewing and observation—going deeper and deeper for longer and longer—help guarantee the validity, the truth of a study.

Participants in qualitative inquiry likewise are seen as conscious individuals, receptacles of knowledge, of stories that reflect the truth of existence waiting to be revealed. In addition, they are assumed to be self-contained and self-aware individuals who not only have a real self but can also step outside it to reflect on it during an interview. And even though social constructionism, much less radical than poststructural theories, grounds much qualitative inquiry, qualitative researchers, in general, continue to view themselves and participants as doers who exist ahead of the deed. Thus, we believe that participants and researchers are separate, intact individuals who exist before the interview, not that they are products, artifacts, of the interview.

The increasing primacy of the interview in qualitative inquiry reflects the age-old and indefatigable power of Platonic phonocentrism that celebrates *voice* as the truest, most authentic data and/or evidence. Poststructuralism, however, alerts us that meaning is always deferred and that language, spoken or written, cannot be trusted to transport meaning from one individual to another as qualitative inquiry suggests. That interviewing can unearth deep, true meaning is highly doubtful. We can interview all we like, but all we can ever get from a participant is today's story, and tomorrow's will no doubt be different. The poststructuralist would claim that that has always been the case.

The point in all this is that qualitative inquiry, as presented in most standard textbooks—even though they may include an introductory chapter on theory—present qualitative methodology (Science) as divorced from epistemology (Philosophy). Note that this is especially true in texts published after the recent installation of scientifically-based or evidence-based research, the phenomenon that restored positivism in social science research during the first decade of the twenty-first century (see, e.g., National Research Council, 2002).

In such texts, after an initial nod to theory, qualitative methodology is presented as just *itself*. It's a stand-alone, instrumental set of research practices that can be organized in different ways (e.g., grounded theory, case study, narrative "research designs"); that describes what counts as data (that which can be textualized in interview transcripts and field notes); that employs two chief methods of data collection (interviewing and observation); that describes what counts as data analysis (usually the quasi-statistical practice of coding of data); that relies heavily on a positivist validity (triangulation, bias, accuracy); that requires representation and a certain kind of representation at that (rich, thick description that assumes the transparency of language); and so on—you know the chapter headings. It is essentially humanist. It assumes the "I" of humanism and, more specifically, of empiricism. Many new qualitative textbooks now forget that early qualitative inquiry borrowed heavily from interpretive anthropology (see, e.g., Geertz, 1973) and set into play both interpretive and critical responses to positivist social science, which had lost its credibility.

To cement qualitative methodology as just itself, we too often teach it as process and technique in a linear sequence of courses—for example, an introductory course, then a course on data collection, and finally a course on data analysis and representation. Doing so separates Science from Philosophy because phenomenology, hermeneutics, existentialism, Marxism, critical race theory, and so on may not agree on what counts as data, as method, as analysis, and so on, and will also rely on different understandings of the humanist individual—the interpreter, the emancipator, and so on. However, we seldom teach courses in which Science and Philosophy are aligned, for example, courses in interpretive qualitative inquiry or critical qualitative inquiry or poststructural feminist qualitative inquiry or race-based qualitative inquiry and so on. Students who may have read deeply in those theories may well experience a disconnect between a theory's assumptions and those that structure conventional humanist qualitative inquiry.

Of course, poststructuralism will refuse qualitative inquiry when it assumes the humanist "I." *In this way, conventional humanist qualitative inquiry and poststructuralism are incommensurable; they cannot be thought together.* A question, then, is how might someone who was trained in conventional humanist qualitative inquiry and who has also studied and taken up poststructural theories inquire? Can one forget qualitative inquiry? Poststructuralists have been practicing the deconstructive strategy of working within/against the structure of conventional humanist qualitative inquiry for decades now, deconstructing its categories one by one—data, voice, reflexivity, validity, interview, and so on. I argue that it's time to practice another deconstructive approach, which is to overturn and leave behind the failed structure so that something else can be thought.

This is the post-qualitative inquiry (see, e.g., St. Pierre, in press) that, as Derrida suggested, is *to-come.* But it is already happening when those who have studied poststructural theories come upon humanist qualitative methodology and resist it. For example, they are leery of interviewing, refuse to "describe" participants, believe words in their literature reviews are as much data as are words in interview transcripts and field notes, refuse to code data, and refuse to write it up. We need to attend to their work, their reinvention of social science inquiry after the posts when the "I" no longer centers inquiry. Now we can rigorously imagine nonsubjective inquiry in entanglement, in assemblage, in the "AND, 'and ... and ... and. ...'" (Deleuze, [1990] 1995, p. 44) of post-inquiry. This is the lure, the work that beckons.

Note

1 See Pillow (2003) for a deconstruction of reflexivity.

References

Barad, K. (2007). *Meeting the universe halfway: Quantum physics and the entanglement of matter and meaning.* Durham, NC: Duke University Press.

Butler, J. (1987). *Subjects of desire: Hegelian reflections in twentieth-century France.* New York: Columbia University Press.

Butler, J. (1990). *Gender trouble: Feminism and the subversion of identity.* New York: Routledge.

Butler, J. (1995). For a careful reading. In S. Benhabib, J. Butler, D. Cornell & N. Fraser (Eds.), *Feminist contentions: A philosophical exchange* (pp. 127–143). New York: Routledge.

Deleuze, G. ([1990] 1995). *Negotiations: 1972–1990.* (M. Joughin, Trans.). New York: Columbia University Press.

Deleuze, G. & Guattari, F. ([1980] 1987). *A thousand plateaus: Capitalism and schizophrenia.* (B. Massumi, Trans.). Minneapolis: University of Minnesota Press.

Derrida, J. ([1966] 1970). Structure, sign and play in the discourse of the human sciences. In R. Macksey & E. Donato (Eds.), *The structuralist controversy: The languages of criticism and the sciences of man* (R. Macksey & E. Donato, Trans.) (pp. 247–272). Baltimore: The Johns Hopkins University Press.

Descartes, R. (1993). *Discourse on method and Meditations on first philosophy.* 4th ed. (D. A. Cress, Trans.). Indianapolis: Hackett. (*Discourse on Method* first published 1637 and *Meditations on First Philosophy* first published 1641.)

Finke, L. A. (1993). Knowledge as bait: Feminism, voice, and the pedagogical unconscious. *College English, 55*, 1, 7–27.

Foucault, M. ([1966] 1970). *The order of things: An archaeology of the human sciences.* (A. M. S. Smith, Trans.). New York: Vintage Books.

Foucault, M. ([1976] 1978). *The history of sexuality, Vol. 1: An introduction.* (R. Hurley, Trans.). New York: Vintage Books.

Foucault, M. (1982). The subject and power. *Critical Inquiry, 8*, 4, 777–795.

Foucault, M. ([1981] 1997a). Sexuality and solitude. In P. Rabinow (Ed.) *Ethics: Subjectivity and truth* (R. Hurley and others, Trans.) (pp. 175–184). New York: The New Press. (Reprinted from *London Review of Books, 3*, 9, 3, 5–6.)

Foucault, M. ([1984] 1997b). The ethics of concern of the self as a practice of freedom. (R. Fornet-Betancourt, H. Becker, & A. Gomez-Müller, Interviewers; P. Aranov & D. McGrawth, Trans.). In P. Rabinow (Ed.), *Ethics: Subjectivity and truth* (pp. 281–301). New York: New Press.

Geertz, C. (1973). *The interpretation of cultures: Selected essays.* New York: Basic Books.

Geertz, C. (1988). Being there: Anthropology and the scene of writing. In *Works and lives: The anthropologist as author* (pp. 1–24). Stanford, CA: Stanford University Press.

Keenan, T. (1997). *Fables of responsibility: Aberrations and predicaments in ethics and politics.* Stanford, CA: Stanford University Press.

Locke, J. ([1690] 1924). *An essay concerning human understanding.* Oxford: Clarendon Press.

National Research Council. (2002). *Scientific research in education.* R. J. Shavelson & L. Towne (Eds.). Committee on Scientific Principles for Education Research. Washington, DC: National Academy Press.

Peshkin, A. (1988). In search of subjectivity—one's own. *Educational Researcher, 17*, 7, 17–22.

Peters, M. A. & Marshall, J. (1993). Beyond the philosophy of the subject: Liberalism, education, and the critique of individualism. *Educational Philosophy and Theory, 25*, 1, 19–39.

Pillow, W. S. (2003). Confession, catharsis, or cure? Rethinking the uses of reflexivity as methodological power in qualitative research. *International Journal of Qualitative Studies in Education, 16*, 2, 175–196.

Rabinow, P. (1997). Introduction: The history of systems of thought. In P. Rabinow (Ed.), *Ethics: Subjectivity and truth* (pp. xi–xlii). New York: New Press.

Rabinow, P. & Sullivan, W. M. (Eds.). (1979). *Interpretive social science: A reader.* Berkeley: University of California Press.

Rajchman, J. (2000). *The Deleuze connections.* Cambridge, MA: MIT Press.

Scott, J. W. (1991). The evidence of experience. *Critical Inquiry, 17*, 4, 773–797.

Spivak, G. C. (1988). Can the subaltern speak? In C. Nelson & L. Grossberg (Eds.), *Marxism and the interpretation of culture* (pp. 271–313). Chicago: University of Chicago Press.

Spivak, G. C. (1999). *A critique of postcolonial reason: Toward a history of the vanishing present.* Cambridge, MA: Harvard University Press.

St. Pierre, E. A. (2000). Poststructural feminism in education: An overview. *International Journal of Qualitative Studies in Education, 13*, 5, 477–515.

St. Pierre, E. A. (in press). Post qualitative research: The coming after and the critique. In N. K. Denzin & Y. A. Lincoln (Eds.). *Handbook of qualitative research.* 4th ed. Thousand Oaks, CA: Sage.

Section II

Politics of Evidence/ Politics of Research

Chapter 6

The Politics of Evidence

Janice M. Morse

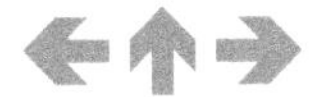

The title that I have used, "The Politics of Evidence,"[1] is an oxymoron. *Evidence* is something that is concrete and indisputable, whereas *politics* refers to "activities concerned with the acquisition or exercise of authority" (Abate, 1996, p. 1152) and is necessarily ephemeral and subjective.

Here, I will examine how the politics of evidence, the politics of ignorance, stigma, and conflicting agendas (which extend to academic and governmental levels) are impediments to health research—and perhaps also educational research—and constrict qualitative inquiry. This oppressive movement is impeding how, when, and to whom qualitative inquiry is taught, contracted, funded, conducted, published, read, and implemented. I will argue that the long debate over the qualitative/quantitative paradigm issues has now gone beyond preferences for a style of approaching research and has become a more serious concern.

> [This] political economy of evidence … is not a question of evidence *or* no evidence, but who controls the definition of evidence and which kind is acceptable to whom. [Larner, 2004, p. 20, emphasis in original]

Originally published in *Qualitative Inquiry and the Conservative Challenge*, edited by Norman K. Denzin and Michael D. Giardina, pp. 79–92. Republished in *Qualitative Inquiry—Past, Present, and Future: A Critical Reader*, edited by Norman K. Denzin and Michael D. Giardina, pp. 121–134. Left Coast Press, Inc.

This Is the Story

A model to evaluate research rigor was introduced in 1972 by Archie Cochrane (1972/1989). In his book *Effectiveness and Efficiency*, he recommended standards for medical research. This model placed randomized control trials as the gold standard for evidence and mere opinion at the lowest level. The model, intended as criteria for the evaluation of drug trials to determine treatment efficacy, has been embraced in medicine as a new standard. The *standards for quality of evidence* were classified by Sackett (1993) as:

> Grade A. Randomized trials with low false positive (alpha) and/or low false negative (beta) errors supported by at least one (preferably more) Level 1 randomized trial.
>
> Grade B. Supported by at least one (preferably more) small randomized trials with high false positive (alpha) and/or high false negative (beta) errors. These are usually inadequate for implementation, but meta-analytic techniques used to analyze the results of 2 or more trials may obtain statistically significant results to move these into Level 1.
>
> Grade C. These consist of Level 3, nonrandomized two-group concurrent cohort comparison (historical control or another site as comparison); Level 4, with no comparison group; and Level 5, opinions of expert committees. Grade C is not recommended to inform practice. Qualitative inquiry is classified as Grade C.

Evidence and *evidence-based practice* have become the new mantras for medical care; they have spawned meta-analyses and the Cochrane Library: a depository of these reviews assessing evidence by evaluating series of trials or replications. This new agenda has resulted in conferences, societies, journals, and databases, and in new approaches to care—evidence-based practice—in which modifications of therapy are made based on its recommendations.

Despite its main criticisms—basically, that the trial conditions are not replicable in day-to-day clinical care and the trial's mean score does little to inform the individual case (Kravitz, Duan, & Braslow, 2004)—evidence-based practice is a trend that is here to stay.

Where Does This Leave Qualitative Inquiry?

Obviously, qualitative inquiry is a poor fit, for it has never purported to be a method that can be used to evaluate the efficacy of drugs or other treatments. But rather than excluding qualitative inquiry from the Cochrane criteria because of the nature of qualitative data, (textual, interviews, conversation, observations), qualitative research was immediately classified as "mere opinion," as Grade C, the lowest level of evidence, not recommended for implementation.[2] Thus, perceived as clinically useless for their agenda of treatment efficacy, it was not taken seriously nor given any credence, until recently.

But my major concern is that disciplines that were the primary users of qualitative inquiry with a mandate for health were virtually excluded from the resources provided for medical research. That is, research from disciplines such as nursing, rehabilitation, occupational therapy, counseling, social work, and the humanistic specialties in medicine, such as family practice and psychiatry, became less credible. Specialties that were not primarily concerned with drug therapy, or that extended beyond this—specialties that valued the *art* of care as well as the science of care, disciplines that were primarily concerned with relationships, interactions, and the context of care—these all slipped from the priority list of medical funding agencies.

The immediate *political* response of many medical granting agencies was to adopt the Cochrane criteria as the standards for evaluating *all* research proposals and, hence, for allocating research funding. In foundations and granting agencies that applied the Cochrane criteria carte blanche, this meant that qualitative research was not considered fundable.

In the United States, nurses had their own funding source in the NIH (National Institutes of Health), NCNR (National Center for Nursing Research) now NINR (The National Institute for Nursing Research), and NIDA (National Institute on Drug Abuse) and they were less affected by this trend. But in Canada, Australia, and New Zealand (and probably the United Kingdom), where the control of health care funding was in the hands of medical researchers, this trend was crippling.

Federal organizations and private foundations that fund research are excellent mirrors of the state of the science. Their health-care priorities and the grants that they fund reveal what research is perceived to be necessary and of outstanding design. Requests for data to both NIH and to CIHR for the percentage of qualitative grants received and funded have bought the response that they do not keep such statistics.[3] Yet, in the United States, since the 1980s, groups of nurses have lobbied consistently to increase the number of qualitative members on the research committees or to establish special committees with the expertise to review qualitative applications.

The agencies' response that other methods do not have special review groups is not exactly correct. Presently, the review groups are predominantly quantitative by default. For instance, the review groups in nutrition understand and respect the methods used by nutritionists, or in engineering, methods used by engineers. There are two problems with the committee structure in NIH for qualitative researchers to get funding. The first problem is the preference that most committee members should have NIH funding, although this is not a requirement. Such a practice perpetuates the status quo and makes it difficult for enough qualitative researchers to establish the track records necessary to "break in." Thus, the second problem is that the membership of these committees is heavily weighted toward quantitative research. In all fairness, if the committee does not have the qualitative expertise needed within the committee membership, another reviewer may be brought in, in person or by phone. But the *dis*advantage of this system is clear. How can one unknown outsider sway a committee (in which friendships and power relations are already established) and, if on the phone, without even the advantages of a personal presence? And it is worse in Canada (from my experience as a reviewer in New Zealand, Australia, Great Britain, and South Africa), where only the external reviewer's written report is considered by the committee, and the "expert" does not have the privilege of listening to and participating in the committee's discussion and debate, nor of voting. These problems continue to this day.

The first response of the qualitative researchers to this inequity in funding in the 1980s and 1990s was an immediate appeal, but their voices were soft. Criticisms were often published in sources that were not on the reading lists of the policy makers. Furthermore, because research is squeezed into most medical curricula—and qualitative inquiry is not usually included in the syllabus—these appeals came from nursing, occupational therapy, speech therapy, and counseling, these being disciplines that were tangential to the mission of the medical foundations, disciplines that were focused on the *person* rather than the therapy and that were not funded as mainstream priorities by the medical review boards. The objections came from stakeholders who were perceived to be outside the core mission of the review boards, so that these complaints were of little concern to the councils approving the funding decisions. And the appeals came over the heads of quantitative health researchers (mainly experimental psychologists and epidemiologists), who were better established, and better funded, and who probably agreed with the medical scientists and decision makers.

The second response of qualitative researchers ("If you can't beat 'em join 'em") was to become a part of the Cochrane movement. A large group of qualitative researchers formed a group that met regularly, with the agenda of including "contextual evidence" in the reviews. Their initial task was methodological—that is, to determine how one should incorporate qualitative findings into the quantitative reviews. Previously, I wrote,

> I am now suggesting that it is time to be honest with ourselves. The assumptions underlying evidence-based medicine are a poor fit with the assumptions of qualitative inquiry. Furthermore, we have contrary research agendas: Whereas the epidemiological and experimental designs for clinical drug trials seek to decontextualize, qualitative research asks them to consider the context. We have different definitions and agendas for "providing care": their focus is on the pill and if it works; our focus is different—why patients might decide whether to swallow the pill or to accept, reject, or modify the prescribed treatment, or how it affects patients' lives. Both perspectives are equally important for "efficacy" but produce complementary information rather than information that may be incorporated into the same reviews. [Morse, 2005, p. 3]

Despite these words, I now believe that this group *has* made headway in raising the consciousness and status of qualitative inquiry. They are making a difference in the way qualitative inquiry is perceived. Some medical journals, such as the *British Medical Journal*, now routinely have a qualitative section, perhaps due, in part, to this lobby. But this is a "side effect" of their work.

The final response was methodological—to develop methods for conducting qualitative meta-analyses. This task itself was onerous, because, of course, textual data are not additive; qualitative studies do not intentionally replicate, and so forth. Following meta-ethnography (Noblit, 1984), the effort was spearheaded by Margarete Sandelowski and her colleagues and is recently completed.. The primary approach followed quantitative meta-analyses: select pertinent studies, critique these studies according to identified standards (Sandelowski & Barroso, 2002), and then use some technique to develop a model according to the major theoretical commonalities (Thorne et al., 2004).

So that is the story to date. But from my perspective, now, in 2005, this *emphasis on evidence* is not going to go away. Indeed, for those of you who are heaving a sigh of relief that you do not do health research or are thanking your lucky stars that you are not entrenched in a health-care discipline, my prediction is that, as it has spread from Britain, to Canada and Australia, and then to the United States, so it will spread laterally, invading other applied disciplines, in particular, education. Politically, qualitative researchers are in for a long and rough ride.

I believe the second problem that we face is not with qualitative inquiry itself but with mainstream medicine's entrapment in clinical drug trials, experimental design, and quantitative analysis—in other words, their perception of their discipline as a biological/physiological rather than a humanistic discipline. I maintain that despite the recent rise of humanistic medicine, their unwavering adherence to randomized drug trials, epidemiological designs, and insistence on the criteria outlined by Cochrane (1972/1989) as The Standard, and fueled by the pharmaceutical industry, is actually occurring in health care at the expense of more significance advances—advances that may make even greater contributions in reducing morbidity and mortality. I maintain that medical granting agencies' limited support for qualitative inquiry, and their limitations in acknowledging, respecting, and funding qualitative modes of inquiry and accepting alternate evidences, will impede advances in health care (Morse, 2006a).

Two factors are driving the health care/medical agenda, and these factors cannot be ignored. The first is that the public lobby for cure is stronger and louder than the public lobby for care. Medical research is expected to reduce morbidity and mortality. The second factor is the political and public lobby of reduced costs, that is, efficiency in care. Medical care is becoming too expensive. These questions are interrelated. Let us ask instead ...

Does Qualitative Research Save Lives?

When I look at the outcomes of most publications in *Qualitative Health Research*, authors claim that their research creates models for practice that "provide insight and understanding" into the experience of patients, families, and caregivers. It is important to be understanding, but in the hardball of everyday life, our "soft" research, with such nebulous outcomes, is not useful to policy planners and those responsible for the health of the nation. From this perspective, our research is not directly relevant to our health care agenda, which is intent on reducing mortality, lowering morbidity, and reducing costs.

Ironically, medical knowledge is dependent on qualitative inquiry. The compendium of signs and symptoms, albeit developed somewhat haphazardly in the eighteenth and nineteenth centuries, was dependent on observations and description. This continues, particularly in the identification of new diseases, for example in the identification of AIDS during the early 1980s. New medical procedures are documented using case study design (consider the evolution of heart transplants). Qualitative research is also being used to explicate symptoms (e.g., the early signs of heart attacks in females; Brink, Karlson, & Hallberg, 2002). But pointing out such obvious inconsistencies is not enough. This basic research (and I use that term deliberately) is not adequate for our critics—they need to see the numbers!

Can We Develop "Proper" Evidence?

Theoretically, we could use a mixed-methods design and calculate any impact on mortality resulting from our research, but in reality our research—when it has an intervention—uses designs that are not relevant to Cochrane (1972/1989) standards. Excellent clinicians (and excellent teachers) do not use behavioral interventions that consist of rigid protocols but, rather, use a blend of science and clinical wisdom. Interventions based on modifying behaviors and working through relationships lack the scientific rigor required by evidence based protocols. Our problems include (a) the impracticality of using double-blind treatment and control groups with replication in at least two independent sites with behavioral interventions (e.g., consider family therapies); (b) the reduction of such interventions to rote and precise rules counters the flexibility in approaches when underlying philosophies and treatment realities require uniqueness when caring for individuals; and (c) an extraordinarily large contextual variation within the presentation of illnesses and needs, and in the contexts, cultures, and expectations of patients. Clearly, another form of evidence must be developed to justify qualitative inquiry as legitimate, appropriate, and desirable.

Alternate Forms of Evidence

What are these "alternative evidences" for demonstrating efficacy? I am thinking of problems that are too chaotic to be explored using experimental design—for example, qualitative problems. I am thinking of demonstrating and extending our findings using *logic* and *common sense*, and, if necessary, our repertoire of *qualitative designs* that have previously not been part of mainstream qualitative health research.

Expanding Qualitative Methods to Expand Types of Evidence

What are these designs?

I am thinking of designs used in the fields of engineering, such as nonhuman models in trials using simulation; also of methods used in biomechanics. I am also thinking of putting interventions in place following a single "near miss," rather than waiting for statistically significant disasters, and the deliberate trialing using *n of 1* research. And I am thinking of legitimizing ethological qualitative microanalysis, used in anthropology, as evidence in its own right.

These research designs are well funded outside of health care but, strangely, are not considered rigorous within health care. How serious is the problem? My own trauma room research has identified "talking through" to help terrified patients with overwhelming pain, when analgesics are ineffective or withheld, to maintain control and not to fight caregivers (Proctor, Morse, & Khonsari, 1996). The efficacy of such human interventions cannot be readily demonstrated in a two-group design, but it could be demonstrated using logic and modeling (*How does resisting/fighting care increase the severity of a head injury?*). Although the intervention is expensive (another nurse is needed), the cost savings in reducing trauma and the severity of head injuries would be remarkable. I could also argue for other advantages—"talking through" synchronizes the trauma team, so that care is actually administered faster. If care is administered with in the first "golden hour" after the accident, mortality is reduced.

Beyond Social Science: Additional Modes of Qualitative Inquiry/Established Types of Evidence

What are these methods?

The first group I have classified as *Qualitative microanalysis.* These are characterized often by a single case, by abduction, and by attention to detail.

1. Forensic designs.

This research is conducted "detective-style" on a single case or incidence, usually following a serious incident or major disaster, including loss of life. The goal of these methods is to identify causation and, hence, prevent recurrence, rather than—as in police work—to convict or—as in journalism—to expose. At the Qualitative Health Research Conference in 2004, Linda Connell (2004), NASA scientist, described the Aviation Safety Reporting System (ASRS), which collects reports on aviation safety events and incidents, and the role of qualitative inquiry in identifying cause: "Black box cockpit recordings are qualitative data." From such research, there are invariably changes of policy and procedure, changes of design of the aircraft, or further investigation into human limitations that may have contributed to the incident. This is a qualitative design that indisputably saves lives.

Forensic designs are used by many disciplines—obviously by police at crime scenes, in cases of sexual assault, domestic violence, missing persons, fraud investigations, and audit procedures. There are also fields of forensic engineering in anthropology and archeology. Of course, when a building has collapsed or a mummy has been discovered, qualitative methods are the only sensible way to proceed, and these techniques are accepted as standard practice.

Nevertheless, according to Connell (2004), the methods used by NASA to "diagnose" aviation errors are now being used in hospitals in the United States to investigate medical errors (Barach & Small, 2000). This is perhaps the most basic of applied research, for it is from examination of these single cases that pattern recognition and principles emerge. This new focus on patient safety will make this one of the most expanding areas of qualitative inquiry, and we should officially embrace these techniques and add them to our repertoire.

Closely associated with the previous aviation model is a new ASRA, NASA Ames Research Center project, in collaboration with the U.S. Department of Veterans Affairs, that evaluates reports describing "near misses." In this case, the "incident" has not actually occurred, but from a single report of "almost," the circumstances are investigated, warning bulletins released, and policy changed. In other words, an intervention is in place before the "problem" becomes an actual event. How to demonstrate efficacy? Just as avoiding a pedestrian at the last minute does not create a statistic, or dodging another vehicle and avoiding a fender bender does not result in actual cost savings, except at the population level and over time, such proven efficacy remains hypothetical.

Because the researchers are not waiting until there is loss of life—they are responding to a hypothetical case—that is the converse of statistical significance: it is hard to claim credit, to demonstrate a drop in mortality. These researchers are working from a theory of causality that states if something *almost* happened once, it could *actually* occur; they are using logic and experience, not experimental design. Their data rely on anonymity in reporting and a guarantee of "no reprisal" to those who report the incidents; hence, they leave no audit trails and cannot demonstrate the validity of their data. But these conditions ensure both that the researchers receive necessary data and that data are as comprehensive as possible; such conditions enhance validity. These are conditions of evidence, of hypothetical outcomes, and are devoid of the quantitative criteria of replication—*the ultimate ethic.*

What do I mean by the ultimate ethic? Simply put, it is to learn from near misses and to modify practices and develop policy from them. Connell's (2004) example of the disregard for this model was a B757 wake turbulence accident at John Wayne Airport in Orange County, California, in December 1993.

The pilot did not know that the air traffic controller had descended a B757 (which has extreme wake [vortex] frequencies [from its wings]) through his intended flight path. The captain was aware of the danger of wake vortices (although he was not told that the preceding aircraft was a B757) and "was acting appropriately, according to what we've all been taught. The Westwind crashed in uncontrolled flight three miles short of the runway" (Pendleton, 2003, para. 10).

At the congressional hearing, the congressman for Orange County, responding to the comment that one near miss was not statistically significant, asked with sarcastic sadness, "And how many bodies on the runway is statistically significant?" (Connell, 2004).

2. Deliberate trial or testing of interventions with n – 1 *research.*

An example of this type of research is the first heart transplant, and may or may not be happening today with human cloning. The design is usually experimental and outcomes unknown or uncertain, and the nature of the trial demands qualitative microanalysis, perhaps combined with some repeated quantitative measures design. Case study design is an inadequate description of this type of research.

This method has tremendous potential in health care for the examination of rare events, such as heart transplantation or the separation of conjoined twins. Are the findings of such research important? I believe Piaget (1954/1999) used this design when he observed and took careful notes observing his infants, and we know the impact his research has had on our understanding of infant behavior.

3. Observation and precise, microanalytic observational description.

This is classic qualitative inquiry, which is not used enough, and it is the method most in need of development in qualitative inquiry. The use of video recordings enables microanalysis of movement, touch, and talk, and examination of the pacing of the care, so that behaviors, interactions, and responses can be examined.

Is this research of any *assistance* to our agenda of saving lives? This method is used in biomechanics and can be used, for example, in observing patient mobility when studying patient falls. This will enable bioengineering solutions, in the form of a safer bed or walking aids, to be developed and trialed.

Video is often used for conducting research with nonverbal patients, such as those with advanced Alzheimer's, or in exploring infants' response to pain, or the study of the breastfeeding dyad, and so forth. Thus, qualitative analysis using videotapes is powerful. It enables us to document, to illustrate our practice, and to communicate our findings, and certainly should be used more often.

4. Simulation.

This is the "crash test dummy" type of research. To reduce risk, simulation replaces people in certain high-risk situations. Despite the use of models used in teaching, I do not know of a single case of this type of research being used in qualitative research. This does not mean, however, that we should forget this option exists.

Developing Qualitative Evidence

As researchers, we are tired of conducting underfunded research that seemingly goes nowhere. Yet, forcing ourselves into a quantitative system does not appear to be the answer. Although we know that our research is significant and addresses problems that may otherwise be declared not researchable, our seemingly insurmountable problem is to convince those who control research funding, curricula, and the publication of texts and mainstream journals that our work is significant. We need to convince them that logic and common sense can produce powerful forms of evidence, and that sometimes we cannot afford, both in terms of morbidity and mortality and of dollars, the cost of quantitative inquiry.

Qualitative researchers sit on the fringes of research, but remember that it is on the fringes where the greatest advances are often made. We are addressing the confusing and chaotic problems that are too difficult to tackle quantitatively. But they are important problems.

Let us look internally, to ourselves, and bring together all our resources, all we know methodologically, and all that we know as professionals. Then, with a united voice, a rising chorus, demand the resources and attention that our research deserves.

Notes

1 This was the opening plenary address presented at the First International Congress of Qualitative Inquiry, May 5–7, 2005, University of Illinois, Urbana-Champaign. Reprinted with permission from Qualitative Health Research, 16 (Morse, 2006b). I am grateful to Linda Connell, M.A., director of ASRS, NASA Ames Research Center, Moffett Field, California, for her comments on an earlier draft.

2 Elsewhere, I suggest that Cochrane (1972/1989) intended to target clinical opinion or clinical judgment regarding treatments in this level, and not qualitative inquiry and the type of problems it addresses, in this categorization. In fact, Cochrane probably did not know anything about qualitative inquiry as it is practiced today (Morse, 2006a). Thus, it is an error—and invalid—to categorize qualitative inquiry into the Cochrane review criteria.

3 NIH-funded applications (with rare exceptions) are in the public domain, but this information could not feasibly be obtained one application at a time.

References

Abate, F. (Ed.). (1996). *The Oxford dictionary and thesaurus: American edition*. New York: Oxford University Press.

Barach, P., & Small, S. D. (2000). Reporting and preventing medical mishaps: Lessons from non-medical near miss reporting systems. *British Medical Journal, 320*, 759–763.

Brink, E., Karlson, B. W., & Hallberg, L. (2002). To be stricken with acute myocardial infarction: A grounded theory study of symptom perception and care-seeking behavior. *Qualitative Health Research, 7*, 533-543.

Cochrane, A. L. (1972/1989). *Effectiveness and efficiency: Random reflections on health services*. London: British Medical Journal.

Connell, L. (2004). Qualitative analysis: Utilization of voluntary supplied confidential safety data in aviation and health care. Presentation to the Qualitative Health Research Conference, Banff, Canada, April/May.

Kravitz, R. L., Duan, N., & Braslow, J. (2004). Evidence-based medicine, heterogeneity of treatment effects, and the trouble with averages. *Milbank Quarterly, 82*(4), 661–687.

Larner, G. (2004). Family therapy and the politics of evidence. *Journal of Family Therapy, 26*, 17–39.

Morse, J. M. (2005). Beyond the clinical trial: Expanding criteria for evidence [Editorial]. *Qualitative Health Research, 15*, 3–4.

Morse, J. M. (2006a). It is time to revise the Cochrane criteria [Editorial]. *Qualitative Health Research, 16*(3).

Morse, J. M. (2006b). The politics of evidence. *Qualitative Health Research, 15*(3), 395–404.

Noblit, G. (1984). *Meta-ethnography: Synthesizing qualitative studies*. Newbury Park, CA: Sage.

Pendleton, L. (2003). *Wake turbulence—An invisible enemy*. Retrieved November 26, 2005, from http://www.avweb.com/news/airman/183095-1.html

Piaget, J. (1954/1999). *The construction of reality in the child*. London: Routledge.

Proctor, A., Morse, J. M., & Khonsari, E. S. (1996). Sounds of comfort in the trauma center: How nurses talk to patients in pain. *Social Sciences & Medicine, 42*, 1669–1680.

Sackett, D. L. (1993). Rules of evidence and clinical recommendations. *Canadian Journal of Cardiology, 9*(6), 487–489.

Sandelowski, M., & Barroso, J. (2002). Reading qualitative studies. *International Journal of Qualitative Methods, 1*(1), Article 5. Retrieved March 10, 2005, from http://www.ualberta.ca/~ijqm/

Thorne, S., Jensen, L., Kearney, M., Noblit, G., & Sandelowski, M. (2004). Qualitative metasynthesis: Reflections on methodological orientation and ideological agenda. *Qualitative Health Research, 14*(10), 1342–1365.

Chapter 7

Building Confidence in Qualitative Research

Engaging the Demands of Policy

Harry Torrance

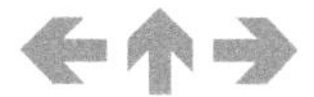

Introduction

Recent U.S. legislation has privileged "scientifically based research" in decisions about funding educational programs and educational research; moreover "scientific" is defined largely in terms of experimental design and methods, especially randomized controlled trials (RCTs), also sometimes known as randomized field trials (Eisenhart, 2006; Eisenhart & Towne 2003). This seems to be related to prior criticism, and review of the quality of educational research (NRC, 2002) has been interpreted as an attack on more qualitative approaches to educational research (Denzin & Giardina, 2006) and one that warrants urgent response from what might loosely be called the "qualitative research community" (St. Pierre & Roulston, 2006).

Attacks on the quality of educational research, particularly qualitative educational research, have their parallels in the United Kingdom (Hargreaves, 1996; Hillage et al., 1998; Tooley & Darby, 1998), have similarly impacted on debate in Australia (Yates, 2004), and are beginning to emerge in the European

Originally published in *Qualitative Inquiry and the Politics of Evidence*, edited by Norman K. Denzin and Michael D. Giardina, pp.55–79. Republished in *Qualitative—Inquiry Past, Present, and Future: A Critical Reader*, edited by Norman K. Denzin and Michael D. Giardina, pp. 135–159. Left Coast Press, Inc.

Union (Bridges, 2005; Brown, 2003). The argument has been that educational research (and, in some respects, social science research more generally) is too often conceived and conducted as a "cottage industry": producing too many small-scale, disconnected, noncumulative studies that do not provide convincing explanations of educational phenomena or how best to develop teaching and learning. There is not a cumulative or informative knowledge base in the field and what is there is characterized as being of both poor quality and limited utility.

Thus, it can be argued that those working in educational research, in general, and in qualitative traditions, in particular, are facing a global movement of neopositivist interest in so-called "evidence-based" policy and practice, where what counts as legitimate evidence is construed very narrowly indeed. This is manifest not only in country-specific initiatives and legislative action (e.g , No Child Left Behind [2001] in the United States and the English National Curriculum and Testing system [Torrance, 2003]), but also in international assessment and evaluation activities such as Trends in International Mathematics and Science Study and the Program for International Student Assessment (Torrance, 2006) and the Campbell Collaboration, which seeks to review and disseminate social science knowledge for policymakers (Davies & Boruch, 2001; Wade et al., 2006). Clearly, these various manifestations differ in their origins, orientations, and specific intentions; they are not a coherent and homogeneous movement. But equally, they do seem to represent a concerted attempt to impose (or perhaps reimpose) scientific certainty and system management on an increasingly complex and uncertain social world.

It is apparent, then, that what is happening in the United States is not unique: It is almost certainly connected to movements elsewhere, and it should probably be understood in these terms (indeed, an exploration of links and policy flows would be a very interesting study). However, the legislative obsession with RCTs does seem to be peculiar to the United States, and I begin by exploring this before moving on to reflect on the British experience of responding to calls for better quality educational research, in particular better quality qualitative research.

The Cases for and against RCTs

The case for RCTs seems to derive from a combination of the methods of natural science with the supposed needs of policy. It is argued that randomized experiments means that any systematic observed differences between the sample that has received the "treatment," and the "control" group that has not must be attributable to the treatment. The design reveals whether there is a "causal link"; the treatment can be said either to "work" or "not work"; and some calculations can be made about the size of the effect: "[T]he experiment is the design of choice for studies that seek to make causal conclusions, and particularly for evaluations of educational innovations" (Slavin, 2002, p. 18).

Of course, experimental design can also be more subtle and complicated than this, with different elements of such designs potentially revealing different aspects of program impact (on different subsamples of students, for example, if the overall sample is large enough), but it is the appeal to certainty about "what works" that is claimed to attract policymakers: "If we implement Program X instead of Program Y, or instead of our current program, what will be the likely outcomes for children?" (Slavin, 2002, p. 18). Such attraction is easy to appreciate. It sounds seductively simple. When charged with dispensing millions of tax dollars on implementing programs and supporting research, one can understand that policymakers would value this sort of help.

This is not the place to discuss all the criticisms (and rejoinders) about the nature of causality and the place of RCTs in understanding social interaction and evaluating human services. They have been well rehearsed in recent issues of *Educational Researcher* (e.g., Burkhardt & Schoenfeld, 2003; Erickson & Gutierrez, 2002; Feuer, Towne, & Shavelson, 2002; Maxwell, 2004; Riehl, 2006; Slavin, 2002). The relevant point about RCTs and policy, particularly when comparing the United States with England, is that so much prior qualitative work has to be accomplished before any RCT might be designed, and much policy is decided well before any RCT might be implemented, let alone the results made public. Thus, Slavin's deceptively simple question about Program X versus Program Y begs many more questions about where Program X and Y come from in the first place. Such decisions are already a long way down the road of policy development and implementation, and often too far down the road for it to be worthwhile doubling back. Prior questions would include how and why have Program X and Y been developed? What sort of perceived problem are they trying to fix? What is the research evidence that indicates the nature of the problem and the specific different approaches to fixing it? These are all questions that require prior investigation of both outcomes (perhaps secondary analysis of test result data) and processes (e.g., ethnographic studies of why the test data are as they are), not to mention value judgments about whether particular practices and/or inconsistencies in the data do indeed indicate the existence of a "problem" that needs to be "solved."

It might be argued that this view of how RCTs are developed renders such earlier investigative work as somehow less "scientific," or even "prescientific" (see Shavelson et al., 2003, p. 28). But we know that RCTs are difficult and expensive to organize (Slavin, 2002) and therefore that the evidence on which the design is based has to be pretty secure in the first place. If various forms of qualitative work can be trusted in this respect, why can't they be trusted in their own right? Certainly in England, although there are criticisms of the quality of educational research and regular calls for more and more rigorously trained quantitative researchers in the social sciences generally (Hillage et al., 1998; OECD, 2002), qualitative studies of the sort indicated above are still funded by government departments and the UK Economic and Social Research Council (ESRC). The value of qualitative studies in exploring the nature of a particular problem is well recognized by government and other research users/sponsors, though their link to policymaking is often indirect: Even when commissioned by government departments, research is not necessarily utilized in the policymaking process in any straightforward way (see below).

Furthermore, the thrust of the evidence-based policy movement in England at present tends to favor *reviews* of research—synthesizing findings from multiple studies—rather than relying on the results of a single study, no matter how well conducted. Arguments in favor of conducting such reviews, particularly those known as "systematic reviews," derive from the critiques of social and educational research outlined earlier: that the findings of empirical studies are often too small-scale, noncumulative, and/or contradictory to be useful (Gough & Elbourne, 2002; Oakley, 2000, 2003). Advocates are closely associated with the Cochrane Collaboration in medical and health care research and the Campbell Collaboration in social science, both of which favor the accumulation and dissemination of research findings based on scientific methods, particularly randomized control trials. As such, systematic reviewing is often associated with criticisms of qualitative research and is very much located within the "evidence-based policy and practice" movement (Davies, 2004).

For these reasons and others, systematic reviewing has its critics in the United Kingdom (e.g., Hammersley, 2001; MacLure, 2005).[2] Nevertheless, for the purposes of the argument here, the development and use of systematic reviewing points to a policy caution about relying on single studies, experimental or otherwise, and further demonstrates the divergent manifestation of apparently similar policy concerns in the United Kingdom and the United States. Moreover, even one of the leading proponents of systematic reviewing and the use of RCTs in England concedes that "RCTs generally find smaller effects than other designs, and the effects of most interventions, whether medical or social, are modest" (Oakley, 2006, p. 76).

This, of course, links with another set of issues: that of the timeliness, cost, and utility of research. It is often incumbent on policymakers to be seen to be doing something about a perceived problem or be acting in response to what seems to be a good idea (be it research based or not) without waiting for the definitive results of science (supposing these can be produced). Even the results of systematic reviews can take months to appear, let alone the results of newly commissioned studies; policymakers in England are just as likely to ask for very rapid reviews of research or rapid evidence assessment (Boaz, Solesbury, & Sullivan, 2004, p. 12), to be conducted over a few days or weeks, and possibly assembled via an expert seminar, as to commission longer term systematic reviews. An investigation of research reviewing by the UK's ESRC-funded Centre for Evidence-based Policy and Practice noted that the shortest period devoted to producing a commissioned research review was fifteen days, whereas the longest period was thirty months (Boaz, Solesbury, & Sullivan, 2007, p. 8).

Similar issues pertain to commissioned studies and evaluations. Colleagues at Manchester Metropolitan University (MMU) are currently involved in several projects evaluating the impact of information and communications technology on schools and teaching in England, including the impact of placing tools such as interactive whiteboards in classrooms (Somekh et al., 2002, 2005). Introducing the latest computer technology into schools is a politically good thing: There is no way that the UK Department for Education and Skills is going to rip out all the whiteboards that have been put into schools if the evaluation is not particularly positive. At the same time, schools and local authorities (school districts) that have not yet had what they would consider to be their "fair share" of this investment are unlikely to be satisfied by a blunt report that simply says it "doesn't work." They want the hardware and the chance to try it out for themselves.[3] Thus, the MMU evaluations are expected to report, through survey, observation, interview, and action research activities with participating teachers, on what *seems* to work and what problems have been encountered; how, and why it works, or not; and what lessons can be learned for future "roll out" of the program to other local authorities, initial training, and continuing professional development activities.

Thus, policy builds, one initiative on another, incrementally over time, with many more issues other than the scientific evidence coming into play. It might be argued that policy shouldn't develop like this, but it does, and in a democracy (rather than a "scientocracy"), it is not clear how it could be otherwise. Scientific evidence is but one element in a democratic policymaking process. Public values and interests influence matters at the macro level of the decision-making process, and the professional judgment of innumerable local actors mediate policy at the micro level.[4]

Interestingly, much of this sort of incremental, practice-oriented research activity seems to be reflected in current debates about design experiments. And, just as criticism of qualitative research is not unique to the United States (although the focus of attention on RCTs seems much sharper there than elsewhere), so, too, the debate about design experiments seems to indicate that RCT advocacy in the United States is not uniquely an attack on the specific field of qualitative research. *All* approaches to research that do not employ RCTs seem to be subject to critical scrutiny. Thus, a recent special issue of *Educational Researcher* (32[1], 2003) devoted to exploring design experiments included a response from Shavelson et al. (2003) that dismissed the approach by asserting that "an entirely different conceptualization of 'evidence-based' education has captured the imagination of federal policymakers" (p. 25). Shavelson and colleagues further asked: "Should we believe the results of design experiments?" (p. 25). In other words, they invoke political power as the determining factor in methodological debate while simultaneously undermining the claims of one particular methodological approach.

Design experiments involve testing hypotheses about learning, embedded in specific materials and pedagogic approaches, in small-scale "real-life" situations (classrooms, after school clubs, etc.); learning the lessons of how the materials and pedagogies work; and trying to "scale up" for more general testing and application. The approach now seems to be associated with psychologists who wanted to "get out of the lab" and conduct field-based experiments (Brown, 1992; The Design Collective, 2003). However, similar approaches have been associated with curriculum research and development and action research for many years (see Elliott, 1989; James, 2006; Stenhouse, 1975) and have parallels in related endeavors such as mixed methods and "deliberative" and "realist" approaches to evaluation (Chatterji, 2005; House & Howe, 1999; Pawson & Tilley, 1997).

A more practical and policy-friendly set of approaches to applied educational research and development is hard to imagine. Yet, such work is dismissed because it relies "on narrative accounts to communicate and justify [its] findings" (Shavelson et al., 2003, p. 25). Shavelson et al. invoke their membership on the NRC Committee (which, interestingly, they describe at one point as "Our committee" [p. 28]) to "scrutinize the knowledge claims from design studies through the lens of the [NRC Report] guiding principles" (p. 26). Shavelson and colleagues conclude that "experiments should [be used] for choices among important design alternatives" (p. 28); by "experiment." in this statement, they mean "randomized experiments" (p. 28). To be fair, design experiments are treated seriously by Shavelson et al.; they are not arbitrarily dismissed, but ultimately they are treated as just another "prescientific" preparatory stage (p. 28) before the "real science" of RCTs begins.

So what is going here? Many different research perspectives and approaches to applied research, curriculum development, and program evaluation cast doubt on RCTs as the "one best way" to conduct educational research and offer convincing evidence that educational progress can be made by other more pragmatic and incremental means (Burkhardt & Schoenfeld, 2003; Chatterji, 2005; Erickson & Gutierrez, 2002; Maxwell, 2004; Riehl, 2006; The Design Collective, 2003).

Yet such arguments appear to be making little headway. Indeed, even those who get directly involved and collaborate in good faith with the What Works agenda may be censored when their findings do not support an apparently previously decided party line (Schoenfeld, 2006). There is not much science in censorship. Equally, exclusive reliance on RCTs is not only not necessary for policymaking, in many key respects it is not desirable, given the diverse constituencies and interests that policymaking must reconcile, the contingent nature of the process, and the contingent nature of local development and implementation of innovative programs. The NRC Report (2002), subsequent reiterations of its main arguments (Feuer, Towne, & Shavelson, 2002; NRC, 2005; Shavelson et al., 2003), and concomitant legislation (Eisenhart & Towne, 2003) seem more like general attempts to discipline educational research and researchers and to produce a general shift in the problematics and topography of educational research rather than to produce better evidence for policymaking.

The Response of Qualitative Research

To recap, the specific focus on RCTs seems peculiar to the United States; advocacy of RCTs seems directed at many different approaches to educational research, not just qualitative research. Nevertheless, criticism of the quality of educational research, in general, and of qualitative research, in particular, is widespread internationally and can certainly be understood as part of a more general move to reassert the preeminence of a natural science model of causality, what counts as evidence in social science, and the primacy of outcome measures in debates about efficiency and effectiveness in human services (Thomas & Pring, 2005; Yates, 2005). In policy terms, the basic issue is that of justifying the overall level and specific content of government expenditure on public services. How can policymakers come to know which programs to invest in and whether they are effective?

As argued above, research evidence can (and should) only ever be one element of such a policymaking process. Equally, there are many good reasons apart from serving policy for qualitative researchers to continue to reflect on the strengths and weaknesses of their field. Nevertheless, the relationship of research to policy is what seems to be driving current concerns and being manifested in reports such as the NRC (2002, 2005), a recent Workshop on Scientific Foundations of Qualitative Research (Ragin et al., 2004), discussion of doctoral programs (Eisenhart & DeHaan, 2005), the new American Educational Research Association (AERA) "guidelines" for reporting research (see http://www.aera.net/opportunities/?id=1850), and so forth. The response to criticism has been to start trying to set standards in qualitative research, particularly qualitative educational research, to reassure policymakers about the quality of qualitative research, and to reassert the contribution that qualitative research can (and should) make to government-funded programs.

The problem, however, is that the field of "qualitative research" or "qualitative inquiry'" is very large and diverse, and there is unlikely to be easy agreement about core standards. Recent meetings of the International Congress of Qualitative Inquiry (University of Illinois 2005, 2006, 2007, and 2008) have attracted up to 1,000 participants on each occasion from fifty-five different countries, working in and across many different disciplines (anthropology, psychology, and sociology, among others), different applied research and policy settings (education, social work, health studies, etc.), and different national environments with their different policy processes and socioeconomic context of action.

It will be difficult to reach agreement; indeed, it is not self-evident that such agreement is desirable even if possible. Nor is this simply a matter of scope and scale, of what might be termed "practical complexity," whereby agreement might eventually be reached, at least in principle. Different disciplines and contexts of action produce different readings and interpretations of apparently common literatures and similar issues. It is the juxtaposition of these readings, the comparing and contrasting within and across boundaries, that allows us to learn about them and reflect on our own situated understandings of our own contexts. Multiplicity of approach and interpretation, and multivocalism of reading and response, is the basis of quality in the qualitative research community and, it might be argued, in the advancement of science more generally. The key issue is to discuss and explore quality across boundaries, thereby continually to develop it, not fix it, as at best a good recipe, at worst a government-issue straight-jacket.

Experience in the United Kingdom

Some attempt at just such fixing has been made in the United Kingdom, and the results are instructive. Recently, for example, independent academics based at the National Centre for Social Research (a not-for-profit organization) were commissioned by the Strategy Unit of the UK government Cabinet Office to produce a report on *Quality in Qualitative Evaluation: A Framework for Assessing Research Evidence* (Cabinet Office, 2003a). The rationale seems to have been that UK government departments are increasingly commissioning policy evaluations in the context of the move toward evidence-informed policy and practice, and it was considered that guidelines for judging the quality of qualitative approaches and methods were necessary.

The report is in two parts: a seventeen-page summary, including the "Quality Framework" itself (Cabinet Office, 2003a), and a 167-page full report (Cabinet Office, 2003b), including discussion of many of the issues raised by the framework. The summary report states that the framework has been

> designed primarily to assess the *outputs* of qualitative enquiry … and … It is also hoped that the framework will have a wider educational function in the preparation of research protocols,

> the conduct and management of research and evaluation and the training of social researchers." (Cabinet Office, 2003a, p. 6, emphasis in the original)

So, the framework is a guide for the commissioners of research when drawing up tender documents and reading reports, but it also has ambitions to influence the conduct and management of research and the training of social researchers.

The problem, however, is that in trying to cover everything, the document ends up covering nothing, or at least nothing of importance. The basic "Quality Framework" begs questions at every turn, and the full 167-page report reads like an introductory text on qualitative research methods. Paradigms are described and issues rehearsed, but all are resolved in a bloodless, technical, and strangely old-fashioned counsel of perfection. The reality of doing qualitative research, and indeed of conducting evaluation, with all the contingencies, political pressures, and decisions that have to be made, is completely absent. Thus, in addition to the obvious need for "Findings/conclusions [to be] supported by data/evidence" (Cabinet Office, 2003b, p. 22), qualitative reports should also include:

- detailed description of the contexts in which the study was conducted (p. 23);
- discussions of how fieldwork methods or settings may have influenced data collected (p. 25);
- descriptions of background or historical developments and social/organizational characteristics of study sites (p. 25);
- description and illumination of diversity/multiple perspectives/alternative positions (p. 26); and
- discussion/evidence of the ideological perspectives/values/philosophies of the research team (p. 27).

And so on and so forth across six pages and seventeen "quality appraisal questions."

No one would deny that these are important issues for social researchers to take into account in the design, conduct, and reporting of research studies. However, simply listed as such, they comprise a banal and inoperable set of standards that beg all the important questions of conducting and writing up qualitative fieldwork: Everything cannot be done; *choices* have to be made; how are they to be made and how are they to be justified?

To be more positive for a moment, it might be argued that if qualitative social and educational research is going to be commissioned, then a set of standards that can act as a bulwark against commissioning inadequate and/or underfunded studies in the first place ought to be welcomed. It might also be argued that this document at least demonstrates that qualitative research is being taken seriously enough within the government to warrant a guidebook being produced for civil servants. This might then be said to confer legitimacy on civil servants who want to commission qualitative work, on qualitative social researchers bidding for such work, and indeed on social researchers more generally, who may have to deal with local research ethics committees [institutional review boards in the United States]) that are predisposed toward a more quantitative natural science model of investigation. But should we really welcome such "legitimacy"? The dangers on the other side of the argument, as to whether social scientists need or should accede to criteria of quality endorsed by the state, are legion. It is not at all clear that, *in principle*, state endorsement of qualitative research is any more desirable than state endorsement of RCTs. *Defining what counts as science is not the state's business.*

Another arena in England where research meets policy is that of systematic reviewing, mentioned above (Oakley, 2003, 2006; Wade et al., 2006). Initially, findings based on RCTs were considered the "gold standard" of systematic reviewing, but this position has been significantly modified as it has encountered considerable scepticism in the United Kingdom and work is now under way to integrate different kinds of research findings, including those of qualitative research, into such reviews. This may be construed as progress of a sort, but it also involves attempts to appraise the quality and thus the "warrant" of individual qualitative research studies and their findings: Are they good enough to be included in a systematic review or not? This, in turn, can lead to absurdly reductionist checklists as the complexity of qualitative work is rendered into an amenable form for instant appraisal. Thus, for example, Attree and Milton (2006) report on a "Quality Appraisal

Checklist ... [and its associated] ... quality scoring system ... [for] "the quality appraisal of qualitative research" (p. 125). Studies are scored on a four-point scale:

A. no or few flaws
B. some flaws
C. considerable flaws, study still of some value
D. significant flaws that threaten the validity of the whole study (p. 125)

Only studies rated A or B were included in the systematic reviews that the authors conducted, and in the paper they attempt to exemplify how these categories are operationalized in their work. But, as with the Cabinet Office example above, their descriptions beg many more questions than they answer. Thus, lengthy appraisal (the Cabinet Office report) leads to a counsel of perfection—researchers are extolled to do everything—whereas rapid appraisal (see Attree & Milton [2006] in the context of systematic reviewing) leads to a checklist of mediocrity. Even the most stunning and insightful piece of qualitative work can only be categorized as having "no or few flaws." Again, to try to be fair to the authors, they indicate that "the checklist was used initially to provide an overview of the robustness of qualitative studies ... to balance the rigor of the research with its importance for developing knowledge and informing policy and practice" (Attree & Milton, 2006, p. 119). But this is precisely the issue: Standards and checklists *cannot* substitute for informed judgment when it comes to balancing the rigor of the research against its potential contribution to policy. This *is* a matter of judgment, both for researchers and for policymakers.

Proponents of systematic reviewing still try to insist on expelling judgment from the process, however, and rendering qualitative work in quantitative terms. As their focus of attention has expanded from a concentration on RCT studies, they bemoan the fact that different reporting traditions and practices in different fields restrict their capacity to evaluate studies and extract data easily. Reporting guidelines have come to be produced with which all empirical studies should accord so that they can more easily be assessed for quality: "draft guidelines for the REPOrting of primary empirical Studies in Education (the REPOSE Guidelines) …" (Newman & Elbourne, 2004, p. 201). Such guidelines are argued to be "relevant to the reporting of any kind of primary empirical research using any type of research design" (Newman & Elbourne 2004, p. 208): an extraordinarily ambitious claim with obvious homogenizing intent. The actual guidelines comprise a two-page checklist of note-type subheadings, including supposedly generic and all-encompassing categories such as "sampling strategy," "data collection," "data analysis," and so forth (p. 211). Individually, they are unobjectionable; taken together, they are yet another counsel of perfection that would require a book-length report to fulfill and, if applied in practice, will always lead to the conclusion that anything short of a book is of poor quality. It is a strange product for a movement ostensibly concerned with utility, as policymakers routinely deal in memos not books.

Developments in the United States

Similar standards and guidelines and checklists are starting to appear in the United States with, I argue, similar results. For example, Ragin et al. (2004) report on a Workshop on Scientific Foundations of Qualitative Research, conducted under the auspices of the National Science Foundation and with the intention of placing "qualitative and quantitative research on a more equal footing … in funding agencies and graduate training programs" (p. 9). The report argues for the importance of qualitative research and thus advocates funding qualitative research *per se*, but by articulating the "scientific foundations," it is arguing for the commissioning of not just qualitative research, but of "proper" qualitative research. Thus, for example, they argue that

> considerations of the scientific foundations of qualitative research often are predicated on acceptance of the idea of 'cases'. … No matter how cases are defined and constructed, in qualitative research they are studied in an in-depth manner. Because they are studied in detail their number cannot be great. (pp. 9–10)

This is interesting and provocative with respect to the idea of standards perhaps acting as a professional bulwark against commissioning inadequate and/or underfunded studies: A quick and cheap survey by telephone interview would not qualify as high-quality, "scientific" qualitative research. But when it comes to the basic logic of qualitative work, Ragin et al. (2004) do not get much further than arguing for a supplementary role for qualitative methods: "Causal mechanisms are rarely visible in conventional quantitative research … they must be inferred. Qualitative methods can be helpful in assessing the credibility of these inferred mechanisms" (p. 15).

In the end, their "Recommendations for Designing and Evaluating Qualitative Research" concludes with another counsel of perfection: "These guidelines amount to a specification of the *ideal* qualitative research proposal [original emphasis]. A strong proposal should include as many of these elements as feasible" (p. 17). But again, that's the point, what is *feasible* is what is important, not what is ideal: How are such crucial choices to be made? Once again, guidelines and recommendations end up as no guide at all, rather they are a hostage to fortune, whereby virtually any qualitative proposal or report can be found wanting.

Perhaps the exemplar *par excellence* of this tendency is the AERA "Standards for Reporting on Empirical Social Science Research in AERA Publications." "The 7,000-plus word document is devoted entirely to "educational research grounded in the empirical traditions of the social sciences.… Other forms of scholarship ... e.g. history, philosophy, literary analysis, arts-based inquiry … are beyond the scope of this document" (p. 1). So we are already alerted to what is *really* important. Even this truncated version of what counts as educational research spawns "eight general areas" (p. 2) of advice, each of which is subdivided into a total of forty subsections, some of which are subdivided still further. Yet only one makes any mention of the fact that research findings should be interesting or novel or significant, and that is the briefest of references under "Problem Formulation," which we are told should answer the question of "why the results of the investigation would be of interest to the research community" (p. 2), though intriguingly, in this context, not the policy community. In this case, then, we are confronted by both a counsel of perfection *and* a checklist of mediocrity. The standards may be of help in the context of producing a book-length thesis or dissertation, but no

5,000 word journal article could meet them all. Equally, however, even supposing that they could all be met, the article might still not be worth reading. It would be "warranted" and "transparent," which are the two essential standards highlighted in the preamble (p. 2), but it could still be boring and unimportant.

It is also interesting to note that words such as "warrant" and "transparency" raise issues of trust. They imply a concern for the very existence of a substantial data-set as well as how it might be used to underpin conclusions drawn. Yet the issue of trust is only mentioned explicitly once, in the section of the standards dealing with "qualitative methods": "It is the researcher's responsibility to show the reader that the report can be trusted" (p. 11). No such injunction appears in the parallel section on "quantitative methods" (pp. 10–11); in fact, the only four uses of the actual word "warrant" in the whole document all occur in the section on "qualitative methods" (pp. 11–12). The implication seems to be that quantitative methods are really trusted—the issue doesn't have to be raised—whereas qualitative methods are not. Standards of probity are only of concern when qualitative approaches are involved.

As is typical of the genre, the standards include an opening disclaimer that "the acceptability of a research report does not rest on evidence of literal satisfaction of every standard. … In a given case there may be a sound professional reason why a particular standard is inapplicable" (p. 1). But once again, this merely restates the problem rather than resolves it: We are confronted by fifteen pages of standards that do not offer any *real* guidance on how *actually* to conduct and report empirical research. The issue, each and every time, is how to choose between alternative courses of action and how to justify that choice.

Toward a Different Approach

It is not that qualitative research has no standards, or even poorly articulated standards. Far from it: The library shelves are stacked with epistemological discussion and methodological advice about the full range of qualitative approaches available, along with what is at stake when fieldwork choices are made and what the implications are of following one course of action rather than another. Reading such sources iteratively and critically, in the context of designing and conducting a study and discussing the implications and consequences with doctoral supervisors, colleagues, or project advisory groups is what maintains and develops standards in qualitative research.

Setting standards in qualitative research, however, is a different matter. It implies the identification of universally appropriate and applicable procedures, which, in turn, involves documentary and institutional realization and compliance. And, as we have seen, the results of such efforts are not helpful to a deliberative process such as research. Moreover, it is not that the committees and research teams that produce such documents are incompetent or malicious, rather the discursive nature of the problem is not resolvable in terms of written standards. Language cannot settle matters of judgment. It can only open up more questions (of ambiguity and specificity: "But what do you mean by ...?"). In turn, the impulse of the committee discussion or the policy workshop is to attempt to answer such questions; but all criteria, pursued in this way, simply "multiply like vermin."[5]

Thus, we cannot legislate judgment out of the process of quality control; rather, our judgments must be educated by discussion, debate, and the testing of ideas and findings in public forums, through the various processes of academic life, both formal and informal. Formerly, such processes have been largely internal to the scientific community, producing self-regulated quality over the long term, though with the possibility that any individual study may fall short of appropriate standards at any particular point in time. This is a situation that governments (and some researchers themselves) no longer seem to want to tolerate. Every study must now be "quality assured" by being "standardized."

At the same time, however, it has been recognized from many different perspectives, including that of the empowerment of research subjects on the one hand, and policy relevance and social utility on the other, that an assumption of scientific disinterest and independence is no longer sustainable. Other voices must be heard in the debate over scientific quality and merit, particularly with respect to applied, policy-oriented research. Thus, for example, Gibbons et al. (1994) distinguish between what they term "Mode 1" and "Mode 2" knowledge, with Mode

1 knowledge deriving from what might be termed the traditional academic disciplines and Mode 2 knowledge deriving from and operating within "a context of application": "[I]n Mode 1 problems are set and solved in a context governed by the, largely academic, interests of a specific community. By contrast, Mode 2 knowledge is carried out in a context of application" (p. 3). Mode 2 knowledge will thus generate solutions to problems as they emerge, in much the same way as the design experiments or action research approaches reviewed above. Such knowledge is "transdisciplinary ... [and] involves the close interaction of many actors throughout the process of knowledge production" (Gibbons et al., 1994, p. vii). In turn, quality must be "determined by a wider set of criteria which reflects the broadening social composition of the review system" (Gibbons et al., 1994, p. 8).

These arguments have been used to underpin a discussion document commissioned by the ESRC on "Assessing Quality in Applied and Practice-Based Educational Research" (Furlong & Oancea, 2005). Although the document falls into the category of yet another "framework" or set of "standards" and largely retains the distinction between scientific merit defined in terms of theory and methodology and social robustness defined in terms of policy relevance and utility, it nevertheless does not simply retreat into science or, perhaps more accurately, a narrow scientism (as does the U.S. advocacy of RCTs, for example). Its production is an acknowledgment that other sources of legitimacy and criteria of quality are important. Thus, the report articulates four dimensions of quality: epistemic, technological, use value for people, and use value for the economy and argues strongly that a restricted, traditional view of scientific quality is no longer tenable.

In practical terms, this means designing studies with collaborating sponsors and participants, including policymakers, and talking through issues of validity, warrant, appropriate focus, and trustworthiness of the results. A significant amount of such work is under way in the United Kingdom at present (see James, 2006; Pollard, 2005, 2006; Somekh & Saunders, forthcoming; Torrance & Coultas, 2004; Torrance et al., 2005). The process is not without its problems or critics, but in essence the argument is that if research is to engage with policy, then research and policymaking must progress, both theoretically and chronologically, in tandem. Neither can claim precedence in the relationship. Research should not simply "serve" policy; equally, policy cannot simply "wait" for the results of research. Research will encompass far more than simply producing policy-relevant findings; policymaking will include far more than research results. Where research and policy do cohere, the relationship must be pursued as an iterative one, with gains on both sides.

Governments and some within the scholarly community itself seem to be seeking to turn educational research into a technology that can be applied to solving short-term educational problems, rather than a system of enquiry that might help practitioners and policymakers think more productively about the nature of the problem and how it might addressed. The latter process will be as beneficial to policy as to research. Producing research results takes time, and the results are unlikely to be completely unequivocal in any case. Drawing policymakers into a discussion of these issues is likely to improve the nature of research questions and research design, while also signaling to them that the best evidence available is unlikely ever to be definitive.

The U.S. policy focus on RCTs is all the more puzzling in light of these developments and arguments in the United Kingdom. Similarly, the more general retreat into trying to define the scientific merit of qualitative research simply in terms of theoretical and methodological standards, rather than in wider terms of social robustness and responsiveness to practice, seems to betray a defensiveness and loss of nerve on the part of the scholarly community. We need to acknowledge and discuss the imperfections of what we do, rather than attempt to legislate them out of existence. We need to embody and enact the deliberative process of academic quality assurance, not subcontract it to a committee. Assuring the quality of research, and particularly the quality of qualitative research in the context of policymaking, must be conceptualized as a vital and dynamic process that is always subject to further scrutiny and debate. The process cannot be ensconced in a single research method or a once-and-for-all set of standards. Furthermore, it should be oriented toward risk taking and the production of new knowledge, including the generation of new questions (some of which may derive from active engagement with research respondents and policymakers), rather than supplication, risk aversion, and the production of limited data on effectiveness for system maintenance (what works). Thus, researchers and, particularly in this context, qualitative researchers, must better manage their relationships with policymakers, rather than their research activities per se. This will involve putting more emphasis on interacting with policy and policymakers and less emphasis on producing guidelines and standards that will only ever be used as a stick with which to beat us.

In the conclusion to a new book on *Knowledge Production: The Work of Educational Research in Interesting Times*, my colleague Bridget Somekh argues that "educational research communities … have been socially constructed as powerless … and have colluded in this process … through an impetus to conformity rather than transgressive speculation" (Somekh & Schwandt, 2007, p. 334). She further argues that engagement with policy and policy making should include the discussion of "speculative knowledge" (i.e., future possibilities emerging out of research), "to improvise the co-construction of new visions" (p. 340). This seems to me to be a much more productive ground for engagement with policymaking. It is not without its threats and challenges, especially with respect to co-option and collusion, but if it is speculative of new policy (and research) and properly cautious about the provisional nature of research knowledge, rather than promising a false certainty and legitimacy for policy, then the dialog could be productive on both sides.

Notes

1 This chapter is based on a paper originally presented to a symposium on Standards of Evidence in Qualitative Inquiry, American Educational Research Association 74th Annual Conference, Chicago, April 9–13, 2007. Direct correspondence to: h.torrance@mmu.ac.uk

2 For example, it is variously argued that the view of knowledge production and accumulation in the social sciences on which systematic reviewing is based is epistemologically flawed and that such reviews are, in any case, not fit for the purpose, taking too long to complete, costing too much, and producing too little by way of useful material for policy. MacLure (2005)

further argues that the technologically driven data-base searches that are employed "degrades the status of reading and writing as scholarly activities" (p. 393) and that the overall approach is animated by a fear of the unknowable (and hence unaccountable) interpretations of researchers inherent in the use of language itself.

3 There are also issues of commercial contracts, government investment in and support of the ICT sector, etc., that need not concern us here, but obviously tie in long-term investment in these and other programs in ways that make a simple "what works" answer untenable and unusable.

4 For a more extensive discussion of these and similar issues, see Hammersley (2005).

5 This exquisitely apposite phrase comes from an article written by Margaret Brown (1988, p. 19) about initial attempts to produce the English National Curriculum and Testing system, which resulted in every member of the subject group writing teams wanting to include everything that they considered important to the subject (see Torrance, 2003).

References

Attree, P., & B. Milton. 2006. Critically appraising qualitative research for systematic review: Defusing the methodological bombs. *Evidence & Policy* *2*(1):109–26.

Boaz, A., W. Solesbury, & F. Sullivan. 2004. *The practice of research reviewing 1: An assessment of 28 review reports.* London: UK Centre for Evidence-Based Policy and Practice, Queen Mary College. http://evidencenetwork.org (accessed November 28, 2007).

Boaz, A., W. Solesbury, & F. Sullivan. 2007. *The practice of research reviewing 2: Ten case studies of reviews.* London: UK Centre for Evidence-Based Policy and Practice, Queen Mary College. http://evidencenetwork.org (accessed November 28, 2007).

Bridges, D. 2005. The international and the excellent in educational research. Paper prepared for the Challenges of the Knowledge Society for Higher Education conference, Kaunus, Lithuania, December 16.

Brown, A. 1992. Design experiments: Theoretical and methodological challenges in creating complex interventions in classroom settings. *Journal of the Learning Sciences* 2(2):141–78.

Brown, M. 1988. Issues in formulating and organising attainment targets in relation to their assessment. In H. Torrance (Ed.), *National assessment and testing: A research response*, pp. 118–34. London: British Educational Research Association.

Brown, S. 2003. Assessment of research quality: What hope of success? Keynote address to European Educational Research Association annual conference, Hamburg, Germany, September 17.

Burkhardt, H., & A. Schoenfeld. 2003. Improving educational research: Toward a more useful, more influential and better-funded enterprise. *Educational Researcher* 32(9):3–14.

Cabinet Office. 2003a. Quality in qualitative evaluation. A framework for assessing research evidence. London: Government Chief Social Researcher's Office. [Report prepared on behalf of the Cabinet Office by L. Spencer, J. Ritchie, J. Lewis, & L. Dillon, National Centre for Social Research.]

Cabinet Office. 2003b. Quality in qualitative evaluation. A framework for assessing research evidence. London: Government Chief Social Researcher's Office. [Report prepared on behalf of the Cabinet Office by L. Spencer, J. Ritchie, J. Lewis, & L. Dillon, National Centre for Social Research.]

Chatterji, M. 2005. Evidence on "What Works": An argument for extended-term mixed-method (ETMM) evaluation designs. *Educational Researcher* 34(5):14–24.

Davies, P. 2004. Systematic reviews and the Campbell Collaboration. In G. Thomas & R. Pring (Eds.), *Evidence-based practice in education*, pp. 21–33. Maidenhead, UK: Open University Press.

Davies, P., & R. Boruch. 2001. The Campbell Collaboration. *British Medical Journal* 323(7308):294–95.

Denzin, N. K., & M. D. Giardina, Eds. 2006. *Qualitative inquiry and the conservative challenge.* Walnut Creek, CA: Left Coast Press, Inc.

Design-Based Research Collective, The. 2003. Design-based research: An emerging paradigm for educational enquiry. *Educational Researcher* 32(1):5–8.

Eisenhart, M. 2006. Qualitative science in experimental time. *International Journal of Qualitative Studies in Education* 19(6):697–708.

Eisenhart, M., & DeHaan, R. L. 2005. Doctoral preparation of scientifically based education researchers. *Educational Researcher* 34(4):3–13.

Eisenhart, M., & L. Towne. 2003. Contestation and change in national policy on "scientifically-based" education research. *Educational Researcher* 32(7):31–38.

Elliott, J. 1989. *Action research for educational change.* Buckingham, UK: Open University Press.

Erickson, F., & K. Gutierrez. 2002. Culture, rigor and science in educational research. *Educational Researcher* 31(8):21–24.

Feuer, M., L. Towne, & R. Shavelson. 2002. Scientific culture and educational research. *Educational Researcher* 31(8)4–14.

Furlong, J., & A. Oancea. 2005. *Assessing quality in applied and practice-based educational research*. Swindon, UK: ESRC.

Gibbons, M., C. Limoges, H. Nowotny, S. Schwartzman, P. Scott, & M. Trow. 1994. *The new production of knowledge*. Thousand Oaks, CA: Sage.

Gough, D., & D. Elbourne. 2002. Systematic research synthesis to inform policy, practice and democratic debate. *Social Policy and Society* 1(3):225–36.

Hammersley, M. 2001. On systematic reviews of research literature: A narrative response. *British Educational Research Journal* 27(4):543–54.

Hammersley, M. 2005. The myth of research-based practice: The critical case of educational inquiry. *International Journal of Social Research Methodology* 8(4):317–30.

Hargreaves, D. 1996. Teaching as a research based profession. TTA annual lecture, April, London, TTA.

Hillage, J., R. Pearson, A. Anderson, & P. Tamkin. 1998. *Excellence in research on school*. DfEE Research Report 74: London: DfEE.

House, E., & K. Howe. 1999. *Values in evaluation and social research*. Thousand Oaks, CA: Sage.

James, M. 2006. Balancing rigour and responsiveness in a shifting context: Meeting the challenges of educational research. *Research Papers in Education* 21(4):365–80.

MacLure, M. 2005. "Clarity bordering on stupidity": Where's the quality in systematic review? *Journal of Education Policy* 20(4)393–416.

Maxwell, J. 2004. Causal explanation, qualitative research and scientific enquiry in education. *Educational Researcher* 33(2):3–11.

National Research Council (NRC). 2002. *Scientific research in education*. Washington, DC: NRC.

National Research Council (NRC). 2005. *Advancing scientific research in education*. Washington, DC: NRC.

Newman, M., & D. Elbourne. 2004. Improving the usability of educational research: Guidelines for the REPOrting of Primary Empirical Research Studies in Education (The REPOSE Guidelines). *Evaluation and Research in Education* 18(4):201–12.

Oakley, A. 2000. *Experiments in knowing*. Cambridge: Polity Press.

Oakley, A. 2003. Research evidence, knowledge management and educational practice: Early lessons from a systematic approach. *London Review of Education* 1(1):21–33.

Oakley, A. 2006. Resistances to new technologies of evaluation: education research in the UK as a case study. *Evidence and Policy* 2(1):63–88.

OECD. 2002. *Educational research and development in England.* OECD Review CERI/CD(2002)10, Paris.

Pawson, R., & N. Tilley. 1997. *Realistic evaluation.* London: Sage.

Pollard, A. 2005. Challenges facing educational research. *Educational Review* 58(3):251–67.

Pollard, A. 2006. So, how then to approach research capacity building? *Research Intelligence* 97(November):18–20.

Ragin, C., J. Nagel, & P. White. 2004. *Workshop on scientific foundations of qualitative research.* http://www.nsf.gov/pubs/2004/nsf04219/start.htm (accessed November, 28, 2007).

Riehl, C. 2006. Feeling better: A comparison of medical research and educational research. *Educational Researcher* 35(5):24–29.

Schoenfeld, A. 2006. What doesn't work: The challenge and failure of the What Works Clearinghouse to conduct meaningful reviews of studies of mathematics curricula. *Educational Researcher* 35(2):13–21.

Shavelson, R., D. Phillips, L. Towne, & M. Feuer. 2003. On the science of education design studies. *Educational Researcher* 32(1):25–28.

Slavin, R. 2002. Evidence-based education policies: Transforming educational practice and research. *Educational Researcher* 31(7):15–21.

Somekh, B. C. Lewin, D. Mavers, C. Harris, K. Haw, T. Fisher, E. Lunzer, A. McFarlane, & P. Scrimshaw. 2002. *ImpaCT2: Pupils' and teachers' perceptions of ICT in the home, school and community.* London: Department for Education and Skills

Somekh, B., Underwood, A. Convery, G. Dillion, T. Harber Stuart, J. Jarvis, C. Lewin, D. Mavers, D. Saxon, P. Twinning, & D. Woodrow. 2005. *Evaluation of the DfES ICT TestBed project.* Coventry, UK: BECTA.

Somekh, B., & L. Saunders. Forthcoming. Developing knowledge through intervention: Meaning and definition of "quality" in research into change. *Research Papers in Education.*

Somekh, B., & T. Schwandt, Eds. 2007. *Knowledge Production: The work of educational research in interesting times.* London: Routledge.

Stenhouse, L. 1975. *An introduction to curriculum research and development.* London: Heinemann Books.

St. Pierre, E., & K. Roulston. 2006. The state of qualitative inquiry: A contested science. *International Journal of Qualitative Studies in Education* 19(6):673–84.

Thomas, G., & R. Pring, Eds. 2005. *Evidence-based practice in education.* Buckingham, UK: Open University Press.

Tooley, J., & D. Darby. 1998. *Educational research: A critique.* London: OfSTED.

Torrance, H. 2003. Assessment of the national curriculum in England. In T. Kellaghan & D. Stufflebeam (Eds.), *International handbook of educational evaluation*, pp. 905–928. Boston: Kluwer.

Torrance, H. 2006. Globalising empiricism: What if anything can be learned from international comparisons of educational achievement? In H. Lauder, P. Brown, J. Dillabough, & A. H. Halsey (Eds.), *Education, globalisation and social change*, pp. 88–98. Oxford: Oxford University Press.

Torrance, H., H. Colley, K. Ecclestone, D. Garratt, D. James, & H. Piper. 2005. *The impact of different modes of assessment on achievement and progress in the learning and skills sector.* London: Learning and Skills Research Centre.

Torrance, H., & J. Coultas. 2004. *Do summative assessment and testing have a positive or negative effect on post-16 learners' motivation for learning in the learning and skills sector?* London: Learning and Skills Research Centre.

Wade, C., H. Turner, H. Rothstein, & J. Lavenberg. 2006. Information retrieval and the role of the information specialist in producing high-quality systematic reviews in the social, behavioural and education sciences. *Evidence and Policy* 2(1):89–108.

Yates, L. 2004. *What is quality in educational research?* Buckingham, UK: Open University Press.

Yates, L. 2005. Is impact a measure of quality? Producing quality research and producing quality indicators of research in Australia. Keynote address for AARE Conference on Quality in Educational Research: Directions for Policy and Practice, Cairns, Australia, July 4–5.

Chapter 8

In the Name of Human Rights

I Say (How) You (Should) Speak (Before I Listen)[1]

Antjie Krog

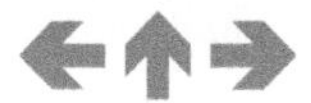

Introduction

It is the year 1872. A Bushman shaman called //Kabbo narrates an incident to a German philologist, Wilhelm Bleek, in Cape Town. In the narration, which took Bleek from April 13 to September 19 to record and translate from /Xam into English, the following two paragraphs describe how a young woman tracks down her nomadic family:

> She (the young widow) arrives with her children at the water hole. There she sees her younger brother's footprints by the water. She sees her mother's footprint by the water. She sees her brother's wife's spoor by the water.
>
> She tells her children: "Grandfather's people's footprints are here; they had been carrying dead springbok to the water so that people can drink on their way back with the game. The house is near. We shall follow the footprints because the footprints are new. We must look for the house. We must follow the footprints. For the people's footprints were made today; the people fetched water shortly before we came." (Lewis-Williams, 2000, p. 61)

Originally published in *Qualitative Inquiry and Human Rights,* edited by Norman K. Denzin and Michael D. Giardina, pp. 125–135. Republished in *Qualitative Inquiry—Past, Present, and Future: A Critical Reader,* edited by Norman K. Denzin and Michael D. Giardina, pp. 160–170. Left Coast Press, Inc.

For more than a hundred years, these words seemed like just another interesting detail in an old Bushmen story, until researcher Louis Liebenberg went to live among modern Bushmen. In his book, *The Art of Tracking: The Origin of Science*, Liebenberg (1990) insists that what seems to be an instinctive capacity to track a spoor, the Bushmen were using intricate decoding, contextual sign analysis to create hypotheses.

Liebenberg distinguishes three levels of tracking among the Bushmen: First, simple tracking just follows footprints. Second, systematic tracking involved the gathering of information from signs until a detailed indication is built up of the action. Third, speculative tracking involves the creation of a working hypothesis on the basis of: (1) the initial interpretation of signs, (2) a knowledge of behavior, and (3) a knowledge of the terrain. According to Liebenberg these skills of tracking are akin to those of Western intellectual analysis and suggests that all science actually started with tracking (Brown, 2006, p. 25).

Returning to the opening two paragraphs, one sees that the young widow effortlessly does all three kinds of tracking identified by Liebenberg. She identifies the makers of the footprints, their coming and going, that they were carrying something heavy and/or bleeding, that they were thirsty, that they drank water on the way back from hunting; she identifies the game as a springbuck; she establishes when the tracks were made and then puts forward a hypothesis of what they were doing and where and how she will find her family that very day.

The question I want to pose here is: Is it justified to regard Wilhelm Bleek (as the recorder of the narration), Louis Liebenberg (as a scholar of tracking), and myself (for applying the tracking theory to the narration) as the scholars/academics while considering //Kabbo (Bushman narrator) and the woman in the story (reading the tracks) as "raw material"?

How does this division respect human right number 19 in the Universal Declaration of Human Rights of the United Nations: "Everyone has the right to freedom of opinion and expression; this right includes freedom to hold opinions without interference *and to seek, receive and impart information and ideas through any media and regardless of frontiers*" (see http://www.un.org/en/documents/udhr/).

Who May Enter the Discourse?

The rights of two groups will be discussed in this chapter: first, the rights of those living in marginalized areas but who produce virtually on a daily basis intricate knowledge systems of survival and second, the rights of scholars coming from those marginalized places, but who can only enter the world of acknowledged knowledge in languages not their own and within discourses based on foreign and estrange-ing structures.

Although Gayatri Spivak describes the first group as subaltern, she deals with both these groups in her famous chapter "Can the Subaltern Speak?" suggesting that the moment that the subaltern finds herself in conditions in which she can be heard "her status as a subaltern would be changed utterly; she would cease to be subaltern" (Landry & Maclean, 1995, pp. 5–6).

Mrs. Konile as Subaltern

During the two years of hearings conducted by the South African Truth and Reconciliation Commission two thousand testimonies were given in public. Instead of listening to the impressive stories of well-known activists, the commission went out of its way to provide a forum for the most marginalized narratives from rural areas given in indigenous languages. In this way, these lives and previously unacknowledged narratives were made audible and could be listened to through translation to become the first entry into the South African psyche of what Spivak (1987) so aptly calls in her piece, "Subaltern Studies: Deconstructing Historiography," "news of the consciousness of the subaltern" (p. 203).

Covering the hearings of the Truth Commission for national radio, one testimony stayed with me as the most incoherent female testimony I had to report on (First TRC Testimony of Mrs. Konile, 1998). I considered the possibility that one needed other tools to make sense of it and wondered whether clarification could be found in the original Xhosa, or was the woman actually mentally disturbed, or was there some vestige of "cultural supremacy" in myself that prevented me from hearing her?

Trying to find her testimony later on the Truth Commission's website was fruitless. There was no trace of her name in the index.

Under the heading of the Gugulethu Seven incident, her surname was given incorrectly as "Khonele," and she was the only mother in this group to be presented without a first name. Her real name was Notrose Nobomvu Konile, but I later found that even in her official identity document her second name was given incorrectly as Nobovu.

One might well ask: Is it at all possible to hear this un-mentioned, incorrectly ID-ed, misspelled, incoherently testifying, translated, and carelessly transcribed woman from the deep rural areas of South Africa?

I asked two colleagues, Nosisi Mpolweni from the Xhosa Department and professor Kopano Ratele from the Psychology Department and Women & Gender Studies, to join me in a reading of the testimony. Ms Mpolweni and Professor Ratele immediately became interested. Using the original Xhosa recording, we started off by transcribing and retranslating. Then we applied different theoretical frameworks (Elaine Scarry, Cathy Garuth, Soshana Felman, Dori Laub, G. Bennington, etc.) to interpret the text and finally, we visited and reinterviewed Mrs. Konile. What started out as a one-off teatime discussion became a project of two and a half years and finally a book: *There Was This Goat: Investigating the Truth and Reconciliation Testimony of Notrose Nobomvu Konile* (Krog, Mpolweni, & Ratele, 2009).

But first, some concepts need to be introduced that play a role the moment the voice of the subaltern becomes audible.

The Fluke of "Raw Material"

I was proud to be appointed by a university that, during apartheid, deliberately ignored the demands of privileged white academia and focused unabashedly on the oppressed communities surrounding the campus. The university prided itself, and rightly so, on being the university of the left and threw all its resources behind the poor.

Since the first democratic election in 1994, South Africa is trying to become part of what is sometimes called "a normal dispensation." So some months after my appointment 5 years ago, I was asked to send a list of what I have published that year. Fortunately, or so I thought, I was quite active: a nonfiction book, poetry, controversial newspaper pieces etc.—so imagine my surprise to receive an email saying that none of the listed writings "counts."

I went to see the dean of research. The conversation went like this:

"Why do my publications not count?

"It's not peer reviewed."

"It was reviewed in all the newspapers!"

"But not by peers."

Wondering why the professors teaching literature would not be regarded as my peers I asked, "So who are my peers?"

"Of course you are peerless," this was said somewhat snottily, "but I mean the people in your field."

"So what is my field?"

"The people working ..." and his hands fluttered "in the areas about which you write."

"Well," I said, "when I look at their work I see that they all quote me."

His face suddenly beamed: "So you see! You are raw material!"

Initially I thought nothing of the remark, but gradually came to realize how contentious, judgmental, and excluding the term "raw material" was. Who decides who is raw material? Are Mrs. Konile and //Kabbo and the Bushman woman raw material? Looking back onto our project, I find myself asking: Why did we three colleagues so easily assume that Mrs. Konile was raw material and not a cowriter of our text? Why are her two testimonies and one interview in which she constructs and analyzes, deducts and concludes less of an academic endeavor than our contribution? Her survival skills after the devastating loss of her son were not by chance but a result of her careful calculations and tested experiences. During our interview, we even asked her to interpret her text. Why should she enter our book and the academic domain as raw material? Should she not be properly credited as a cotext producer on the cover like the three of us?

I began wondering: What would another Gugulethu mother ask Mrs. Konile? Or to move to another realm: How would one cattle herder interview another cattle herder? How would one cattle herder analyze and appraise the words of a fellow cattle herder? How would such an interview differ from me interviewing that cattle herder? And, finally, how can these experiences enter the academic discourse *without* the conduit of a well-meaning scholar? How shall we ever enter any new realm if we insist that all information must be processed by ourselves for ourselves?

The Fluke of Discipline

After being downgraded to raw material, I duly applied to attend a workshop on how to write unraw material so as to meet one's peers through unread but accredited journals. The workshop was organized by the university after it became clear that our new democratic government wants universities to come up with fundable research. We were obliged to compete with the established and excellently resourced former white universities and their impressive research records.

I walked into this organized workshop. There were about forty of us. I was the only white person. During smoke breaks the stories poured out.

A professor in math told me the following:

> One Sunday a member of the congregation told me that he was installing science laboratories in the schools of the new South Africa, that it was very interesting because every school was different. So this went on every Sunday until I said to him that he should write it down. So after I had completely forgotten about it, he pitched up with a manuscript this thick (about four inches) and joked: Is this not a MA thesis? I looked and indeed it was new, it was methodically researched and systematically set out and riveting to read. So where to now? I said it was not math so he should take it to the science department. Science said it was more history than science. History said no, … and so forth.

Those who attended the workshop were by no means subaltern, but first-generation educated men and women from formerly disadvantaged communities in apartheid South Africa. As we attended subsequent workshops in writing academic papers, we became aware of how the quality of "on the ground experience" was being crushed into a dispirited nothingness through weak English and the specific format of academic papers. We learned how easily an important story died within the corset of an academic paper; how a crucial observation was nothing without a theory; and how a valuable experience dissolved outside a discipline.

The Fluke of Theory

The last story is about a seminar on the black body that I attended. Opening the seminar, the professor said that when he was invited he thought that the paper he was preparing would already have been accepted by an accredited journal and the discussion could then have taken place together with the peer reviews. The journal had, however, rejected the piece, so ... maybe the discussion should start from scratch.

The paper he presented was indeed weak. As he was speaking, one had the distinct feeling of seeing a little boat rowing with all its might past waves and fish and flotillas and big ships and fluttering sails to a little island called Hegel. The oar was kept aloft until, until ... at last, the oar touched Hegel. Then the rowing continued desperately until the oar could just touch the island called Freud or Foucault. In the meantime, you want to say forget these islands, show us what's in your boat, point out the fish that you know, how did you sidestep that big ship, where did you get these remarkable sails?

The discussion afterward was extraordinary. Suddenly, the professor was released from his paper and the black students and lecturers found their tongues and it became a fantastic South African analysis. Afterward I asked the professor: "Why didn't you write what you have just said?" He answered:

> Because I can't find a link between what I know and existing literature. It's a Catch 22 situation: I cannot analyze my rural mother if it is assumed that there is no difference between her mind and the average North American or Swedish mind. On the other hand, my analysis of my rural mother will only be heard and understood if it is presented on the basis of the North American and Swedish mind.

Academics from Marginalized Communities

Both of my colleagues, Nosisi Mpolweni and Prof. Kopano Ratele, were the first in their families to be tertiary educated, whereas I was the fourth generation of university-educated women. Right through our collective interpretative analysis on the testimony of Mrs. Konile, the power relations among us changed. The project started with my initiative, but I quickly became the one who knew the least. Prof. Ratele was the best educated of us three and had already published academically. Nosisi provided invaluable input with her translations and knowledge about Xhosa culture. I could write well, but not academically well. English was our language, but only Prof. Ratele could speak it properly. During our field trip to interview Mrs. Konile, the power swung completely to Nosisi, and I, not understanding Xhosa, had no clout during our fieldwork excursions.

However, during our discussions, I became aware that while we were talking, my colleagues had these moments of perfect formulation, a sort of spinning toward that sentence that finally says it all. We would stop and realize: Yes, this was it! This was the grasp we were working toward. But when we returned with written texts, these core sentences were nowhere to be seen in their work.

For the next discussion, I brought a tape recorder. We were discussing why Mrs. Konile so obsessively uses the word "I" within her rural collective worldview. I transcribed the conversation and sent everybody these chunks; here is the text returned by Prof. Ratele:

> Mrs. Konile dreamt about the goat the night before she heard that her son was killed. The TRC however was not a forum for dreams, but for the truth about human rights abuses. I suggest that through telling about the dream, Mrs. Konile was signaling to the TRC her connection to the ancestral worlds.
>
> The dream revealed that she was still whole, that she was in contact with the living and the dead and she clearly experienced little existential loneliness. … Her son's death is what introduced her to a loneliness, a being, an "I." She had become an individual through the death of her son—selected, cut off, as it were, to

> become an individual. She was saying: "I am suffering, because I had been forced to become an individual." The word "I" was not talking about her real psychological individuality. Mrs. Konile was using "I" as a form of complaint. She was saying: "I don't want to be I. I want to be us, but the killing of my son, made me into an 'I.'" (Krog, Mpolweni, & Ratele, 2009, pp. 61–62)

As a white person steeped in individuality, I initially didn't even notice the frequency of the word "I," but when I did it merely confirmed to me that the notion of African collective-ness was overrated, despite the emphasis it receives from people like Nelson Mandela and Archbishop Desmond Tutu. The conclusion Prof. Ratele came to, however, was the opposite and it was a conclusion I could not have come to, and up until now neither has any other white TRC analyst.

For me this was the big breakthrough, not only in the book, not only in TRC analysis, but also in our method of working. The confidence of the spoken tone, a confidence originating from the fact that somebody was talking from within and out of a world she knows intimately, had been successfully carried over on to paper. Prof. Ratele was crossing "frontiers" to get past all the barriers lodged in education, race, background, structure, language, and academic discipline to interpret his own world from out of its postcolonial, postmodern past, and racial awarenesses with a valid confidence that speaks into and even beyond exclusive and prescriptive frameworks.

My guess is that my colleague would never have been able to write this particular formulation without first talking it, and talking it to us—a black woman who understood him and a white woman who didn't.

We wrote an essay about Mrs. Konile's dream in our three different voices but the piece was rejected by a South African journal for allowing contradictory viewpoints to "be" in the essay, for having a tone that seems oral, for not producing any theory that could prove that Mrs. Konile was somehow different from other human beings, etc. The piece was, however, I'm glad to say, accepted by Norman Denzin, Yvonna Lincoln, and Linda Tuhiwai Smith (2007) for their *Handbook of Critical and Indigenous Methodologies*.

Conclusion: Research as Reconciliatory Change

These examples, ranging from a Bushman shaman to a black professor in psychology, expose the complexities of doing research in a country emerging from divided histories and cultures. It also poses some ethical questions about the conditions we set for people to enter academic discourse. Spivak (1988) indeed stresses that ethics is not a problem of knowledge but a call of relationship. When she claims that the subaltern "cannot speak," she means that the subaltern as such cannot be heard by the privileged of either the First or Third Worlds. If the subaltern was able to make herself heard then her status as a subaltern would be changed utterly; she would cease to be subaltern. But isn't the goal of our research "that the subaltern, the most oppressed and invisible constituencies, as such might cease to exist" (Landry & Maclean, 1995, p. 6).

French philosopher Gilles Deleuze rightly remarks that the power of minorities "is not measured by their capacity to enter into and make themselves felt within the majority system." At the same time, Deleuze points out that it is precisely these different forms of minority-becoming that provide the impulse for change, but change can only occur to the extent that there is adaptation and incorporation on the side of the standard or the majority (Deleuze & Guattari 1987, p. 520).

We have to find ways in which the marginalized can enter our discourses in their own genres and their own terms so that we can learn to hear them. They have a universal right to impart information and ideas through any media and regardless of frontiers, and we have a duty to listen and understand them through engaging in new acts of becoming.

Note

1 This chapter extends and inserts itself in the discussion of *testimonio* as given in John Beverley, 2005, pp. 547–558.

References

Beverley, J. (2005). Testimonio, subalternity, and narrative authority. In N. K. Denzin and Y. S. Lincoln (Eds.), *Handbook of qualitative research* (3rd ed., pp. 547–558). Thousand Oaks, CA: Sage.

Brown, D. (2006). *To speak of this land—Identity and belonging in South Africa and beyond,* Scottsville, South Africa: University of KwaZulu Natal Press.

Denzin, N. K., Lincoln, Y.S., & Smith, L. T. (Eds.) (2007). *Handbook of critical and indigenous methodologies*. Thousand Oaks, CA: Sage.

Deleuze, G., & Guattari, F. (1987). *Thousand plateaus: Capitalism and schizophrenia* (B. Massumi, Trans.). Minneapolis: University of Minnesota Press.

First TRC Testimony of Mrs. Konile. 1998. http://www.doj.gov.za/trc/hrvtrans/heide/ct00100.htm (accessed March 12, 2009).

Krog, A, Mpolweni, N., & Ratele, K. (2009). *There was this goat—Investigating the Truth Commission testimony of Notrose Nobomvu Konile*. Scottsville, South Africa: University of KwaZulu-Natal Press.

Landry, D., & Maclean, G. (1995). Introduction: Reading Spivak. In D. Landry and G. Maclean (Eds.) *Selected works of Gyatri Chakravorty Spivak* (pp. 1-13). New York: Routledge.

Lewis-Williams, J. D. (Ed). (2000). *Stories that float from afar: Ancestral folklore of the San of Southern Africa*, Cape Town: David Philip.

Liebenberg, L. (1990). *The art of tracking: The origin of science*. Cape Town: David Philip.

Spivak, G. C. (1987). Subaltern studies: Deconstructing historiography. *In other worlds: Essays in cultural politics* (pp. 197–221). London: Routledge.

Spivak, G. C. (1988). "Can the subaltern speak?" In C. Nelson and L. Grossberg (Eds.), *Marxism and the interpretation of culture* (pp. 271–313). Basingstoke, UK: Macmillan Education.

Chapter 9

Education Research in the Public Interest[1]

Gloria Ladson-Billings

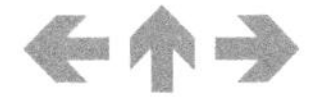

I watched Katrina from the other side of the Atlantic Ocean. I was attending a conference in London when news from the BBC and CNN International arrived about the strength of the hurricane, the devastation of an area the size of the United Kingdom, and the utter despair of the poor, elderly, and black citizens of the Gulf Coast region. What could we say about the public interest when it appeared that the public institutions most responsible for responding to the most needy segments of the public had almost no interest in them?

The strange contrast between the response to September 11, 2001, and Hurricane Katrina left a sickening feeling in the pit of my stomach. Let me be clear: These are not equivalent events. September 11 was an attack of foreign terrorists that made us all feel confused, horrified, and vulnerable. The nation mourned the death of so many Americans and lifted up the heroism of hundreds of brave first responders. We rallied around a president whose competence (and legitimacy) many of us questioned. New York, the city that never sleeps, became a place that was home to us all. I worried if my family members who live in New York

Originally published in *Qualitative Inquiry and Social Justice*, edited by Norman K. Denzin and Michael D. Giardina, pp.124–138. Republished in *Qualitative Inquiry—Past, Present, and Future: A Critical Reader*, edited by Norman K. Denzin and Michael D. Giardina, pp. 171–185.

were safe. I heard scores of stories about New Yorkers exhibiting their best selves. There were reports of merchants who handed out sneakers to women who were walking through Manhattan in high-heeled shoes because the transportation system was crippled. There were other reports of children passing out bottles of water to the stunned commuters. Help for victims of 9/11 came in many forms from around the country and throughout the world.

Hurricane Katrina was a natural disaster. It was not contained to a few buildings in New York, Washington, DC, and a field in Pennsylvania. The storm could not be prevented. Indeed, the last few years have seen a number of devastating tropical storms and hurricanes. The state of Florida alone was battered by three or four major storms in the 2004 hurricane season. The shock of Katrina was the way so many U.S. citizens were left to fend for themselves. In an administration that claimed to leave no child behind, large numbers of poor, elderly, and black citizens *were* left behind. Our horror was not over the path of destruction the storm left but rather the gaping hole in the safety net left by twenty-five years of public neglect.

The spectacle that became the Hurricane Katrina crisis forces me to ask: "Which public(s) command our interest and what, if anything, can we say about those publics that we regularly and systematically ignore?" Over forty years ago, Michael Harrington (1962) published the book, *The Other America*, which is credited with launching the "War on Poverty." In it, Harrington described the social and economic isolation that millions of poor urban and rural citizens experience in America. He also described their relative invisible status in the American psyche. During the 2004 presidential campaign, Democratic vice-presidential candidate, John Edwards (D-NC), tried to bring an awareness of the persistence of two Americas to the consciousness of the American electorate:

> Today, under George W. Bush, there are two Americas, not one: One America that does the work, another that reaps the reward. One America that pays the taxes, another America that gets the tax breaks. One America—middle-class America—whose needs Washington has long forgotten, another America—a narrow-interest America—whose every wish is Washington's

> command. One America that is struggling to get by, another America that can buy anything it wants, even a Congress and a president. (available online at (http://en.wikiquote.org/wiki/John_Edwards, accessed October 6, 2005)

But even Edwards was not referencing the poorest of the poor. His appeal was to the middle class that was slowly but surely feeling the impact of stagnant wages and increasing health care costs. The desperately poor who emerged across our media or were perhaps "washed up" after Katrina represented an entirely new magnitude of poverty to which too many had become insensitive and unaware. Katrina's gift was its in-your-face confrontation of how we are going to define the public and its interests.

Some might question the relevance of Hurricane Katrina to the discourse of education research and the public interest. However, in the aftermath of Katrina—where many cities and small towns are still attempting to pull their lives back together some three years later—we can again witness examples of how the inequities continue to manifest. The hurricane was an equal opportunity destroyer. Million-dollar beachfront homes and casinos were destroyed alongside housing projects, tenements, and "shotgun" houses. But the process of reconstruction reveals very different patterns. Evacuees from the wealthier communities have been able to place their children in private schools or attend public schools outside the urban community of New Orleans. Evacuees from the infamous lower 9th Ward and most of New Orleans proper have been told that their public schools may not reopen for some time.

The public interest aspect of education research is linked to the increasing public *involvement* in education. Since the *Brown v. Board of Education* decisions (1954, 1955), it has been clear that there is a national interest in education. The contour of that interest has shifted with the political winds. There have been times when education barely registered on the national agenda. Ronald Reagan was determined to dismantle the Department of Education. His disdain for what he termed "big government" caused him to urge policies such as school choice vouchers, character education, and an emphasis on back to basics curriculum such as reading, mathematics, and history. However, we must recall that it was during Reagan's administration that the agenda for federal intervention in education was reset. The release of *A Nation at Risk: The Imperative for Educational Reform* (1983) by the National Commission on Excellence in Education set the direction for education reform. This report was followed by a spate of documents and initiatives decrying the terrible state of the nation's educational system.

The response to the alarm that education was failing on all fronts was to raise the bar and depend primarily on standardized assessments to measure academic progress. During the first term of the George W. Bush administration, the Elementary and Secondary Education Act was due for reauthorization. Instead of focusing the reauthorization solely on the compensatory aspects of Title I, the Bush White House made it an omnibus act that impacted all public school. They called their program "No Child Left Behind" (NCLB: Public Law 107-110) and required schools to test students regularly, hire what was termed "highly qualified" teachers, and use "scientifically proven" teaching methods. Unfortunately, these grand plans were not matched with adequate funding from the federal government.

As shortsighted as I think NCLB is, I do think there are aspects of it that do exactly what education needs. For example, NCLB forces schools to disaggregate their data by racial/ethnic group. This is particularly important in suburban and metropolitan districts where so-called good schools were guilty of masking the poor academic performance of students of color by the much greater numbers of their white middle-class students. However, the real genius of NCLB was to include all students—not just Title I students—in the reauthorization. This approach forced many educators off of the sidelines and into the fray. We were no longer talking simply about "other people's children" (Delpit, 1995); we now had to think about our own children. But those points do not outweigh the serious flaws in the legislation or its unfunded mandates.

New Orleans and the Perfect Storm

I reflect back on New Orleans and the aftermath of the hurricane because New Orleans provides a perfect example of what happens when *everything* goes wrong. Before Katrina, the statistics on Orleans Parrish painted a grim picture of life for many of its citizens. According to the U.S. Census Bureau (2000), New Orleans had a population of 484,674 before the hurricane. Sixty-seven percent of that population was African American, with 23.7 percent of the total population living below the poverty line, and 35 percent of the African American population living below the poverty line. More than 40,000 New Orleanians had less than a ninth-grade graduation, and 56,804 residents had between ninth- and twelfth-grade educations without diplomas. A telling statistic is that 96.1 percent of the public school population was African American, which means that most of the white families with school-aged children send their children to private schools. Thirteen percent of the public school teachers in the state were uncertified.

Education clearly was not working for those in New Orleans who depended on public schools. It was not working long before the streets were flooded and the roofs were blown away. A well-known Norman Rockwell painting shows a little African American girl walking between federal marshals on her way to school. That depiction represents Ruby Bridges, who, in 1960, was the first African American to integrate New Orleans' schools. Wells (2004) details the history of resistance by white communities bordering New Orleans to allowing African American students to enter their schools. Bridges's story, although compelling, is even more extraordinary in light of the context of school desegregation in New Orleans. Out of 137 African American students who applied to attend formerly all white schools, only four were selected. One of the four was Ruby Bridges. She attended the William Frantz Elementary School; all of the white students then boycotted the school. Only one teacher, a white woman from New York, was willing to teach Ruby. As a consequence of her attending the previously all-white school, Ruby's father was fired from his job and her grandparents were evicted from their tenant farm.

For most of us, the story of Ruby Bridges is a story of courage and heroism—and it is. But the deeper story is the story of how America's fatal flaw—racism—continues to distort and destroy the promise on which the nation claimed to be founded. The same mentality that allowed white citizens to barricade themselves from school desegregation in the 1960s was present among white citizens who armed themselves to prevent desperate black citizens of New Orleans in the midst of the hurricane disaster from seeking refuge from the floodwaters. Which public are we referencing when, in 2005 a public official (a sheriff) points a gun at destitute evacuees and says, "You're not coming in here" and leaves them to wither on a freeway overpass (Glass, 2005)?

This history of New Orleans school desegregation is a part of a larger history of not just educational access denied but rather the history of citizenship denied. Limiting education is just one of the ways to create second-class citizenship. However, it is one of the more effective ways because once a people are *mis*-educated and/or undereducated, society can claim the need to use "merit" as the standard by which decisions for post-secondary decisions (e.g., college admission, job placement) will be made. New Orleans is a municipality where people were *systematically* excluded from social benefits—housing, health, employment, and education: Hurricane Katrina brought to the surface the horror that existed in New Orleans for more than a century.

The horror of Hurricane Katrina is made more frustrating by the history of flooding in the Gulf Coast region. In the great Mississippi flood of 1927, Louisiana officials deliberately flooded African American neighborhoods (allegedly to prevent greater flooding in other parts of the city). Officials dynamited the Poydras levee, which led ultimately to 700,000 people—half of them African Americans—being displaced. More horrific than the flood (which killed about 246 people) were the conditions in the evacuation camps.

Now, almost eighty years later, we see an eerily similar situation. The poor are abandoned and displaced, and we seem to have learned little from the lessons of history. What, if anything, can education research tell us about what we should do to ensure that the rebuilding process in New Orleans does not reproduce the substandard education that had become emblematic of the city?

In many ways, New Orleans has the opportunity to do exactly what Anyon (2005) argues must be done to improve urban schools. The schools must be reformed in tandem with improvements to the entire city. In the case of New Orleans, everything has to be rebuilt and the schools have an opportunity to emerge anew. Unfortunately, some disturbing rumblings have already emerged. The city's power elite, civic leaders, developers, and speculators plan to build a "different" New Orleans—one with fewer poor people and presumably fewer African Americans. Because so many of the city's displaced residents are poor, it is unlikely that they will be able to quickly pick up and return to the city. If they have been fortunate enough to find housing, employment, and decent schooling in another city, we cannot expect them to return to New Orleans. With fewer residents returning to the city, the school population will be smaller. The smaller school population can provide an opportunity for smaller schools (and it is hoped smaller classrooms).

With a smaller school population, New Orleans has an opportunity to be more selective in the hiring of teachers and other school personnel. They even have the opportunity to create a new school district that is not limited to the geographic confines of Orleans Parish. Orfield and Eaton (1996) point out that one of the major problems that school desegregation addresses is the concentration of poverty. A new school district configuration can address that. Delpit (1995), Foster (1997), Hilliard (2000), Irvine (2002), and Siddle-Walker (1996) all address the point that African Americans do know how to educate themselves. Anderson (1988) and Willis (2002) detail the historical pattern of African Americans creating, building, maintaining, and sustaining educational institutions. A new New Orleans school district has the opportunity to build on this legacy of success.

It is important to acknowledge that schools are not the sole site of community and individual development. Rothstein (2004) has consistently argued that in addition to school improvement, policymakers and educators must pursue expanded notions of schooling that include out-of-school experiences, and "social and economic policies that will enable children to attend school more equally ready to learn" (p. 109). The policies that Rothstein references, similar to Anyon (2005), include expanded and affordable health services and housing along with jobs that allow people to make a true living wage. Rubinowitz and Rosenbaum (2000) documented the ability of low-income African Americans to "move to opportunity" by integrating into suburban communities. Comparisons between the people who moved to suburban communities and those who moved within the city show significant differences. Forty percent of the students who attended schools in the suburbs were enrolled in college-track curricula compared to the 24% enrolled in college-tracks in the city. Fifty-four percent of the African American students who moved to the suburbs enrolled in some type of postsecondary education, 27% of whom enrolled in a four-year college. Their city counterparts enrolled in postsecondary programs at the rate of 21%, with only 4% enrolled in a four-year college. On the economic front, 75% of the mothers who moved to the suburbs were working, compared to just 41% of their peers who remained in the city.

But all was not positive in the suburbs. African American students had higher rates of special education placement in the suburbs, with 19% of students placed in special needs categories versus 7% in the city. This special education disproportionality is consistent with Skiba et al.'s (in press) findings on black students in special education placement and discipline referrals.

I recount these figures to point toward the troubling attitudes and behaviors that are likely to emerge even if New Orleans has the opportunity to start over and create a new city that truly provides equal opportunities for all of its residents. Unfortunately, as a critical race theorist I am not optimistic about the likelihood of a just resolution to the reconstruction of New Orleans. If I were forced to predict the outcome of the reconstruction it would resemble the following scenario:[2]

> It is the near-future, and with my eyes closed and ears wide open I can tell I am in New Orleans. The aroma is a mix of savory and sweet—hot and languid. I can smell the down home gumbo, the tangy jambalaya, and a wonder shrimp etouffee simmering on the collective stoves of French Quarter restaurants. My sweet tooth is tickled by the prospect of luscious hot bread pudding and Bananas Foster. Yes, my nose tells me I am in New Orleans. My ears also tell me that I am in the "Big Easy." I hear the strains of Dixieland coming from one street corner and Zydeco coming from another. There is no other town where this music is

so prominent and evident in everyday living. However, it is when I open my eyes that I begin to doubt myself. Some aspects of the city are immediately recognizable. I see Jackson Square with the lovely Cathedral of St. Louis on one side and the Mississippi River on the other. The shops of the French Quarter are humming with activity. Tourists are browsing the many souvenir shops. Every now and then I see someone with a t-shirt attesting to their experience of having survived "Katrina."

As I look down Poydras I can see that the horror of the Superdome and the New Orleans Convention Center have been replaced by a new sports and convention center complex. A gleaming new Hyatt Hotel sits between the two. I decide to grab the trolley on Canal Street and head out toward the zoo. I recognize the grandeur of the Garden District. Organizations like National Historic Preservation have worked hard to make sure the stately mansions were brought back to their timeless beauty. Looking at this community you would never guess that a hurricane and flooding had ever occurred. I step off the trolley at Tulane University where I see a bustling campus, beautifully appointed and clearly a center of academic activity. It looks like the new New Orleans is better than ever.

I return downtown so that I can head toward the places I know best. I want to check out Congo Square in Louis Armstrong Park. I want to see if someone dusted off Marie Laveaux's tomb. I want to see how Xavier, Dillard, and Southern universities came through the disaster. I am buoyed by what I have seen at both Tulane and Loyola. When I get hungry I will probably sneak into Dooky Chase to eat some things that have not been on my diet for years, but Leah Chase is an institution, having cooked at that location since 1946, has earned a special place in my heart. One year while my family and I were in New Orleans for the Sugar Bowl game we had dinner at Dooky Chase. It was late on a Sunday evening and there wasn't much foot traffic. The food was not particularly outstanding but I wanted my teenaged daughter to go to a black New Orleans institution. Some days after we returned home I noticed that my credit card was missing. In attempting to retrace my steps I realized that the last time I used the card was at the restaurant. A quick phone call to New Orleans got me in touch with the maître d', who informed me that he had found the card but did not know how to get in touch with me. In a matter of minutes the card was destroyed and canceled.

Louis Armstrong Park is just where it was. It has been cleaned up and the maker for Congo Square remains. This is the place where former enslaved Africans spent their Sunday afternoons. Their stories of resistance and survival were formulated here. To me, it is sacred ground. I breathe a sigh of relief, but my relief is short-lived. My visits to Dillard, Xavier, and Southern universities are much less satisfying. Both Dillard and Xavier have had to merge with two of the city's predominately white institutions—Xavier with Loyola and Dillard with Tulane. Southern (or SUNO) has closed and moved its operation to Baton Rouge. The state has decided it can no longer afford to have two branches of the Southern campus.

I decide to pick up my spirits with a shrimp po'boy at Dooky Chase's but when I turn down Orleans Street I barely recognize it. Gone are the ramshackle public housing units and in their place there is nothing. Just as it is in North Philadelphia, Detroit, South Central Los Angeles, East Oakland, East St. Louis, and countless other U.S. cities, there has been no attempt to rebuild in this area. The infamous 9th Ward that was home to a large number of the city's poor and African American community lays fallow. It is caught between the greedy land developers from the east coast and the holier-than-thou environmentalists from the west coast. The two groups are mired in litigation while squeezed in the middle are the poorest of the poor who would like to return but have nowhere to live.

Without a 9th Ward, Orleans parish schools were a very different place. Instead of 60,000 students it now had less than half that number with about 28,000 students. When the first residents returned to repopulate the city, those with school-aged children were offered vouchers to take to private schools because the public system was not yet fully online. By the time the city was up and running, the damage that this diversion of students from the public system had taken its toll. The failure to bring all segments of the community back into the city means that there was a smaller tax base upon which to build a school system.

The booming downtown area was deceptive. Yes, there were gleaming new hotels and department stores. In fact, several corporate headquarters had relocated to the newly reconstructed New Orleans. These companies were able to make sweet deals with the city fathers. They were promised tax credits and a variety of workplace waivers that allowed them to hire people for their low level jobs (e.g. janitors, cafeteria workers, clerks) without providing full benefits. Housing was at a premium in the new city. Condos and town homes dominated the downtown area. The stately mansions remained in the hands of the city's 'old money' families. The poor were locked out. A few of the poor were able to find some housing across the river in the Algiers section of the city but there is not much in the rebuilt city that can accommodate people of modest means.

For many months New Orleans was known as the "childless city" (MSNBC, 2005). Those poor families with children did not return because they did not want to risk moving their children out of the somewhat stable school environments they had found in other communities. Others worried that the level of contamination caused by the sewage, standing water, and lack of sanitation created a toxic environment that they could not risk with their children and still others recognized that the limited social services—day care, after school, community centers—meant that there was not enough community infrastructure in which their children could flourish.

New Orleans had become a city of odd demographics. It reminded me of the District of Columbia. It was a place where almost no families sent their children to public schools. Private schools were springing up all over the place. In a nod to its French heritage the city became home to several lyceums attended by the wealthiest residents. The public schools, although smaller, were not much better than before the disaster. Few "highly qualified" teachers returned to the system. Most of the newer teachers had found jobs in other communities. Large numbers of veteran teachers retired. This smaller school system had its share of "competent" teachers but a better assessment was that most of the system's teachers were mediocre.

The pattern of racism seemed clear to me but I was assured that race had nothing to do with how the city was reconstructed. I was shown how a variety of old line (read: Creole) families were an integral part of the rebuilding. Indeed, the mayor was black. No, racism had no place in New Orleans. The city was just adamant about not allowing an unsavory element to repopulate the new city. I had been in this place before. Every time someone said the words "urban renewal," I witnessed the dissolution of poor African American communities, the loss of community control, the influx of high-end homes, and the disappearance of strong public schools.

The new New Orleans is an adult city—a kind of Las Vegas south. The needs of low- to moderate-income families are not taken into consideration. There is a need for some low-income people to do service work in the hotels and growing number of casinos that jumpstarted the economy after the hurricane. Many of these workers are migrant and undocumented. They rarely demand social services for fear of being harassed by government officials regarding their immigrant status. Many of these workers work two (and sometimes three) jobs.

The strange thing about this new New Orleans is that so many people are so positive about the reconstruction. The newspapers are filled with good news stories about new hotels, restaurants, and businesses opening. The Bureau of Tourism is thriving, and conventions and meetings are at an all-time high. As a part of the redevelopment, the city provides huge discounts for organizations to book their conferences and conventions in New Orleans. The voices of the suffering poor are muted and their advocates are regularly dismissed. The only thing they can hope for is another devastating hurricane. Then the nation will be forced to gaze on them once again.

Coda

Some might argue that the chronicle I detailed is far-fetched and has no basis in reality. However, the story has a basis in the historical reality of generations of New Orleans families. In both the flood of 1927 and Hurricane Betsy, the African American community was the most vulnerable. Rumors of deliberate levee breaches and slow responses (or responses primarily motivated by the possibility of political gain) have kept African Americans suspicious and distrustful of their governments at all levels—local, state, and federal.

The one thing that many planners and reconstruction gurus have not understood is the incredible pull of family in the African American community in New Orleans. Many of the residents of the 9th Ward have not lived anywhere other than New Orleans. With family members deceased and dispersed because of Hurricane Katrina, many African Americans have lost their moorings. Their extended families provided the safety net that kept them from starvation and homelessness. The complex and vital social networks of mothers, grandmothers, aunts, uncles, and cousins are what kept people connected to and functioning in the city, no matter how marginal those existences were.

What, then, can education research offer to a place of such utter devastation and despair? My initial response is nothing. But as I think about our work, I am convinced that the hurricane also gave us an opportunity to recapture our humanity. Our work is not merely about data points and effect sizes. It is also about what difference our work can make in the lives of real people. Hurricane Katrina brings shame on us all. We have no excuse for our ignorance about poverty. We cannot keep writing about schools as some idyllic, romantic places where a few students are failing. The work we have to do must be done in the public interest. We cannot hide behind notions of neutrality or objectivity when people are suffering so desperately. The questions we pursue, the projects we choose, the agenda we champion have to be about more than career advancement. If education research is going to matter, we have to make it matter in the lives of real people around real issues. It is just too bad that we had to have a disaster to make this clear to us.

Notes

1 This chapter draws from and reworks arguments in the introduction to my recent book *Education Research in the Public Interest: Social Justice, Education, and Policy*, coedited with William F. Tate (Teachers College Press, 2006).

2 Critical race theory relies heavily on storytelling and counter-storytelling. Here I am using Derrick Bell's (1987) notion of the chronicle to set this scenario.

References

Anderson, J. D. (1988). *The education of Blacks in the South, 1860–1935*. Chapel Hill: University of North Carolina Press.

Anyon, J. (2005). *Radical possibilities: Public policy, urban education and a new social movement*. New York: Routledge.

Bell, D. (1987). *And we are not saved: The elusive quest for justice*. New York: Basic Books.

Delpit, L. (1995). *Other people's children: Cultural conflict in the classroom*. New York: The Free Press.

Foster, M. (1997). *Black teachers on teaching*. New York: The New Press.

Glass, I. (Ed.). (2005). After the flood. This American Life, Public Radio Broadcast. Available online at http://www.thislife.org/pdf/296.pdf (accessed October 15, 2005).

Harrington, M. (1962). *The other America: Poverty in the United States*. New York: Macmillan.

Hilliard, A. G. (2000). Excellence in education versus high stakes testing. *Journal of Teacher Education*, 51, 293–304.

Irvine, J. J. (2002). *In search of wholeness: African American teachers and their culturally specific classroom practices*. New York: Palgrave/St. Martin's Press.

MSNBC. (2005). New Orleans faces months without children. Available online at http://msnbc.msn.com/id/9480718/ (accessed October 16, 2005).

National Commission on Excellence in Education. (1983). *A nation at risk: The imperative for education reform. A report to the nation and the Secretary of Education, University States Department of Education*. Washington, DC: Government Printing Office.

Oliver Brown et al. v. Board of Education of Topeka et al. (a.k.a *Brown v. Board of Education*). (1954). 347 U. S. 483. Appeal from the United States District Court for the District of Kansas. No. 1. Argued December 9, 1952. Reargued December 8, 1953. Decided May 17, 1954.

Oliver Brown et al. v. Board of Education of Topeka et al. (a.k.a *Brown v. Board of Education II*, or *Brown II*) (1955). 349 U.S. 294. Appeal from the United States District Court for the District of Kansas. Reargued on the question of relief April 11–14., 1955. Opinion and judgments announced May 31, 1955.

Orfield, G. & Eaton, S. (1996). *Dismantling desegregation: The quiet repeal of Brown v. Board of Education*. New York: The New Press.

Rothstein, R. (2004). A wider lens on the black-white achievement gap. *Phi Delta Kappan*, 86, 105–110.

Rubinowitz, L. S. & Rosenbaum, J. E. (2000). *Crossing the class and color lines: From public housing to white suburbia*. Chicago: University of Chicago Press.

Siddle-Walker, V. (1996). *Their highest potential: An African American community in the segregated South*. Chapel Hill: University of North Carolina Press.

Skiba, R. J., Michael, R. S., Nardo, A. C., & Peterson, R. (in press). The color of discipline: Sources of racial and gender disproportionality in school punishment. *Urban Review*.

U.S. Census Bureau. (2000). *Census 2000*. Washington, DC: Government Printing Office.

Wells, A. (2004). Good neighbors? Distance, resistance, and desegregation in metropolitan New Orleans. *Urban Education*, 39, 408–427.

Willis, A. I. (2002). Literacy at Calhoun Colored School, 1892–1943. *Reading Research Quarterly*, 37(1), 8–44.

Chapter 10

"I Read the News Today, Oh Boy …"

The War on Public Workers[1]

H. L. (Bud) Goodall, Jr.

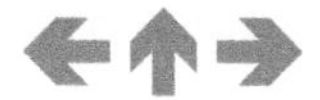

Every day I read the news and every day the news I read is worse. American higher education is under siege. It's a war out there. Battle lines have been drawn from sea to shining sea as Republican governors and their legislatures no longer make a secret of their ambition, which is to defund public education, end tenure, and rid the land of the scourge known as the cultural elite.

ALEC, which is the well-funded conservative group responsible for writing template-based legislation to attain those ends, no longer makes a secret of its existence, much less of its funding, which comes directly from wealthy families, such as the notorious Koch brothers, and wealthy corporations, such as many of those whose profits have never been healthier due to two long wars, the Wall Street bailout, and deregulation carried out by the Bush administration.

Tenure is under siege, too. Think of attacks on it as attacks on the supply lines that feed higher education. Without tenure, who in their right mind would choose this line of work? But that, of course, is exactly the point. Without the supply lines, the troops in the field starve. And the hungry easily lose political commitment or are willing to trade it in for the semi-security of annual contracts.

Originally published in *Qualitative Inquiry and the Politics of Advocacy*, edited by Norman K. Denzin and Michael D. Giardina, pp. 237–244. Republished in *Qualitative Inquiry—Past, Present, and Future: A Critical Reader*, edited by Norman K. Denzin and Michael D. Giardina, pp. 186–193. Left Coast Press, Inc.

Universities, havens of the so-called cultural elite, are under siege, too from within and without. The big book of shame published this year, Robert Arum and Josipa Roksa's (2011) *Academically Adrift*, argues that students in state universities and colleges aren't learning anything, which only underscores the dogma of right-wing commentators who claim that most professors don't teach, or at least don't teach anything of value, probably because we are too preoccupied with converting students to communism and atheism. In Texas, Governor Rick Perry has introduced a plan to stop funding for higher education in the traditional way and replace it with a voucher system that allows each student—heretofore defined as a consumer—to choose which professors to support with their enrollment.

But wait, it gets better: Faculty bonuses are to replace merit raises, and those bonuses will be based entirely on student evaluations. In Arizona, where I teach, as elsewhere, draconian cuts to higher education budgets—in our case, back to a 1960 level, back when we had 20,000 students instead of today's 74,000 and no real research agenda—means much larger classes, fewer faculty, no new tenure-earning hires, and tuition increases that have almost doubled what it costs to attend our state university, making a college education untenable for a substantial population of our state's poor, minority, and/or immigrant population.

When universities don't have money they have to find it. Guess what? The Koch brothers again. I read in the news just last week, oh boy, that two faculty positions in economics at Florida State University (and others at Clemson University, and still others at other places) were funded by the Koch brothers with the stipulation that they are dedicated to the advocacy of free market capitalism. And the faculty had no real say in who was hired for those positions. As Stanley Fish (2011)—no friend to changing the political world in the classroom—wrote just this week, that decision was, in fact, a textbook violation of academic freedom, as well as an insult to any sense of due process in academic hiring. The cultural elite cry foul! But the economic elite are buying the game.

I could go on.

We all could go on.

← ↑ →

We are fiddling with evaluation metrics while the university burns. We are hiding behind the very traditions that are under attack and we are largely opting out of service in a war whose outcome, if we lose it, will eventually imprison us.

The fact is that after years of doing mostly nothing publicly to combat the growing Republican narrative that demeans our profession, as well as casts cynical doubt on the value of an educated person to a free society, most academics find that we now don't know what to do.

Write letters to the editor?

Take a look at the public responses.

Get up a petition for the legislature?

Uh-huh, go ahead.

Write a blog?

Look at mine, read the right-wing trolls who daily attack it, and see if you have the stomach for the fight.

How about organize a protest?

Or a boycott?

Sure, we can do that, but so far none of the places where that strategy has been tried has produced change. Except in Wisconsin, where it might, but the verdict is still out and a lot of damage has already been done.

Retreat into our offices and wait for the storm to blow over?

I think that is what most of us do. We have been conditioned to do little else. Nor do we have the financial resources to stand up against billionaires and millionaires and state legislatures or even a hoodwinked electorate. We are the cultural elite, not the economic elite. And it takes money, big money, to win a campaign or to counter propaganda.

If you wanted to write a script for a movie or a novel about a right-wing conspiracy to systematically dumb down a populace so that "divide and conquer" fanatical sound bites and mean-spirited slogans, campaigns based on fear and lies and fueled by big moneyed interests whose only real interest is maintaining power through media spectacles, war narratives, and coordinated civic control, you could do no better than what we have right here in River City.

Except no one would believe it.

This truth is not only stranger than fiction; it's a truth that denies the possibility of fiction.

We are late to this fight.

Maybe too late.

I don't know.

But what I do know is that we are losing this war. We are losing it in the streets and we are losing it at the ballot box. We are losing it in legislative votes and in congressional action. Even our president, who says he is one of us, is unable or unwilling to stand up for us other than in the most symbolic of ways. Some of us hope that will change if he wins a second term. Some of us doubt it will. And the rest of us?

One thing I've noticed while dreaming of a brighter future for higher education is that most of us on the left have lost sight of two important things. First, we have lost sight of a vital historical and cultural truth about labor: *This is class war and our enemy is not ever going to save us or speak up for our rights.* They hate us. Literally hate us. And they use, abuse, and eventually discard what they hate. I wrote a piece for Norman Denzin on this subject and here is the gist of the rich Republican attack on us, an attack based on a very simple premise:

> If we were rich, we would become Republicans. ... We would, if we were wealthy, embrace a rich white man's—or rich white woman's—Republican values. Which is to say we would understand that there is something wrong with people who don't translate the freedoms and liberties, the low taxes and lack of government regulation of this great nation into vast personal wealth. We must be either stupid or lazy. It's really that simple. We only have ourselves to blame.

So why should our enemy support us? Did Caesar free the slaves? Did the bosses take pity on the workers who went on strike? Did our Congress, making claims about the threat posed by the enormity of our national debt, see fit to raise taxes on the rich? Is your college president creating a fund for all the lecturers she or he has laid off?

The second principle we have lost sight of is there are far more of us than there are of them. United we stand, divided we fall. Their strategy—a time-honored first principle of propaganda—is to divide the public from the private, then to subdivide the public into the unionized and the non-unionized, then further divide those who make $41,000 a year as firefighters from those who make $61,000 as assistant professors, and so on. Cast doubt on the patriotism, the loyalty, the honor, and/or the work ethic of those who are in every other way our brothers and sisters in arms, and you slowly but surely divide and conquer.

Finally, we are *not* the cultural elite. We are working-class intellectuals. We don't come from money and we don't have money. The cultural elite was a rhetorical bon bon created and distributed by Wall Street to dangle before status-starved college professors, knowing that we would grab them. But there is a big difference, as Thomas Frank argued years ago, between a cultural elite and an economic elite.

Here's that bon bon. Now swallow it. Meanwhile, the rich get richer, buy elections, cut their own taxes, create subprime mortgages, build hedge funds, manipulate markets, and quietly convince themselves that they are the smart ones as well as the rich ones. Doubt it? Read Karen Ho's (2009) devastating ethnography of Wall Street, *Liquidated*. And the further removed they are from main street, from university drive, from college avenue, the louder they laugh at our expense. I mean, we make really bad choices. It's our own fault.

And what has been our response? So what if we make less than a living wage for many years? We are the cultural elite. We are cool. Smart. Proud of our poverty and proud of how distanced we are from mainstream values and habits. What if once we get a job in one of the most competitive arenas on planet Earth we are paid less and owe more than any of our colleagues in Business, Engineering, or the medical sciences? We are the cultural elite, though. Right?

Oh man, oh woman, what were you thinking when you swallowed that sweet slice of status covering a much deeper cultural sin? Didn't we see it coming? Divide and conquer. Create a category that irks the vast majority of citizens who hated high school, flunked the hard courses in college, and couldn't get into grad school—which is to say, about 75 percent of the voting public—and then get those college professors to parade around in those fancy tenured robes owning that class-based cultural elite rhetoric, I mean, what did we expect? That we would be loved?

Do you love those you don't understand and who you feel have oppressed or made fun of you?

Revenge in a capitalist society is best represented in cold hard cash. It's that Protestant ethic that makes us this way. And with the evangelical zeal of the new "prosperity gospel" that remakes Jesus into the veritable image of conservative Republican values, we end up with a reverse Kenneth Burke: The rich are no longer guilty for being "up" while others are "down"; in fact, it's the opposite. The rich are saved by their prosperity gospel, and everyone else is suspect because, really, we don't seem to be making the right choices for a capitalist America.

How much money do you make? Where do you live? What kind of car do you drive? Where do you vacation? And please, don't tell me you prefer to be relatively poor, or that your values prevent you from seeking wealth and influence. In America, my friend, there are only two right answers to any question regarding money: More is better than less, and sooner is better than later. If you don't know that, then what, really do you know? That is of any value, I mean.

Who knows that lesson better than college presidents? Or overpriced provosts? Or bloated deans? You want something close to a cultural elite, that's where you ought to look. My University president makes $725,000 a year in addition to a generous housing, entertainment, and car allowance. He enjoys unlimited free travel worldwide. And as long as he meets his metrics for enrollment growth (never mind that there is no corresponding faculty growth) and retention, he gets an annual increase somewhere in the neighborhood of a new BMW 7-series. *Which, by the way, he drives.*

His message to the newly minted doctoral class last week was emblematic of his privilege. He said, and I quote: "Stop arguing. Stop it. Just go out there and do something." In other words, fuggedabout politics; make me some money!

And you would be surprised, or maybe not, at how many tenured faculty nodded their heads.

William Deresiewicz, writing in *The Nation* (2011), puts the crisis in higher education this way:

> What we have in academia, in other words, is a microcosm of the American economy as a whole: a self-enriching aristocracy, a swelling and increasingly immiserated proletariat, and a shrinking middle class. The same devil's bargain stabilizes the system: the middle, or at least the upper middle, the tenured professoriate, is allowed to retain its prerogatives—its comfortable compensation packages, its workplace autonomy and its job security—in return for acquiescing to the exploitation of the bottom by the top, and indirectly, the betrayal of the future of the entire enterprise.

So I wasn't surprised to learn from reading the news in May 2011 that according to a new Pew Center/*Chronicle of Higher Education* Study, 69 percent of the college presidents who are supposed to be leading the charge for us are themselves no longer supportive of tenure (Stripling, 2011). More than half say that higher education is heading in the wrong direction. And most of them admit they haven't a clue what to do about it.

That's the bottom line, my friends.

It's the *story* that fuels the revolution.

And we don't yet have one.

Note

1 The title of this chapter is inspired by "A Day in the Life" from The Beatles' *Sgt. Pepper's Lonely Hearts Club Band.*

References

Arum, R., & Roksa, J. (2011). *Academically adrift: Limited learning on college campuses.* Chicago: University of Chicago Press.

Deresiewicz, W. (2011). Faulty towers: The crisis in higher education. *The Nation,* May 4. http://www.thenation.com/article/160410/faulty-towers-crisis-higher-ducation?page=full (accessed February 4, 2012).

Fish, S. (2011). Sex, the Koch brothers, and academic freedom. *The New York Times,* May 16. http://opinionator.blogs.nytimes.com/2011/05/16/sex-the-koch-brothers-and-academic-freedom/ (accessed February 4, 2012).

Ho, K. (2009). *Liquidated: An ethnography of Wall Street.* Durham, NC: Duke University Press.

Stripling, J. (2011). Most presidents prefer no tenure for majority of faculty. *The Chronicle of Higher Education,* May 15. http://chronicle.com/article/Most-Presidents-Favor-No/127526/ (accessed February 4, 2012).

Chapter 11

Public Intellectuals Against the Neoliberal University

Henry A. Giroux

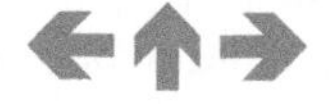

I want to begin with the words of the late African-American poet, Audre Lorde, who was in her time a formidable writer, educator, feminist, gay rights activist, and public intellectual who displayed a relentless courage in addressing the injustices she witnessed all around her. She writes:

> Poetry is not a luxury. It is a vital necessity of our existence. It forms the quality of the light within which we predicate our hopes and dreams toward survival and change, first made into language, then into idea, then into more tangible action. Poetry is the way we help give name to the nameless so it can be thought. The farthest horizons of our hopes and fears are cobbled by our poems, carved from the rock experiences of our daily lives. (Lorde, 1984, p. 38)

And while Lorde refers to poetry here, I think a strong case can be made that the attributes she ascribes to poetry can also be attributed to higher education—a genuine higher education.[1] In this case, an education that includes history, philosophy, all of the arts and humanities, the criticality of the social sciences, the

Originally published in *Qualitative Inquiry Outside the Academy,* edited by Norman K. Denzin and Michael D. Giardina, pp. 35–60. Republished in *Qualitative Inquiry—Past, Present, and Future: A Critical Reader,* edited by Norman K. Denzin and Michael D. Giardina, pp. 194–219. Left Coast Press, Inc.

world of discovery made manifest by science, and the transformations in health and in law wrought by the professions which are at the heart of what it means to know something about the human condition. Lorde's defense of poetry as a mode of education is especially crucial for those of us who believe that the university is nothing if it is not a public trust and social good; that is, a critical institution infused with the promise of cultivating intellectual insight, the imagination, inquisitiveness, risk-taking, social responsibility, and the struggle for justice. At best, universities should be at the "heart of intense public discourse, passionate learning, and vocal citizen involvement in the issues of the times" (Scott, 2012). It is in the spirit of such an ideal that I first want to address those larger economic, social, and cultural interests that threaten this notion of education, especially higher education.

Across the globe, the forces of casino capitalism are on the march. With the return of the Gilded Age and its dream worlds of consumption, privatization, and deregulation, not only are democratic values and social protections at risk, but the civic and formative cultures that make such values and protections crucial to democratic life are in danger of disappearing altogether. As public spheres, once enlivened by broad engagements with common concerns and multiple voices, are being transformed into spectacular spaces of consumption, the flight from mutual obligations and social responsibilities intensifies and has resulted in what Tony Judt identifies as a "loss of faith in the culture of open democracy" (quoted in Foley, 2010, para. 2). This loss of faith in the power of public dialogue and dissent is not unrelated to the diminished belief in higher education as central to producing critical citizens and a crucial democratic public sphere in its own right. At stake here is not only the meaning and purpose of higher education, but also civil society, politics, and the fate of democracy itself. Thomas Frank (2012) is on target when he argues that "over the course of the past few decades, the power of concentrated money has subverted professions, destroyed small investors, wrecked the regulatory state, corrupted legislators en masse and repeatedly put the economy through the wringer. Now it has come for our democracy itself." And, yet, the only questions being asked about knowledge production, the purpose of education, the nature of politics, and our understanding of the future are determined largely by market forces.

The mantras of neoliberalism are now well known: government is the problem; society is a fiction; sovereignty is market-driven; deregulation and commodification are vehicles for freedom; and higher education should serve corporate interests rather than the public good. In addition, the yardstick of profit has become the only viable measure of the good life, while civic engagement and public spheres devoted to the common good are viewed by many politicians and their publics as either a hindrance to the goals of a market-driven society or alibis for government inefficiency and waste.

In a market-driven system in which economic and political decisions are removed from social costs, the flight of critical thought and social responsibility is further accentuated by what Zygmunt Bauman calls "ethical tranquillization" (McCarthy, 2007). One result is a form of depoliticization that works its way through the social order, removing social relations from the configurations of power that shape them, substituting what Wendy Brown (2006, p. 16) calls "emotional and personal vocabularies for political ones in formulating solutions to political problems." Consequently, it becomes difficult for young people too often bereft of a critical education to translate private troubles into public concerns. As private interests trump the public good, public spaces are corroded and short-term personal advantage replaces any larger notion of civic engagement and social responsibility.

Under such circumstances, to cite C. Wright Mills (2008, p. 200), we are witnessing the breakdown of democracy, the disappearance of critical intellectuals, and "the collapse of those public spheres which offer a sense of critical agency and social imagination." Mills's prescient comments amplify what has become a tragic reality. Missing from neoliberal market societies are those public spheres—from public and higher education to the mainstream media and digital screen culture—where people can develop what might be called the civic imagination. For example, in the last few decades, we have seen market mentalities attempt to strip education of its public values, critical content, and civic responsibilities as part of its broader goal of creating new subjects wedded to consumerism, risk-free relationships, and the disappearance of the social state in the name of individual, expanded choice. Tied largely to instrumental ideologies and measurable paradigms, many institutions of higher education are now committed almost exclusively to economic goals, such as preparing students for the workforce—all done as part of an appeal to rationality, one that eschews matters of inequality, power, and the ethical grammars of suffering (Wilderson III, 2012, p. 2). Many universities have not only strayed from their democratic mission, they also seem immune to the plight of students who face a harsh new world of high unemployment, the prospect of downward mobility, and debilitating debt.

The question of what kind of education is needed for students to be informed and active citizens in a world that increasingly ignores their needs, if not their future, is rarely asked (Aronowitz, 2008, p. xii). In the absence of a democratic vision of schooling, it is not surprising that some colleges and universities are increasingly opening their classrooms to corporate interests, standardizing the curriculum, instituting top-down governing structures, and generating courses that promote entrepreneurial values unfettered by social concerns or ethical consequences. For example, one university is offering a Master's degree to students who, in order to fulfill their academic requirements, have to commit to starting a high-tech company. Another university allows career officers to teach capstone research seminars in the humanities. In one of these classes, the students were asked to "develop a 30-second commercial on their 'personal brand'" (Zernike, 2009). This is not an argument against career counselling or research in humanities seminars, but the confusion in collapsing the two.

Central to this neoliberal view of higher education in the United States and United Kingdom is a market-driven paradigm that seeks to eliminate tenure, turn the humanities into a job preparation service, and transform most faculty into an army of temporary subaltern labor. For instance, in the United States out of 1.5 million faculty members, 1 million are "adjuncts who are earning, on average, $20K a year gross, with no benefits or healthcare, no unemployment insurance when they are out of work" (Scott, 2012). The indentured service status of such faculty is put on full display as some colleges have resorted to using "temporary service agencies to do their formal hiring" (Jaschik, 2010).

There is little talk in this view of higher education about the history and value of shared governance between faculty and administrators, nor of educating students as critical citizens rather than potential employees of Walmart. There are few attempts to affirm faculty as scholars and public intellectuals who have a measure of both autonomy and power. Instead, faculty members are increasingly defined less as intellectuals than as technicians and grant writers. Students fare no better in this debased form of education and are treated as either clients or as restless children in need of high-energy entertainment—as was made clear in the 2012 Penn State University scandal. Such modes of education do not foster a sense of organized responsibility fundamental to a democracy. Instead, they encourage what might be called a sense of organized irresponsibility—a practice that underlies the economic Darwinism and civic corruption at the heart of a debased politics.

Higher Education and the Crisis of Legitimacy

In the United States and, increasingly, in Canada, many of the problems in higher education can be linked to diminished funding, the domination of universities by market mechanisms, the rise of for-profit colleges, the intrusion of the national security state, and the diminished role of faculty in governing the university, all of which both contradict the culture and democratic value of higher education and make a mockery of the very meaning and mission of the university as a democratic public sphere. Decreased financial support for higher education stands in sharp contrast to increased support for tax benefits for the rich, big banks, the military, and mega corporations. Rather than enlarge the moral imagination and critical capacities of students, too many universities are now encouraged to produce would-be hedge fund managers, depoliticized students, and modes of education that promote a "technically trained docility" (Nussbaum, 2010, p. 142). Increasingly, pedagogy is reduced to learning reified methods, a hollow mechanistic enterprise divorced from understanding teaching as a moral and intellectual practice central to the creation of critical and engaged citizens. This reductionist notion of pedagogy works well with a funding crisis that is now used by conservatives as an ideological weapon to defund certain disciplines, such as history, English, sociology, anthropology, minority studies, gender studies, and language programs. While there has never been a golden age when higher education was truly liberal and democratic, the current attack on higher education by religious fundamentalists, corporate power, and the apostles of neoliberal capitalism appears unprecedented in terms of both its scope and its intensity.[2]

Universities are losing their sense of public mission, just as leadership in higher education is being stripped of any viable democratic vision. In the United States, college presidents are now called CEOs and move without apology between interlocking corporate and academic boards. With few exceptions, they are praised as fundraisers but rarely acknowledged for the quality of their ideas. It gets worse. As Adam Bessie (2013) points out,

> the discourse of higher education now resembles what you might hear at a board meeting at a No.2 pencil-factory, [with its emphasis on]: productivity, efficiency, metrics, data-driven value, [all of] which places utter, near-religious faith in this highly technical, market-based view of education [which] like all human enterprises, can (and must) be quantified and evaluated numerically, to identify the 'one best way,' which can then be 'scaled up,' or mass-produced across the nation, be it No. 2 pencils, appendectomies, or military drones.

In this new Gilded Age of money and profit, academic subjects gain stature almost exclusively through their exchange value on the market. Pharmaceutical companies determine what is researched in labs and determine whether research critical of their products should be published. Corporate gifts flood into universities, making more and more demands regarding what should be taught. Boards of trustees now hire business leaders to reform universities in the image of the marketplace. For-profit universities offer up a future image of the new model of higher education, characterized by huge salaries for management, a mere "17.4 per cent of their annual revenue spent on teaching, while 20 per cent was distributed as profit (the proportion spent on marketing [is] even higher)" (Collini, 2013). Large numbers of students from many of these for-profit institutions—offering subprime degrees and devoid of any sense of civic purpose—never finish their degree programs and are saddled with enormous debts. As Stefan Collini (2013) observes, at the University of Phoenix, owned by the Apollo Group,

> 60 percent … of their students dropped out within two years, while of those who completed their courses, 21 per cent defaulted on paying back their loans within three years of finishing. [Moreover], 89 per cent of Apollo's revenue comes from federal student loans and [Apollo] spends twice as much on marketing as on teaching.

What happens to education when it is treated like a corporation? What are we to make of the integrity of a university when it accepts a monetary gift from powerful corporate interests or a rich patron demanding as part of the agreement the power to specify what is to be taught in a course or how a curriculum should be shaped? Some corporations and universities now believe that what is taught in a course is not an academic decision but a market consideration. In addition, many disciplines are now valued almost exclusively with how closely they align with what might be euphemistically called a business culture. One egregious example of this neoliberal approach to higher education is on full display in Florida where Governor Rick Scott's task force on education is attempting to implement a policy that would lower tuition for degrees friendly to corporate interests in order to "steer students toward majors that are in demand in the job market" (Alvarez, 2012, para. 3). Scott's utterly instrumental and anti-intellectual message is clear: "Give us engineers, scientists, health care specialists and technology experts. Do not worry so much about historians, philosophers, anthropologists and English majors" (Alvarez, 2012).

Not only does neoliberalism undermine both civic education and public values and confuse education with training, it also wages a war on what might be called the radical imagination. For instance, thousands of students in both the United States and Canada are now saddled with debts that will profoundly impact their lives and their futures, likely forcing them away from public service jobs because the pay is too low to pay off their educational loans. Students find themselves in a world in which heightened expectations have been replaced by dashed hopes and a world of onerous debt.[3] For those struggling to merely survive, the debt crisis represents a massive assault on the imagination by leaving little or no room to think otherwise in order to act otherwise. David Graeber is right in insisting that the student loan crisis is part of a war on the imagination. He writes:

> Student loans are destroying the imagination of youth. If there's a way of a society committing mass suicide, what better way than to take all the youngest, most energetic, creative, joyous people in your society and saddle them with $50,000 of debt so they have to be slaves? There goes your music. There goes your culture. ... And in a way, this is what's happened to our society. We're a society that has lost any ability to incorporate the interesting, creative and eccentric people. (Kelly, 2013)

Questions regarding how education might enable students to develop a keen sense of prophetic justice, utilize critical analytical skills, and cultivate an ethical sensibility through which they learn to respect the rights of others are becoming increasingly irrelevant in a market-driven university in which the quality of education is so dumbed down that too few students on campus are really learning how to think critically, engage in thoughtful dialogue, push at the frontiers of their imagination, employ historical analyses, and move beyond the dreadful, mind-numbing forms of instrumental rationality being pushed by billionaires such as Bill Gates, Amazon's Jeff Bezos, Facebook's Mark Zuckerberg, and Netflix's Reed Hastings. In this world, "all human problems are essentially technical in nature and can be solved through technical means" (Bessie, 2013). As the humanities and liberal arts are downsized, privatized, and commodified, higher education finds itself caught in the paradox of claiming to invest in the future of young people while offering them few intellectual, civic, and moral supports (Nussbaum, 2010).

Higher education has a responsibility not only to search for the truth regardless of where it may lead, but also to educate students to be capable of holding authority and power accountable while at the same time sustaining "the idea and hope of a public culture" (Scialabba, 2009, p. 4). Though questions regarding whether the university should serve *strictly* public rather than private interests no longer carry the weight of forceful criticism as they did in the past, such questions are still crucial in addressing the purpose of higher education and what it might mean to imagine the university's full participation in public life as the protector and promoter of democratic values. Toni Morrison (2001, p. 278) is instructive in her comment:

> If the university does not take seriously and rigorously its role as a guardian of wider civic freedoms, as interrogator of more and more complex ethical problems, as servant and preserver of deeper democratic practices, then some other regime or ménage of regimes will do it for us, in spite of us, and without us.

What needs to be understood is that higher education may be one of the few public spheres left where knowledge, values, and learning offer a glimpse of the promise of education for nurturing public values, critical hope, and what my late friend Paulo Freire called "the practice of freedom." It may be the case that everyday life is increasingly organized around market principles, but confusing a market-determined society with democracy hollows out the legacy of higher education, whose deepest roots are philosophical, not commercial. This is a particularly important insight in a society where the free circulation of ideas is not only being replaced by mass mediated ideas but where critical ideas are increasingly viewed or dismissed as liberal, radical, or even seditious.

In addition, the educational force of the wider culture, dominated by the glorification of celebrity life-styles and a hyper-consumer society, perpetuates a powerful form of mass illiteracy and manufactured idiocy, witness the support for Ted Cruz and Michelle Bachmann in American politics, if not the racist, reactionary, and anti-intellectual Tea Party. This manufactured stupidity does more than depoliticize the public. To paraphrase Hannah Arendt, it represents an assault on the very possibility of thinking itself. Not surprisingly, intellectuals who engage in dissent and "keep the idea and hope of a public culture alive" (Scialabba, 2009, p. 4) are often dismissed as irrelevant, extremist, elitist, or un-American. As a result, we now live in a world in which the politics of disimagination dominates; public discourses that bears witness to a critical and alternative sense of the world are often dismissed because they do not advance economic interests.

In a dystopian society, utopian thought becomes sterile and, paraphrasing Theodor Adorno, thinking becomes an act of utter stupidity. Anti-public intellectuals now define the larger cultural landscape, all too willing to flaunt co-option and reap the rewards of venting insults at their assigned opponents while being reduced to the status of paid servants of powerful economic interests. But the problem is not simply with the rise of a right-wing cultural apparatus dedicated to preserving the power and wealth of the rich and corporate elite. As Stuart Hall recently remarked, the state of progressive thought is also in jeopardy in that, as he puts it, "the left is in trouble. It's not got any ideas, it's not got any independent analysis of its own, and therefore it's got no vision. It just takes the temperature. … It has no sense of politics being educative, of politics changing the way people see things" (Williams, 2012). Of course, Hall is not suggesting the left has no ideas to speak of. He is suggesting that such ideas are removed from the larger issue of what it means to address education and the production and reception of meaningful ideas as a mode of pedagogy that is central to politics itself.

The issue of politics being educative, of recognizing that matters of pedagogy, subjectivity, and consciousness are at the heart of political and moral concerns, should not be lost on academics. Nor should the relevance of education being at the heart of politics be lost on those of us concerned about inviting the public back into higher education and rethinking the purpose and meaning of higher education itself. Democracy places civic demands upon its citizens, and such demands point to the necessity of an education that is broad-based, critical, and supportive of meaningful civic values, participation in self-governance, and democratic leadership. Only through such a formative and critical educational culture can students learn how to become individual and social agents, rather than disengaged spectators or uncritical consumers, able both to think otherwise and to act upon civic commitments that "necessitate a reordering of basic power arrangements" (Wolin, 2010, p. 43) fundamental to promoting the common good and producing a strong democracy. This is not a matter of imposing values on education and in our classrooms. The university and the classroom are already defined through power-laden discourses and a myriad of values that are often part of the hidden curriculum of educational politics and pedagogy. A more accurate position would be, as Toni Morrison (2001, p. 276) points out, to take up our responsibility "as citizen/scholars in the university [and] to accept the consequences of our own value-redolent roles." She continues, "Like it or not, we are paradigms of our own values, advertisements of our own ethics—especially noticeable when we presume to foster ethics-free, value-lite education."

Dreaming the Impossible

Reclaiming higher education as a democratic public sphere begins with the crucial recognition that education is not solely about job training and the production of ethically challenged entrepreneurial subjects, but also about matters of civic engagement, critical thinking, civic literacy, and the capacity for democratic agency, action, and change. It is also inextricably connected to the related issues of power, inclusion, and social responsibility.[4] For example, Martin Luther King, Jr. (1967/1991, p. 644), recognized clearly that when matters of social responsibility are removed from matters of agency and politics, democracy itself is diminished.

> When an individual is no longer a true participant, when he no longer feels a sense of responsibility to his society, the content of democracy is emptied. When culture is degraded and vulgarity enthroned, when the social system does not build security but induces peril, inexorably the individual is impelled to pull away from a soulless society.

If young people are to develop a deep respect for others, a keen sense of social responsibility, as well as an informed notion of civic engagement, pedagogy must be viewed as the cultural, political, and moral force that provides the knowledge, values, and social relations to make such democratic practices possible. Central to such a challenge is the need to position intellectual practice "as part of an intricate web of morality, rigor and responsibility" that enables academics to speak with conviction, enter the public sphere to address important social problems, and demonstrate alternative models for bridging the gap between higher education and the broader society (Roy, 2001, p. 1). Connective ties are crucial in that it is essential to develop intellectual practices that are collegial rather than competitive, refuse the instrumentality and privileged isolation of the academy, link critical thought to a profound impatience with the status quo, and connect human agency to the idea of social responsibility and the politics of possibility.

Increasingly, as universities are shaped by an audit culture, the call to be objective and impartial, whatever one's intentions, can easily echo what George Orwell called the 'official truth' or the establishment point of view. Lacking a self-consciously democratic political focus, teachers are often reduced, or reduce themselves, to the role of a technician or functionary engaged in formalistic rituals, unconcerned with the disturbing and urgent problems that confront the larger society or the consequences of one's pedagogical practices and research undertakings. Hiding behind appeals to balance and objectivity, too many scholars refuse to recognize that being committed to something does not cancel out what C. Wright Mills once called 'hard thinking.' Teaching needs to be rigorous, self-reflective, and committed not to the dead zone of instrumental rationality but to the practice of freedom, to a critical sensibility capable of advancing the parameters of knowledge, addressing crucial social issues, and connecting private troubles and public issues.

In opposition to the instrumental model of teaching, with its conceit of political neutrality and its fetishization of measurement, I argue that academics should combine the mutually interdependent roles of critical educator and active citizen. This requires finding ways to connect the practice of classroom teaching with important social problems and the operation of power in the larger society while providing the conditions for students to view themselves as critical agents capable of making those who exercise authority and power answerable for their actions.

Higher education cannot be decoupled from what Jacques Derrida calls a 'democracy to come,' that is, a democracy that must always "be open to the possibility of being contested, of contesting itself, of criticizing and indefinitely improving itself" (Boradorri, 2004, p. 121). Within this project of possibility and impossibility, critical pedagogy must be understood as a deliberately informed and purposeful political and moral practice, as opposed to one that is either doctrinaire or instrumentalized, or both. Moreover, a critical pedagogy should also gain part of its momentum in higher education among students who will go back to the schools, churches, synagogues, and workplaces in order to produce new ideas, concepts, and critical ways of understanding the world in which young people and adults live. This is a notion of intellectual practice and responsibility that refuses the professional neutrality and privileged isolation of the academy. It also affirms a broader vision of learning that links knowledge to the power of self-definition and to the capacities of students to expand the scope of democratic freedoms, particularly those that address the crisis of education, politics, and the social as part and parcel of the crisis of democracy itself.

In order for critical pedagogy, dialogue, and thought to have real effects, they must advocate that all citizens, old and young, are equally entitled, if not equally empowered, to shape the society in which they live. This is a commitment we heard articulated by the brave students who fought against tuition hikes and the destruction of civil liberties and social provisions in Quebec and to a lesser degree in the Occupy Wall Street movement. If educators are to function as public intellectuals, they need to listen to young people who are producing a new language in order to talk about inequality and power relations, attempting to create alternative democratic public spaces, rethinking the very nature of politics, and asking serious questions about what democracy is and why it no longer exists in many neoliberal societies. These young people who are protesting against the 'one percent' recognize that they have been written out of the discourses of justice, equality, and democracy and are not only resisting how neoliberalism has made them expendable, they are also arguing for a collective future very different from the one that is on display in the current political and economic systems in which they feel trapped. These brave youth are insisting that the relationship between knowledge and power can be emancipatory, that their histories and experiences matter, and that what they say and do counts in their struggle to unlearn dominating privileges, productively reconstruct their relations with others, and transform, when necessary, the world around them.

Although there are still a number of academics, such as Noam Chomsky, Angela Davis, John Rawlston Saul, Bill McKibben, Germaine Greer, and Cornel West, who function as public intellectuals, they are often shut out of the mainstream media or characterized as marginal, unintelligible, and sometimes as unpatriotic figures. At the same time, many academics find themselves laboring under horrendous working conditions that either don't allow for them to write in a theoretically rigorous and accessible manner for the public because they do not have time—given the often intensive teaching demands of part-time academics and increasingly of full-time, non-tenured academics as well. Or they retreat into a kind of theoreticism in which theory becomes lifeless, detached from any larger project or the realm of worldly issues. In this instance, the notion of theory as a resource, if not theoretical rigor itself, is transformed into a badge of academic cleverness shorn of the possibility of advancing thought within the academy or reaching a larger audience outside of academic disciplines.

Consequently, such intellectuals often exist in hermetic academic bubbles cut off from both the larger public and the important issues that impact society. To no small degree, they have been complicit in the transformation of the university into an adjunct of corporate power. Such academics run the risk of not only becoming incapable of defending higher education as a vital public sphere, but also of having any say over the conditions of their own intellectual labor. Without their intervention as public intellectuals, the university defaults on its role as a democratic public sphere willing to produce an informed public, enact and sustain a culture of questioning, and enable a critical formative culture capable of producing citizens "who are critical thinkers capable of putting existing institutions into question so that democracy again becomes society's movement" (Castoriadis, 1997, p. 10).

Before his untimely death, Edward Said, himself an exemplary public intellectual, urged his colleagues in the academy to confront directly those social hardships that disfigure contemporary society and pose a serious threat to the promise of democracy.[5] He urged them to assume the role of public intellectuals, wakeful and mindful of their responsibilities to bear testimony to human suffering and the pedagogical possibilities at work in educating students to be autonomous, self-reflective, and socially responsible. Said rejected the notion of a market-driven pedagogy that, lacking a democratic project, was steeped in the discourse of instrumental rationality and fixated on measurement. He insisted that when pedagogy is taken up as a mechanistic undertaking, it loses any understanding of what it means for students to "be thoughtful, layered, complex, critical thinker[s]" (Cunningham-Cook, 2013). For Said, such methodological reification was antithetical to a pedagogy rooted in the practice of freedom and attentive to the need to construct critical agents, democratic values, and modes of critical inquiry. On the contrary, he viewed it as a mode of training more suitable to creating cheerful robots and legitimating organized recklessness and legalized illegalities.

The famed economist, William Black, goes so far as to argue that such stripped down pedagogies are responsible for creating what he calls 'criminogenic cultures,' especially in business schools and economics departments at a number of Ivy League universities. An indication of this crowning disgrace can be found in the Oscar winning documentary, *Inside Job,* which showed how Wall Street bought off high profile economists from Harvard, Yale, MIT, and Columbia University. For instance, Glenn Hubbard, Dean of Columbia Business School, and Martin Feldstein of Harvard got huge payoffs from a number of financial firms and wrote academic papers or opinion pieces favoring deregulation, while refusing to declare that they were on the payroll of Met Life, Goldman Sachs, or Merrill Lynch.[6]

In opposition to such a debased view of educational engagement, Said argued for what he called a 'pedagogy of wakefulness.' In defining and expanding on Said's pedagogy of wakefulness, and how it shaped his important consideration of academics as public intellectuals, I begin with a passage that I think offers tremendous insight on the ethical and political force of much of his writing. This selection is taken from his memoir, *Out of Place,* which describes the last few months of his mother's life in a New York hospital and the difficult time she had falling asleep because of the cancer that was ravaging her body. Recalling this traumatic and pivotal life experience, Said's meditation moves between the existential and the insurgent, between private pain and worldly commitment, between the seductions of a "solid self" and the reality of a contradictory, questioning, restless, and at times, uneasy sense of identity. He writes:

> 'Help me to sleep, Edward,' she once said to me with a piteous trembling in her voice that I can still hear as I write. But then the disease spread into her brain—and for the last six weeks she slept all the time—my own inability to sleep may be her last legacy to me, a counter to her struggle for sleep. For me sleep is something to be gotten over as quickly as possible. I can only go to bed very late, but I am literally up at dawn. Like her I don't possess the secret of long sleep, though unlike her I have reached the point where I do not want it. For me, sleep is death, as is any diminishment in awareness... Sleeplessness for me is a cherished state to be desired at almost any cost; there is nothing for me as invigorating as immediately shedding the shadowy half-consciousness of a night's loss than the early morning, reacquainting myself with or resuming what I might have lost completely a few hours earlier. I occasionally experience myself as a cluster of flowing currents. I prefer this to the idea of a solid self, the identity to which so many attach so much significance. These currents, like the themes of one's life, flow along during the waking hours, and at their best, they require no reconciling, no harmonizing. They are 'off' and may be out of place, but at least they are always in motion, in time, in place, in the form of all kinds of strange combinations moving about, not necessarily forward, sometimes against each other, contrapuntally yet without one central theme. A form of freedom, I like to think, even if I am far from being totally convinced that it is. That skepticism too is one of the themes I particularly want to hold on to. With so many dissonances in my life I have learned actually to prefer being not quite right and out of place. (Said, 2000, pp. 294–299)

Said posits here an antidote to the seductions of conformity and the lure of corporate money that insures, as Irving Howe (1990, p. 27) once pointed out caustically, "an honored place for the intellectuals." For Said, it is a sense of being awake, displaced, caught in a combination of contradictory circumstances that suggests a pedagogy that is cosmopolitan and imaginative—a public affirming pedagogy that demands a critical and engaged interaction with the world we live in mediated by a responsibility for challenging structures of domination and for alleviating human suffering. This is a pedagogy that addresses the needs of multiple publics. As an ethical and political practice, a public pedagogy of wakefulness rejects modes of education removed from political or social concerns, divorced from history and matters of injury and injustice. Said's notion of a pedagogy of wakefulness includes "lifting complex ideas into the public space," recognizing human injury inside and outside of the academy, and using theory as a form of criticism to change things (Said, 2000, p. 7). This is a pedagogy in which academics are neither afraid of controversy nor the willingness to make connections between private issues and broader elements of society's problems that are otherwise hidden.

For Said, being awake becomes a central metaphor for defining the role of academics as public intellectuals, defending the university as a crucial public sphere, engaging how culture deploys power, and taking seriously the idea of human interdependence, while always living on the border—one foot in and one foot out, an exile and an insider for whom home was always a form of homelessness. As a relentless border crosser, Said embraced the idea of the "traveler" as an important metaphor for engaged intellectuals. As Stephen Howe, referencing Said, points out, "It was an image which depended not on power, but on motion, on daring to go into different worlds, use different languages, and 'understand a multiplicity of disguises, masks, and rhetorics. Travelers must suspend the claim of customary routine in order to live in new rhythms and rituals ... the traveler crosses over, traverses territory, and abandons fixed positions all the time'" (Howe, 2003). And as a border intellectual and traveler, Said embodied the notion of always "being quite not right," evident by his principled critique of all forms of certainties and dogmas and his refusal to be silent in the face of human suffering at home and abroad.

Being awake meant refusing the now popular sport of academic bashing or embracing a crude call for action at the expense of rigorous intellectual and theoretical work. On the contrary, it meant combining rigor and clarity, on the one hand, and civic courage and political commitment, on the other. A pedagogy of wakefulness meant using theoretical archives as resources, recognizing the worldly space of criticism as the democratic underpinning of publicness, defining critical literacy not merely as a competency, but as an act of interpretation linked to the possibility of intervention in the world. It pointed to a kind of border literacy in the plural in which people learned to read and write from multiple positions of agency; it also was indebted to the recognition forcibly stated by Hannah Arendt (1977, p. 149) that "without a politically guaranteed public realm, freedom lacks the worldly space to make its appearance."

I believe that Said was right in insisting that intellectuals have a responsibility to unsettle power, trouble consensus, and challenge common sense. The very notion of being an engaged public intellectual is neither foreign to nor a violation of what it means to be an academic scholar, but central to its very definition. According to Said (2001, p. 504), academics have a duty to enter into the public sphere unafraid to take positions and generate controversy, functioning as moral witnesses, raising political awareness, making connections to those elements of power and politics often hidden from public view, and reminding "the audience of the moral questions that may be hidden in the clamor and din of the public debate." Said (2004, p. 70) also criticized those academics that retreat into a new dogmatism of the disinterested specialist that separates them "not only from the public sphere but from other professionals who don't use the same jargon." This was especially unsettling to him at a time when complex language and critical thought remain under assault in the larger society by all manner of anti-democratic and anti-intellectual forces. But there is more at stake here than a retreat into discourses that turn theory into a mechanical act of academic referencing, there is also the retreat of intellectuals from being able to defend the public values and democratic mission of higher education. Or, as Irving Howe (1990, p. 36) put it, "Intellectuals have, by and large, shown a painful lack of militancy in defending the rights which are a precondition of their existence."

The view of higher education as a democratic public sphere committed to producing capable young people willing to expand and deepen their sense of themselves, to think the "world" critically, "to imagine something other than their own well-being," to serve the public good, take risks, and struggle for a substantive democracy has been in a state of acute crisis for the last thirty years.[7] When faculty assume, in this context, their civic responsibility to educate students to think critically, act with conviction, and connect what they learn in classrooms to important social issues in the larger society, they are hounded by those who demand "measurable student outcomes," as if deep learning breaks down into such discrete and quantifiable units. What do the liberal arts and humanities amount to if they do not teach the practice of freedom, especially at a time when training is substituted for education? Gayatri Spivak (2010, p. 8) provides a context for this question with her comment: "Can one insist on the importance of training in [higher education] in [a] time of legitimized violence?"

In a society that remains troublingly resistant to or incapable of questioning itself, one that celebrates the consumer over the citizen, and all too willingly endorses the narrow values and interests of corporate power, the importance of the university as a place of critical learning, dialogue, and social justice advocacy becomes all the more imperative. Moreover, the distinctive role that faculty play in this ongoing pedagogical project of shaping the critical rationalities through which agency is defined and civic literacy and culture produced, along with support for the institutional conditions and relations of power that make them possible, must be defended as part of a broader discourse of excellence, equity, and democracy.

Higher education represents one of the most important sites over which the battle for democracy is being waged. It is the site where the promise of a better future emerges out of those visions and pedagogical practices that combine hope, agency, politics, and moral responsibility as part of a broader emancipatory discourse. Academics have a distinct and unique obligation, if not political and ethical responsibility, to make learning relevant to the imperatives of a discipline, scholarly method, or research specialization. But more importantly, academics as engaged scholars can further the activation of knowledge, passion, values, and hope in the service of forms of agency that are crucial to sustaining a democracy in which higher education plays an important civic, critical, and pedagogical role.

C. Wright Mills (2000, p. 181) was right in contending that higher education should be considered a "public intelligence apparatus, concerned with public issues and private troubles and with the structural trends of our time underlying them." He insists that academics in their roles as public intellectuals ought to transform personal troubles and concerns into social issues and problems open to critique, debate, and reason. Matters of translation, connecting private troubles with larger systemic considerations were crucial in helping "the individual become a self-educating [person], who only then would be reasonable and free" (Mills, 2000, p. 186). Yet, Mills also believed, rightly, that that criticism is not the only responsibility of public intellectuals. As Archon Fung (2011) points out, they can "also join with other citizens to address social problems, aid popular movements and organizations in their efforts to advance justice, and sometimes work with governments to construct a world that is more just and democratic."

Academics as public intellectuals can write for multiple audiences, expand those public spheres, especially the many sites opening up online, to address a range of important social issues. A small and inclusive list would include the relationship between the attack on the social state and the defunding of higher education. Clearly, in any democratic society, education should be viewed as a right, not an entitlement, and suggests a reordering of state and federal priorities to make that happen. For instance, the military budget can be cut by two thirds and the remaining funds can be invested in public and higher education. There is nothing utopian about this demand given the excessive nature of military power in the United States. Addressing this task demands a sustained critique of the militarization of American society and a clear analysis of the damage it has caused both at home and abroad. Brown University's Watson Institute for International Studies, along with a number of writers such as Andrew Bacevich, has been doing this for years, offering a treasure trove of information that could be easily accessed and used by public intellectuals in and outside of the academy. Relatedly, as Angela Davis, Michelle Alexander, and others have argued, there is a need for public intellectuals to become part of a broader social movement aimed at dismantling the prison-industrial complex and the punishing state, which drains billions of dollars in funds to put people in jail when such funds could be used to fund public and higher education. The punishing state is a dire threat to both public and higher education and to democracy itself. It is the pillar of the authoritarian state, undermining civil liberties, criminalizing a range of social behaviors related to concrete social problems, and intensifying the legacy of Jim Crow against poor minorities of color. The American public does not need more prisons; it needs more schools.

Second, academics, artists, journalists and other cultural workers need to connect the rise of subaltern, part-time labor in both the university and the larger society with the massive inequality in wealth and income that now corrupts every aspect of American politics and society. Precarity has become a weapon to both exploit adjuncts, part-time workers, and temporary laborers and to suppress dissent by keeping them in a state of fear over losing their jobs. Insecure forms of labor increasingly produce "a feeling of passivity born of despair" (Standing, 2011, p. 20). Multinational corporations have abandoned the social contract and any vestige of supporting the social state. They plunder labor and perpetuate the mechanizations of social death whenever they have the chance to accumulate capital. This issue is not simply about restoring a balance between labor and capital, it is about recognizing a new form of serfdom that kills the spirit as much as it depoliticizes the mind. The new authoritarians do not ride around in tanks, they have their own private jets, they fund right-wing think tanks, they lobby for reactionary policies that privatize everything in sight while filling their bank accounts with massive profits. They are the embodiment of a culture of greed, cruelty, and disposability.

Third, academics need to fight for the rights of students to get a free education, be given a formidable and critical education not dominated by corporate values, and to have a say in the shaping of their education and what it means to expand and deepen the practice of freedom and democracy. Young people have been left out of the discourse of democracy. They are the new disposables who lack jobs, a decent education, hope, and any semblance of a future better than the one their parents inherited. They are a reminder of how finance capital has abandoned any viable vision of the future, including one that would support future generations. This is a mode of politics and capital that eats its own children and throws their fate to the vagaries of the market. If any society is in part judged by how it views and treats its children, American society by all accounts has truly failed in a colossal way and, in doing so, provides a glimpse of the heartlessness at the core of the new authoritarianism.

Finally, there is a need to oppose the ongoing shift in power relations between faculty and the managerial class. Too many faculty are now removed from the governing structure of higher education and as a result have been abandoned to the misery of impoverished wages, excessive classes, no health care, and few, if any, social benefits. This is shameful and is not merely an education issue but a deeply political matter, one that must address how neoliberal ideology and policy has imposed on higher education an anti-democratic governing structure that mimics the broader authoritarian forces now threatening the United States.

Conclusion

In conclusion, I want to return to my early reference to the global struggles being waged by many young people. I believe that while it has become more difficult to imagine a democratic future, we have entered a period in which students and disenfranchised youth all over the world are protesting against neoliberalism and its instrumentalized pedagogy and politics of disposability. Refusing to remain voiceless and powerless in determining their future, these young people are organizing collectively in order to create the conditions for societies that refuse to use politics as an act of war and markets as the measure of democracy. And while such struggles are full of contradictions and setbacks, they have opened up a new conversation about politics, poverty, inequality, class warfare, and ecological devastation. The ongoing protests in the United States, Canada, Greece, and Spain make clear that this is not—indeed, *cannot be*—only a short-term project for reform, but a political movement that needs to intensify, accompanied by the reclaiming of public spaces, the progressive use of digital technologies, the development of public spheres, the production of new modes of education, and the safeguarding of places where democratic expression, new identities, and collective hope can be nurtured and mobilized.

Academics, artists, journalists, and other cultural workers can play a crucial role in putting into place the formative cultures necessary to further such efforts through the production and circulation of the knowledge, values, identities, and social relations crucial for such struggles to succeed. Writing in 1920, H. G. Wells insisted that "history is becoming more and more a race between education and catastrophe" (Braindash). I think Wells got it right, but what needs to be acknowledged is that there is more at stake here than the deep responsibilities of academics to defend academic freedom, the tenure system, and faculty autonomy, however important. The real issues lie elsewhere and speak to preserving the public character of higher education and recognizing that defending it as a public sphere is essential to the very existence of critical thinking, dissent, dialogue, engaged scholarship, and democracy itself. Universities should be subversive in a healthy society, they should push against the grain, and give voice to the voiceless, the unmentionable, and the whispers of truth that haunt the apostles of unchecked power and wealth. These may be dark times, as Hannah Arendt once warned, but they don't have to be, and that raises serious questions about what educators are going to do within the current historical climate to make sure that they do not succumb to the authoritarian forces circling the university, waiting for the resistance to stop and for the lights to go out. Resistance is no longer an option, it is a necessity.

Acknowledgment

This chapter was originally published as Giroux, H. A. (2013, October 29), Public Intellectuals Against the Neoliberal University, in *Truthout.* It is reprinted here with permission.

Notes

1 I have taken this idea of linking Lorde's notion of poetry to education from Smith (2011), "Humanities Are a Manifesto," pp. 48–55.

2 For a series of brilliant analyses on public education, inequality, read everything that Michael Yates writes. He is one of our national treasures.

3 See Fraser (2013), "Politics of Debt in America." On the history of debt, see Graeber (2012), *Debt: The First 5,000 Years.*

4 On this issue, see the brilliant essay by Giroux (2012), "On the Civic Function of Intellectuals Today," pp. ix–xvii.

5 I have used this example in other pieces, and I use it again because of its power and insight.

6 This issue is taken up in great detail in Ferguson (2012), *Predator Nation.*

7 See, especially, Newfield (2008), *Unmaking the Public University.*

References

Alvarez, L. (2012). Florida may reduce tuition for select majors. *New York Times.* Retrieved from www.nytimes.com/2012/12/10/education/florida-may-reduce-tuition-for-select-majors.html

Arendt, H. (1977). *Between past and future: Eight exercises in political thought.* New York: Penguin.

Aronowitz, S. (2008). *Against schooling: Education and social class.* Boulder, CO: Paradigm.

Bessie, A. (2013). The answer to the great question of education reform? The number 42. *Truthout.* Retrieved from truth-out.org/opinion/item/19356-the-answer-to-the-great-question-of-education-reform-the-number-42

Borradori, G. (2004). Autoimmunity: Real and symbolic suicides—A dialogue with Jacques Derrida. In G. Borradori (Ed.), *Philosophy in a time of terror: Dialogues with JurgenHabermas and Jacques Derrida* (pp. 121). Chicago: University of Chicago Press.

Braindash. (n.d.). *H. G. Wells.* Retrieved from www.braindash.com/quotes/h_g_wells/human_history_becomes_more_and_more_a_race between_education_and_catastrophe

Brown, W. (2006). *Regulating aversion: Tolerance in the age of identity and empire.* Princeton, NJ: Princeton University Press.

Castoriadis, C. (1997). Democracy as procedure and democracy as regime. *Constellations, 4*(1),10.

Collini, S. (2013, October). Sold Out. *London Review of Books. 35*, 20–24. www.lrb.co.uk/v35/n20/stefan-collini/sold-out

Cunningham-Cook, M. (2013). Re-imagining dissent. *Guernica Magazine.* Retrieved from www.guernicamag.com/interviews/re-imagining-dissent

Ferguson, C. H. (2012). *Predator nation: Corporate criminals, political corruption, and the hijacking of America.* New York: Crown Press.

Foley, S. (2010, March 24). Tony Judt: 'I am not pessimistic in the long run.' *The Independent* (London). Retrieved February 1, 2014, from www.independent.co.uk/arts-entertainment/books/features/tony-judt-i-am-not-pessimistic-in-the-very-long-run-1925966.html

Frank, T. (2012). It's a rich man's world: How billionaire backers pick America's candidates. *Harper's Magazine.* Retrieved from harpers.org/archive/2012/04/0083856

Fraser, S. (2013). The politics of debt in America: From debtor's prison to debtor nation. *TomDispatch.com.* Retrieved from www.tomdispatch.com/dialogs/print/?id=175643

Fung, A. (2011). The constructive responsibility of intellectuals. *Boston Review.* Retrieved from www.bostonreview.net/BR36.5/archon_fung_noam_chomsky_responsibility_of_intellectuals.php

Giroux, S. S. (2012). On the civic function of intellectuals today. In G. Olson & L. Worsham (Eds.), *Education as civic engagement: Toward a more democratic society* (pp. ix–xvii). Boulder, CO: Paradigm.

Graeber, D. (2012). *Debt: The first 5,000 years.* New York: Melville House.

Howe, I. (1990). *This age of conformity. Selected writings 1950–1990.* New York: Harcourt Brace Jovanovich.

Howe, S. (2003). Edward Said: The traveller and the exile. *Open Democracy.* Retrieved from www.opendemocracy.net/articles/ViewPopUpArticle.jsp?id=10&articleId=1561

Jaschik, S. (2010). Making adjuncts temps—Literally. *Inside Higher Ed.* Retrieved from www.insidehighered.com/news/2010/08/09/adjuncts

Kelly, A. R. (2013). David Graeber: 'There has been a war on the human imagination.' *Truthdig.* Retrieved from www.truthdig.com/avbooth/item/david_graeber_there_has_been_a_war_on_the_human_imagina tion_20130812.

King, Jr., M. L. (1991). The trumpet of conscience. In J. M. Washington (Ed.), *The essential writings and speeches of Martin Luther King, Jr.* (p. 644). New York: Harper Collins.

Lorde, A. (1984). Poetry is not a luxury. In *Sister outsider: Essays and speeches.* Freedom, CA: Crossing Press.

McCarthy, G. (2007). The social edge interview: Zygmunt Bauman. *The Social Edge.* Retrieved January 6, 2013, from webzine.thesocialedge.com/interviews/the-social-edge-interview-sociologist-and-author-zygmunt-bauman

Mills, C. W. (2000). On politics. In *The Sociological Imagination.* New York: Oxford UniversityPress.

Mills, C. W. (2008). *The politics of truth: selected writings of C. Wright Mills.* New York: Oxford University Press.

Morrison, T. (2001). How can values be taught in this university. *Michigan Quarterly Review* (Spring), 276–278.

Newfield, C. (2008). *Unmaking the public university: The forty-year assault on the middle class.* Cambridge, MA: Harvard University Press.

Nussbaum, M. C. (2010). *Not for profit: Why Democracy needs the humanities.* Princeton, NJ: Princeton University Press.

Roy, A. (2001). *Power politics.* Cambridge, MA: South End Press.

Said, E. (2000). *Out of place: A memoir.* New York: Vintage.

Said, E. (2001). On defiance and taking positions. In *Reflections on exile and other essays.* Cambridge, MA: Harvard University Press.

Said, E. (2004). *Humanism and democratic criticism.* New York: Columbia University Press.

Scialabba, G. (2009). *What are intellectuals good for?* Boston: Pressed Wafer.

Scott, D. L. (2012). How the American university was killed, in five easy steps. *The Homeless Adjunct Blog.* Retrieved from junctrebellion.wordpress.com /2012/08/12/how-the-american-university-was-killed-in-five-easy-steps

Smith, M. N. (2011). The humanities are a manifesto for the twenty-first century. *LiberalEducation* (Winter), 48–55.

Spivak, G. C. (2010). Changing reflexes: Interview with Gayatri Chakravorty Spivak. *Works and Days, 55/56* (Vol. 28), 8.

Standing, G. (2011). *The precariat: The new dangerous class.* New York: Bloomsbury.

Wilderson III, F. B. (2012). Introduction: Unspeakable ethics. In *Red, White, & Black.* London: Duke University Press.

Williams, Z. (2012). The saturday interview: Stuart Hall. The *Guardian.* Retrieved from www.guardian.co.uk/theguardian/2012/feb/11/saturday-interview-stuart-hall

Wolin, S. S. (2010). *Democracy, Inc.: Managed democracy and the specter of inverted totalitarianism.* Princeton, NJ: Princeton University Press.

Zernike, K. (2009). Making college 'relevant.' *New York Times.* Retrieved from www.nytimes.com/2010/01/03/education/edlife/03careerism-t.html?pagewanted=all&_r=0

Section III

Methodological Imperatives

Chapter 12

Interviewing and the Production of the Conversational Self

Svend Brinkmann

We live in a world of crises. Economic, climate, war, and poverty crises all affect our world on a global scale. Our problems are complex, but many of the world's troubles undoubtedly stem from a Western consumerist culture that seems to be out of control (Bauman, 2007). Unlike the society of producers, sometimes referred to as "industrial society," which had an economy that fundamentally worked by producing goods, the current consumer society primarily produces needs and desires in consumers. A culture that valorized stable selves is giving way to one that valorizes flexible selves that are able to change and develop in accordance with market needs. Not only are citizens increasingly seen as consumers, which threatens our political (Barber, 2007) and moral (Bauman, 2008) practices, but the exclusionist practices in the society of consumers are stricter and harsher than in the society of producers because almost all life problems and forms of failure are now seen as the outcome of individual faults (Bauman, 2007, p. 56). Consumer society is thoroughly psychologized. Furthermore, it seems that members of the society of consumers are themselves becoming consumer commodities (Bauman, 2007, p. 57), acknowledged mainly in

Originally published in *Qualitative Inquiry and Global Crises*, edited by Norman K. Denzin and Michael D. Giardina, pp. 56–74. Republished in *Qualitative Inquiry—Past, Present, and Future: A Critical Reader*, edited by Norman K. Denzin and Michael D. Giardina, pp. 223–241.

terms of their "saleability" on the different markets (economic, romantic, etc.) (Brinkmann, 2009).

The relationships between social science, *in casu* qualitative inquiry, and the social and cultural worlds in which inquiry is practiced, are multifaceted. One legitimate reading of the current popularity of interview research in particular, however, focuses on the cultural change from industrial society with harsh objectifying means of control and power, to consumer society and its softer seductive forms of power through dialog, narrative, empathy, and intimacy (Brinkmann & Kvale, 2005). Undoubtedly, interviewing people about their lives, opinions, and experiences and allowing them freedom of expression in telling their stories is a powerful method of understanding people's life worlds (Kvale & Brinkmann, 2008). Without denying the genuine knowledge-producing potentials of interviewing, we must not remain blind to the fact that the modern consumer society is an interview society (Atkinson & Silverman, 1997). This is a society that knows itself through the conversations that circulate in the media, ranging from talk shows, radio phone-ins, and political interviews to focus group interviews for commercial purposes. However valuable interviewing may be for research purposes, as a social technique it is also part of what Denzin (1995, p. 191) has called a "pornography of the visible," or, to paraphrase in interview terms, a pornography of the *audible*. As a social technique it serves to make visible and uncover, and, like journalism, its close ally and nineteenth-century predecessor, it serves to realize "the dream of a transparent society," to borrow Foucault's words (2001, p. 190).

To stay with Foucault's analytics, it seems reasonable to think of qualitative research interviewing as a central technology of the self in a postmodern consumerist culture, where nothing is or must remain hidden, and where selves are commodified conversational products. In this chapter, I argue that we, as qualitative interview researchers, must continuously reflect on how we stage and handle interviews if this social technique is to give us something different than a simple reflection of the consumer society that is a significant cause of the world's global crisis.

Interviewing in a Conversational Reality

In a philosophical sense, all human research must be understood as conversational, since we are linguistic creatures and language is best understood in terms of the figure of conversation (Mulhall, 2007). For discourse theorists, it has long been acknowledged that "The primary human reality is persons in conversation" (Harré, 1983, p. 58). Our cultures are constantly produced, reproduced, and revised in dialogs among their members (Mannheim & Tedlock, 1995, p. 2). The same is true of the cultural investigation of cultural phenomena, or what we call social science. We should see language and culture as emergent properties of conversations rather than the other way around. Conversations—dialogs—are not several monologs that are added together, but the basic, primordial form of associated human life. In other words, "we live our daily social lives within an ambience of conversation, discussion, argumentation, negotiation, criticism and justification; much of it to do with problems of intelligibility and the legitimation of claims to truth" (Shotter, 1993, p. 29).

Not just our interpersonal social reality is constituted by conversations. It also applies to the self. Charles Taylor (1989) argues that the self exists only within what he calls "webs of interlocution" (p. 36). We are selves only in relation to certain interlocutors with whom we are in conversation and from whom we gain a language of self-understanding. In referring to Heidegger's concept of *Dasein*—or human existence—philosopher Stephen Mulhall (2007), author of the aptly entitled book *The Conversation of Humanity*, states that "Dasein is not just the locus and the precondition for the conversation of humankind; it is itself, because humankind is, a kind of enacted conversation" (p. 58). We understand ourselves as well as others only because we can speak, and "being able to speak involves being able to converse" (Mulhall, 2007, p. 26). Human reality is a conversational reality—humankind is an enacted conversation, as are particular selves.

The idea that humankind is a kind of enacted conversation gives the interview a privileged position in producing knowledge about the social world. The processes of our lives—actions, thoughts, and emotions—are nothing but physiology if considered as isolated elements outside of conversations and interpretative contexts. A life, as Paul Ricoeur (1991) has said, "is no more than a biological phenomenon as long as it has not been interpreted" (p. 28). The phenomena of our lives must be seen as interpretive *responses* to people, situations, and events. As responses they are conversational and dialogical, for, to quote Alasdair MacIntyre (1985), "conversation, understood widely enough, is the form of human transactions in general" (p. 211). When people are talking (e.g., in interviews), they are not simply putting preconceived ideas into words, but are dialogically responding to each other's expressions and trying to make sense by using the narratives and discourses that are available (Shotter, 1993, p. 1).

If conversations are the stuff that human life is made of, it becomes pertinent to study the specific qualities of our conversations and ask what kinds of persons we become through different forms of conversation. If one believes—as I do—that the conversational approach gives us a fruitful way of understanding the human predicament, we must consider the quality of our conversations, for who we are will (to some extent) depend on the conversations in which we engage, and our values and self-understandings will depend on the subject positions into which our conversations invite us. If true, it means that social scientists and others who conduct interviews are engaged in the production of human subjectivity. Below, I distinguish between different types of interviews and describe some of the subject positions that these types entail. I will argue that too many interviews today are conducted based on what I shall refer to as a spectator's stance—a voyeur's epistemology or an epistemology of the eye—which, through the analytic perspective of Foucault, seems to be part of "the disciplinary society" and its "mobile panoptic eye, an eye that could hear and see everything that was going on in the social world" (Denzin, 1995, p. 206). Against this, I will posit the need for thinking about interviewing in more active, performative, or participatory terms—based on what I have elsewhere referred to as an epistemology of the hand (Brinkmann & Tanggaard, 2010).

Interviewing and the Spectator's Stance

Based on readings of current interview studies and textbooks instructing researchers how to interview, it is my impression that qualitative interviewers today are often acting as either pollsters, who passively record people's attitudes, opinions, and experiences, or as probers who aim to enter the private worlds of the interviewees to uncover concealed aspects of their lives (for a more thorough analysis, see Brinkmann, 2007); for example, by working with what has been called "a method of friendship" (Fontana & Frey, 2005). In both cases, the practice is based on what John Dewey ([1929] 1960) criticized as the spectator theory of knowledge: The theory that true knowledge arises through passive observation of reality, which allegedly is as it is in independence of being observed (p. 23).

In the first case of the pollster, a receptive, nondirective practice is followed, where the implicit model of the interviewer resembles Carl Rogers (1945), who developed client-centered therapy and nondirective interviewing in the 1940s. In more postmodern approaches, this practice is sometimes conceptualized as polyphonic interviewing "where the voices of the respondents are recorded with minimal influence from the researcher" (Fontana & Prokos, 2007, p. 53).

In the second case of the prober, a therapeutic practice of intimacy is followed, where the probing interviewer sometimes appears in the guise of a psychoanalyst. Both of these spectator forms are, as I shall explain, doxastic (*doxa* is Greek for opinion), in being concerned with the individual's experiences, attitudes, and narratives. My argument, presented in greater detail elsewhere (Brinkmann, 2007), is that by simply recording their respondents' experiences and opinions (the *doxa*), interview researchers are often engaged in what seems like a time-consuming kind of opinion-polling, for which quantitative instruments such as questionnaires often appear to be much more efficient.

Rogers is a clear and classic example of an interviewer working with a spectator's epistemology. His early "non-directive method as a technique for social research" (Rogers, 1945) was meant to sample the respondent's attitudes toward herself: "Through the non-directive interview we have an unbiased method by which we may plumb these private thoughts and perceptions of the individual" (p. 282). In contrast to psychoanalytic practice, the respondent in client-centered therapy/research is a client rather than a patient, and the client is the expert. Although often framed in different terms, I believe that many contemporary interview researchers conceptualize the research interview in line with Rogers's humanistic, nondirective approach, valorizing the respondents' private experiences, narratives, opinions, beliefs, and attitudes, which can be captured with the concept of *doxa*.

"Empathetic interviewing" (Fontana & Frey, 2005), for example, involves taking a stance in favor of the persons being studied, not unlike the positive regard displayed by Rogerian therapists, and the approach is depicted as at once a "method of friendship" and a humanistic "method of morality because it attempts to restore the sacredness of humans before addressing any theoretical or methodological concerns" (p. 697). In line with an implicit therapeutic metaphor, the interview is turned "into a walking stick to help some people get on their feet" (p. 695). This is a laudable intention, but there seems to be significant limitations to such forms of interviewing as well, not least that it becomes difficult to interview people with whom one disagrees and does not want to help (e.g., neo-Nazis).

Attempts to include the researcher's experience in interview research (e.g., as described by Ellis and Berger [2003]) also often focus on doxastic experience, and the interviewer is presented in a therapeutic vein as someone who "listens empathically" and "identifies with participants, and shows respect for participants' emotionality" (pp. 469–470). Ellis and Berger also refer to a number of interview researchers who "emphasize the positive therapeutic benefits that can accrue to respondents and interviewers who participate in interactive interviews" (p. 470), and one experiential form of qualitative inquiry in particular, "mediated co-constructed narratives," is presented as "similar to conjoint marital therapy" (p. 477), in which a couple jointly constructs an epiphany in their relationship, with the interviewer/therapist acting as moderator. In doxastic interviews that focus on experiences, opinions, and attitudes, knowing the experiencing self is seen as presupposed in knowing as such. A key point in these forms of interviewing is that *"Understanding ourselves is part of the process of understanding others"* (Ellis & Berger, 2003, p. 486; emphasis added). This can be interpreted as analogous to therapists' own need for therapy in their professional development. As Rogers knew, the most efficient way of eliciting private doxastic elements is by engaging in a warm and accepting relationship, in line with the principles of client-centered psychotherapy (Rogers advocated what he called "unconditional positive regard").

I believe that we may read the spread of Rogers's humanistic interviews as a reflection of the contemporary consumer society where the client is always right, where his or her experiences and narratives are always interesting *because* they are some individual's experiences and narratives, and where the interviewer acts as a mirror of the respondent's feelings, attitudes, and beliefs. Consumer society is an *experience society*, to quote the German sociologist, Gerhard Schulze (1992), and the interview is a central technology for sampling and circulating experiences, not just in research contexts, but also in confessional talk shows and marketized focus groups (Kvale, 2006).

There are other and much more theoretically informed conceptualizations of the interview and the interviewee that share the psychologistic, spectator's stance. A good example comes from Wendy Hollway and Tony Jefferson (2000). In their psychoanalytic eyes, the qualitative interview researcher is always closer to the truth than the research subject (whom they call a "defended subject"), for "subjects are motivated *not* to know certain aspects of themselves and ... they *produce* biographical accounts which avoid such knowledge" (p. 169; emphases in the original). In this perspective, the respondents can give away only *doxa*, and the researcher-therapists are in a unique position to obtain true knowledge, given their superior theoretical knowledge and psychoanalytic training. The model for the relation between interviewer and interviewee consequently becomes that of psychotherapist and patient, where the patient is cast in the experiencing, suffering position and the therapist in the seeing and (therefore) knowing position.

A critique of what I here refer to as doxastic interviews is not new. In the 1950s, David Riesman warned against the tendency to use the level of "rapport" in an interview to judge its qualities concerning knowledge. He thought it was a prejudice, "often based on psychoanalytic stereotypes, to assume the more rapport-filled and intimate the relation, the more 'truth' the respondent will vouchsafe" (Riesman & Benney, 1956, p. 10). Rapport-filled interviews often spill over with "the flow of legend and cliché" (p. 11), according to Riesman's verdict, where interviewees adapt their responses to what they take the interviewer expects from them (see Lee, 2008; and, for a related analysis that puts weight on participants' objections during the interview, see Tanggaard, 2008).

Interviewing and the Participant's Stance

What, then, are the alternatives to the spectators' doxastic interviews? To answer this question, it may be useful to look at other writings on the subject and other terminologies. Wengraf (2001), for example, does not talk about *doxa* but about "receptive interviewing" and opposes this to "assertive" styles. He also aligns the receptive practice with Rogers's model of psychotherapy, which seeks to empower the informant (p. 154), and the assertive practice with legal interrogations where the interviewer is in control and seeks to provoke and illuminate self-contradictions (p. 155). Wengraf cites Holstein and Gubrium's (1995) "active interviewing" as a form of assertive interviewing practice (but, like most researchers, he favors the receptive style). Holstein and Gubrium have long argued that interviews are unavoidably interpretively active, meaning-making practices. Interviews are not simply practices of "seeing" the other, but processes of meaning construction (i.e., of "doing" something together). The interviewer here appears as a participant rather than spectator, but active interviews are to some extent still dominated by the spectator's stance, and researchers are encouraged to experiment "with alternative representational forms that they believe can convey respondents' experience more on, if not in, their own terms" (Holstein & Gubrium, 2003, p. 20).

For some time, I have been interested in how conversations can help us produce knowledge in the sense of *episteme* (the Greek term for knowledge that has been arrived at through dialectical processes of questioning).[1] The greatest epistemic interviewer in history was no doubt Socrates, who will serve as my main inspiration for an alternative to doxastic forms of interviewing. Plato's dialogs, in which Socrates appears as "interviewer," were designed as ways of testing whether the conversation partners have knowledge (i.e., whether they are capable of adequately justifying their beliefs, and if they cannot [which is normally the case], if their beliefs are unwarranted, the dialogs unfold as dialectical processes of refining their beliefs)—their *doxa*—in light of good reasons, in order to approach *episteme*.

To illustrate more concretely what I mean by epistemic interviews, I shall give a simple and very short example from Plato's *The Republic*. It elegantly demonstrates epistemically that no moral rules are self-applying and self-interpreting but must always be understood contextually. Socrates is in a conversation with Cephalus, who believes that justice (*dikaiosune*)—here "doing right"—can be stated in universal rules, such as "tell the truth" and "return borrowed items":

> "That's fair enough, Cephalus," I [Socrates] said. "But are we really to say that doing right consists simply and solely in truthfulness and returning anything we have borrowed? Are those not actions that can be sometimes right and sometimes wrong? For instance, if one borrowed a weapon from a friend who subsequently went out of his mind and then asked for it back, surely it would be generally agreed that one ought not to return it, and that it would not be right to do so, not to consent to tell the strict truth to a madman?"
>
> "That is true," he [Cephalus] replied.
>
> "Well then," I [Socrates] said, "telling the truth and returning what we have borrowed is not the definition of doing right." (Plato, 1987, pp. 65–66)

Here, the conversation is interrupted by Polemarchus who disagrees with Socrates' preliminary conclusion, and Cephalus quickly leaves to go to a sacrifice. Then Polemarchus takes Cephalus's position as Socrates' discussion partner and the conversation continues as if no substitution had happened.

Initially, we may notice that Socrates violates almost every standard principle of qualitative research interviewing. First, we see that he talks much more than his respondent. There is some variety across the dialogs concerning how much Socrates talks in comparison with the other participants, but the example given here, where Socrates develops an absurd conclusion from the initial belief voiced by Cephalus, is not unusual, although the balance is much more equal in other places. Second, Socrates has not asked Cephalus to "describe a situation in which he has experienced justice" or "tell a story about doing right from his own experience" or a similar concretely descriptive question, probing for "lived experience." Instead, they are talking about the definition of an important general concept. Third, Socrates contradicts and challenges his respondent's view. He is not a warm and caring conversationalist, working with "a methodology of friendship." Fourth, there is no debriefing or attempt to make sure that the interaction was a "pleasant experience" for Cephalus. Fifth, the interview is conducted in public rather than private, and the topic is not private experiences or biographical details, but justice, a theme of common human interest, at least of interest to all citizens of Athens.

Sixth, and perhaps most importantly, the interview here is radically anti-psychologistic and anti-individualist. Interestingly, it does not make much of a difference whether the conversation partner is Cephalus or Polemarchus—and the discussion continues in exactly the same way after Cephalus has left. The crux of the discussion is whether the participants are able to give good reasons for their belief in a public discussion, not whether they have this or that biographical background or defense mechanism, for example. The focus is on *what* they say—and whether it can be normatively justified—not on dubious psychological interpretations concerning *why* they say it, neither during the conversation, nor in some process of analysis after the conversation. In the words of Norwegian philosopher Hans Skjervheim (1957), the "researcher" (Socrates) is a *participant*, who takes seriously what his fellow citizen says ("what does he say?")—seriously enough to disagree with it in fact—he is not a *spectator* who objectifies the conversation partner and his arguments by ignoring the normative claims of the statements, or looks at them in terms of the causes (psychological or sociological) that may have brought the person to entertain such beliefs ("why does he say that?").

Socrates' "method" is not a method in the conventional sense, but an *elenchus*, a Greek term that means examining a person and considering his or her statements normatively (Dinkins, 2005). The Socratic conversation is a mode of understanding, rather than a method in any mechanical sense (see Gadamer, 1960). Sometimes, the conversation partners in the Platonic dialogs settle on a definition, but more often the dialog ends without any final, unarguable definition of the central concept (e.g., justice, virtue, love). This lack of resolution—*aporia* in Greek—can be interpreted as illustrating the open-ended character of our conversational reality, including the open-ended character of the discursively produced knowledge of human social and historical life generated by (what we today call) the social sciences. If humankind is a kind of enacted conversation, the goal of social science should not be to arrive at "fixed knowledge" once and for all, but to help human beings constantly improve the quality of their conversational reality, to help them know their own society and debate the goals and values that are important in their lives (Flyvbjerg, 2001).

Michel Foucault (2001) also discussed Socrates' conversational practices in some of his last writings, and the quotation below nicely brings out the normative and epistemic dimensions of Socratic interviewing. When Socrates asks people to give accounts, "what is involved is not a confessional autobiography," Foucault makes clear (p. 97). Instead:

> In Plato's or Xenophon's portrayals of him, we never see Socrates requiring an examination of conscience or a confession of sins. Here, giving an account of your life, your *bios*, is also not to give a narrative of the historical events that have taken place in your life, but rather to demonstrate whether you are able to show that there is a relation between the rational discourse, the *logos*, you are able to use, and the way that you live. Socrates is inquiring into the way that *logos* gives form to a person's style of life. (Foucault, 2001, p. 97)

Socrates was engaged in conversational practices where people, in giving accounts of themselves, exhibited the logos by which they lived (Butler, 2005, p. 126). The conversation partners were thus positioned as responsible citizens, accountable to each other with reference to the normative order in which they acted, and the conversational topic would therefore not be the narrative of the individual's life, or his or her experiences, but rather people's epistemic practices of justification. In short, people are approached as accountable citizens rather than as consumers/clients that are always right.

Epistemic Interviews Today

It seems pertinent to ask whether this approach to interviewing is possible today, or whether it should be considered as an ancient Hellenic practice that is no longer viable. I support the former idea and believe that it is possible to point to a number of significant interview studies that have employed some version of the Socratic approach, perhaps not in a pure form, but nonetheless in a form that seeks to distance itself from doxastic interviewing.

What Bellah and coworkers (1985) referred to as "active interviews" in their classic *Habits of the Heart* correspond, for example, quite well to epistemic interviews, and they represent one worked-out alternative to the standard doxastic interviews that probe for private meanings and opinions. In the appendix to their study of North American values and character, the researchers spell out their view of social science and its methodology, summarized as "social science as public philosophy." The empirical material for their book consisted of interviews with more than 200 participants, some of whom were interviewed more than once. In contrast to the interviewer as a friend or therapist, probing deeply in the private psyche of the interviewee, Bellah and coworkers practiced active interviews, which were intended to generate public conversation about societal values and goals. Such active interviews do not necessarily aim for agreement between interviewer and interviewee, so there is no danger of instrumentalizing the researcher's feelings to obtain good rapport. The interviewer is allowed to question and challenge what the interviewee says. In this example, the interviewer, Steven Tipton, tries to discover at what point the respondent would take responsibility for another human being:

Q: So what are you responsible for?

A: I'm responsible for my acts and for what I do.

Q: Does that mean you're responsible for others, too?

A: No.

Q: Are you your sister's keeper?

A: No.

Q: Your brother's keeper?

A: No.

Q: Are you responsible for your husband?

A: I'm not. He makes his own decisions. He is his own person. He acts his own acts. I can agree with them or I can disagree with them. If I ever find them nauseous enough, I have a responsibility to leave and not deal with it any more.

Q: What about children?

A: I ... I would say I have a legal responsibility for them, but in a sense I think they in turn are responsible for their own acts. (Bellah et al., 1985, p. 304)

Here, Tipton repeatedly challenges the respondent's claim of not being responsible for other human beings. With the Socratic principles in mind, we can see the interviewer pressing for a contradiction between the respondent's definition of responsibility, involving the idea that she is only responsible for herself, and her likely feeling of at least some (legal) responsibility for her children. The individualist notion of responsibility is almost used *ad absurdum*, but the definition apparently plays such a central role in the person's life that she is unwilling to give it up. I would argue that this way of interviewing, although not asking for concrete descriptions or narratives, gives us important knowledge *primarily* about the doxastic individualist beliefs of Americans in the mid-1980s, but *secondarily* about the idea of responsibility in a normative-epistemic sense. For most readers would appreciate the above sequence as implying the argument that the respondent is wrong—she *is* responsible for other people, most clearly her children. At the very least, the reader is invited into an epistemic discussion not just about beliefs, but also about citizenship, virtue, responsibility, and ethics. The authors of *Habits of the Heart* conclude that unlike "poll data" generated by fixed questions that "sum up the *private* opinions," active (epistemic) interviews "create the possibility of *public* conversation and argument" (Bellah et al., 1985, p. 305). We are far away from the pollster and the traditional doxastic view of social science interviews, portraying these as ways of understanding what people privately think, feel, and want.

Concluding Ethico-Political Thoughts

The project of developing the epistemic potentials of interviewing is allied, I believe, with other recent explorations of alternative interview forms, for example Denzin's (2001) idea of performance interviews in the "cinematic-interview society." Denzin formulates "a utopian project," searching for a new form of the interview, which he calls "the reflexive, dialogic, or performative interview" (p. 24). The utopian project of epistemic interviewing outlined above, however, has a more explicit emphasis on civic responsibility. Qualitative researchers are increasingly becoming aware that interviewing, as Charles Briggs (2003, p. 497) has argued, is "a 'technology' that invents both notions of individual subjectivities and collective social and political patterns." Different conversational practices, including research interviews, produce and activate different forms of subjectivity and social life. Thus, ethico-political issues are always internal to practices of interviewing. Epistemic interviews position respondents as accountable, responsible citizens, which I have presented as an alternative to experience-focused, psychologized interviews that position respondents as clients or patients. And epistemic interviews position interviewers as participants rather than spectators.

According to the view of social science that goes back to Plato and Aristotle (1976), the social sciences are *practical* sciences that should ideally enable the creation of a knowledgeable citizenry capable of discussing matters of communal value (this was also Dewey's view; see Brinkmann, 2004). Social science should serve the political community in the sense of engaging this community in conversations about ethical, political, and other normative issues. Qualitative social science, according to this view, should not just serve to bring forth privatized narratives or other intimate aspects of people's lives. It should also serve the *Res Publica* (i.e., the ethical and political relations between human beings that are not constituted by intimacy) (Sennett, 1977).

In *The Fall of Public Man*, Richard Sennett warned against seeing society as a grand, psychological system (Sennett, 1977, p. 4), where the question "Who am I?" is constantly pursued, and where psychological categories invade and destroy public life, making us forget that political questions cannot be dealt with alone through trust, empathy, warmth, and a disclosure of private opinions (p. xvii). Under the conditions Sennett describes as "the tyranny of intimacy," public, social, civic, and political phenomena are transformed into questions of personality, biography and individual narratives (p. 219). As an antidote, Sennett calls for more "impersonal" forms of action in public arenas (p. 340).

My worry is that some of the social science interviews, which I have referred to as doxastic, can be said to uncritically reproduce and reinforce the view of social life as reducible to psychology in the form of people's experiences and opinions. Here, the researcher is a spectator, a voyeur, who observes, sees, and hears the intimate details of the respondents. What Sennett said of contemporary life in general also applies to much interview research: "Each person's self has become his principle burden; to know oneself has become an end, instead of a means through which one knows the world" (Sennett, 1977, p. 4). Current doxastic interviews are often about getting to know people's selves, which is often portrayed as an end in itself in the contemporary "interview society" (Atkinson & Silverman, 1997), and I would echo Sennett's claim that we need a forum "in which it becomes meaningful to join with other persons without the compulsion to know them as persons" (Sennett, 1977, p. 340)—also in the contexts of qualitative inquiry. No doubt, we also often need to know others "as persons," and here doxastic interviews have been very efficient, but if we genuinely want to examine ethical and political issues for the sake of the public good, one way could be to add epistemic interviews to the repertoire of qualitative inquiry to a larger extent.

Still, we may ask, if the practice of Socratic interviews involves challenging respondents and confronting them with the task of giving reasons and normative accounts, isn't this ethically problematic? I would counter this by arguing that epistemic interviews have the potentials for at least as great a transparency of its power relations as doxastic interviews and do not commodify or instrumentalize human feeling, friendship, and empathy (Brinkmann & Kvale, 2005). Certainly, like all other human practices, epistemic interviews come with certain ethical challenges that should be taken into consideration. Nevertheless, I believe that the active and assertive style in epistemic interviews in many ways enable researchers to proceed ethically in qualitative knowledge production. As shown in the epistemic interviews above, the interviewers do not try to suck as much private information out of the respondents as possible without themselves engaging in the conversation with all the risks that are involved in this. Interviewers become participants in, rather than spectators of, the production of social life.

In conclusion, I want to make clear that the purpose of this chapter has definitely not been to invalidate the use of phenomenological or narrative interviews that focus on experiences and opinions—the *doxa*. Rather, my aim has been to argue that other kinds of human conversations can also be practiced with the goal of reaching knowledge, as classically illustrated by Socrates in the role of epistemic interviewer. Socrates is never content to hear what people believe or how they experience the world. He is always interested in examining whether people's beliefs and experiences can be justified, and his dialectical method (his *elenchus*) was developed to bring human beings from a state of being opinionated to a state of knowing. In what I have called epistemic interviews, the analysis is in principle carried out *in* the conversation, together with the accountable respondents involved, since the analysis mainly consists of testing, questioning, and justifying what people say. Such interviews involve a co-construction of conversational reality *in situ*. In Plato's dialogs, we do not hear about Socrates continuing his analyses in solitude after the public meetings. In conventional research interviews, on the other hand, the analysis is typically carried out after the interview has taken place, often informed by the researcher's theoretical preferences that may be totally alien to the participants. I believe that researchers ought to experiment more with testing their own and their respondents' statements in public discussion in the course of the interview, rather than just seeing this as something to be carried out behind closed doors. I believe that this could often improve the analyses and perhaps also create more interesting interviews. Often, the use of challenging and confronting questions in epistemic interviews generates more readable interview reports compared with the long monologs that sometimes result from phenomenological and narrative approaches.

The epistemic interviewer is not a spectator, gazing at a research subject and consuming his stories, but a participant in the creation of our conversational reality. His "intrusion" into the conversation is not thought of as a source of error, or as something unnatural. On the contrary, if knowledge and subjectivity are produced in conversations, it is an epistemic virtue to become visible as a questioner in the interview.

Note

1 The ensuing discussion reworks parts of Brinkmann, 2007.

References

Aristotle. (1976). *Nichomachean ethics.* London: Penguin.

Atkinson, P. & Silverman, D. (1997). Kundera's immortality: The interview society and the invention of the self. *Qualitative Inquiry, 3*, 3, 304–325.

Barber, B. (2007). *Consumed: How markets corrupt children, infantilize adults, and swallow citizens whole.* New York: W.W. Norton.

Bauman, Z. (2007). *Consuming life.* Cambridge: Polity Press.

Bauman, Z. (2008). *Does ethics have a chance in a world of consumers?* Cambridge, MA: Harvard University Press.

Bellah, R. N., Madsen, R., Sullivan, W. M., Swidler, A., & Tipton, S. M. (1985). *Habits of the heart: Individualism and commitment in American life.* Berkeley: University of California Press.

Briggs, C. L. (2003). Interviewing, power/knowledge, and social inequality. In J. A. Holstein & J. F. Gubrium (Eds.), *Inside interviewing: New lenses, new concerns* (pp. 495–506). Thousand Oaks, CA: Sage.

Brinkmann, S. (2004). Psychology as a moral science: Aspects of John Dewey's psychology. *History of the Human Sciences, 17*, 1, 1–28.

Brinkmann, S. (2007). Could interviews be epistemic? An alternative to qualitative opinion-polling. *Qualitative Inquiry, 13*, 8, 1116–1138.

Brinkmann, S. (2009). Literature as qualitative inquiry: The novelist as researcher. *Qualitative Inquiry, 15*, 8, 1376–1394.

Brinkmann, S., & Kvale, S. (2005). Confronting the ethics of qualitative research. *Journal of Constructivist Psychology, 18*, 2, 157–181.

Brinkmann, S., & Tanggaard, L. (2010). Toward an epistemology of the hand. *Studies in Philosophy and Education, 29*, 3, 243–257.

Butler, J. (2005). *Giving an account of oneself.* New York: Fordham University Press.

Denzin, N. K. (1995). *The cinematic society: The voyeur's gaze.* Thousand Oaks, CA: Sage.

Denzin, N. K. (2001). The reflexive interview and a performative social science. *Qualitative Research, 1*, 1, 23–46.

Dewey, J. ([1929] 1960). *The quest for certainty.* New York: Capricorn Books.

Dinkins, C. S. (2005). Shared inquiry: Socratic-hermeneutic interpre-viewing. In P. Ironside (Ed.), *Beyond Method: Philosophical conversations in healthcare research and scholarship* (pp. 111–147). Madison: University of Wisconsin Press.

Ellis, C., & Berger, L. (2003). Their story/my story/our story: Including the researcher's experience in interview research. In J. A. Holstein & J. F. Gubrium (Eds.), *Inside Interviewing: New lenses, new concerns* (pp. 467–493). Thousand Oaks, CA: Sage.

Flyvbjerg, B. (2001). *Making social science matter—Why social inquiry fails and how it can succeed again.* Cambridge: Cambridge University Press.

Fontana, A., & Frey, J. H. (2005). The interview: From neutral stance to political involvement. In N. K. Denzin & Y. S. Lincoln (Eds.) *The Sage handbook of qualitative research* (3rd ed., pp. 695–727). Thousand Oaks, CA: Sage.

Fontana, A., & Prokos, A. H. (2007). *The interview: From formal to postmodern.* Walnut Creek, CA: Left Coast, Inc.

Foucault, M. (2001). *Fearless speech.* (J. Pearson, Ed.). New York: Semiotext(e).

Gadamer, H. G. (1960). *Truth and method.* (2nd revised edition, 2000). New York: Continuum.

Harré, R. (1983). *Personal being.* Oxford: Basil Blackwell.

Hollway, W., & Jefferson, T. (2000). Biography, anxiety and the experience of locality. In P. Chamberlayne, J. Bornat, & T. Wengraf (Eds.), *The turn to biographical methods in social science* (pp. 167–180). London: Routledge.

Holstein, J. A., & Gubrium, J. F. (1995). *The active interview.* London: Sage.

Holstein, J. A., & Gubrium, J. F. (2003). Inside interviewing: New lenses, new concerns. In J. A. Holstein & J. F. Gubrium (Eds.), *Inside interviewing: New lenses, new concerns* (pp. 3–30). Thousand Oaks, CA: Sage.

Kvale, S. (2006). Dominance through interviews and dialogues. *Qualitative Inquiry, 12*, 3, 480–500.

Kvale, S., & Brinkmann, S. (2008). *InterViews: Learning the craft of qualitative research interviewing*. Thousand Oaks, CA: Sage.

Lee, R. M. (2008). David Riesman and the sociology of the interview. *The Sociological Quarterly, 49*, 2, 285–307.

MacIntyre, A. (1985). *After virtue*. (2nd ed., with postscript). London: Duckworth.

Mannheim, B., & Tedlock, B. (1995). Introduction. In D. Tedlock & B. Mannheim (Eds.), *The dialogic emergence of culture* (pp. 1–32). Urbana: University of Illinois Press.

Mulhall, S. (2007). *The conversation of humanity*. Richmond: University of Virginia Press.

Plato (1987). *The republic*. London: Penguin.

Ricoeur, P. (1991). Life in quest of narrative. In D. Wood (Ed.), *On Paul Ricoeur: Narrative and interpretation* (pp. 20–33). London: Routledge.

Riesman, D., & Benney, M. (1956). The sociology of the interview. *Midwestern Sociologist, 18*, 1, 3–15.

Rogers, C. (1945). The non-directive method as a technique for social research. *The American Journal of Sociology, 50*, 2, 279–283.

Schulze, G. (1992). *Die Erlebnisgesellschaft: Kultursoziologie Der Gegenwart* [The experience society: A cultural sociology of the present]. Frankfurt: Campus.

Sennett, R. ([1977] 2003). *The fall of public man*. London: Penguin.

Shotter, J. (1993). *Conversational realities: Constructing life through language*. London: Sage.

Skjervheim, H. (1957). *Deltaker og tilskodar* [Participant and spectator]. Oslo: Oslo University Press.

Tanggaard, L. (2008). Objections in research interviewing. *International Journal of Qualitative Methods, 7*, 1, 15–29.

Taylor, C. (1989). *Sources of the self*. Cambridge: Cambridge University Press

Wengraf, T. (2001). *Qualitative research interviewing*. Thousand Oaks, CA: Sage.

Chapter 13

Remix Cultures, Remix Methods

Reframing Qualitative Inquiry for Social Media Contexts

Annette Markham

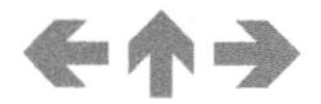

In early 2011, I started getting all of my news of the world exclusively through my social media networks, specifically Twitter and Facebook. I wanted to immerse myself in the premise that "while people using media are simultaneously and instantaneously connected with large and multiple groups and networks, they are also increasingly ascribed with a deeply individualized and self-centered value system" (Deuze et al., 2012, para. 28). Homophily, a concept describing the way people tend to flock toward similar others, is one way to describe how our understandings of the world are idiosyncratic, narrowly channeled through our social networks, and therefore polarized.

Not only did I experience homophily, but I soon found myself saturated in situations that I would not otherwise experience. I saw certain tragedies very up close and personal, like the Queensland floods and the New Zealand earthquakes (two of my colleagues lived in Brisbane, Australia; one lived in Christchurch, New Zealand). I learned a lot about the music scene in Britain (I followed a musician who tweeted a lot and lived only one time zone away from me). I watched a lot of Rachel Maddow

Originally published in *Global Dimensions of Qualitative Inquiry,* edited by Norman K. Denzin and Michael D. Giardina, pp. 63–81. Republished in *Qualitative Inquiry—Past, Present, and Future: A Critical Reader,* edited by Norman K. Denzin and Michael D. Giardina, pp. 242–260. Left Coast Press, Inc.

and Jon Stewart (as most of my friends in both Facebook and Twitter would forward these clips). I read scholarly articles that were posted when I was awake (and, since I was in Denmark, this meant my stream was primarily European).

As Deuze et al. (2012) write, "the whole of the world and our lived experience in it can and perhaps should be seen as framed by, mitigated through, and made immediate by pervasive and ubiquitous media" (para 3). This became clearer to me on January 25, as the Egyptian Revolution started to flood my Twitter streams. The speed at which tweets flowed on hashtags like #jan25 limited me to quick flashes of statements before they disappeared. Clicking on links became a fairly random act, but led to some amazing pathways of meaning. On January 27, 2011, my mom watched MSNBC News on her TV, listening to the anchor talk about growing concerns about rioters getting ready for a "day of rage," while a video clip over the anchor's shoulder showed crowds of rioters shouting with fires visible in the distance. She learned that rioters had injured eighty-seven police officers and that one was killed (Bloggit, 2011). Meanwhile, halfway around the world, I cried as I watched a remix created by Tamar Shaaban (2011) that clipped footage from various news agencies as well as on-the-ground local video clips. Over a stirring soundtrack, I heard the passionate and committed voices of the Egyptian people, bloodied on the streets of Cairo.[1]

We are witnessing a startling transformation in the way cultural knowledge is produced and how meaning is negotiated. The digital era does not mark the beginning of this sort of activity by any means, yet it has facilitated a remarkable acceleration toward deprivileging expert knowledge, decentralizing culture production, and unhooking cultural units of information from their origins. One way to think about this is through the lens of remix. Although remix has long been associated with hip hop music forms, it is now a general term referring to the processes and products of taking bits of cultural material and, through the process of copy/paste and collage, producing new meaning to share with others. As I experience social reality that has been remixed by my interactions with my social media networks, I gain a particular understanding of the world, remix it again, and distribute this to others.

Inspired by my experiment of saturating myself in the way our understanding of the world is remixed by our engagement with social media,[2] I have been thinking about the ways in which remix is a powerful tool for thinking about qualitative, interpretive research practice. The form and cultural practice of remix offers a lens through which we may be able to better grapple with the complexity of social contexts characterized by ubiquitous Internet, always-connected mobile devices, dense global communication networks, fragments of information flow, and temporal and ad hoc community formations.

Rather than inventing new methods, a remix approach offers a different way of thinking about what we do when we engage with particular methods to make sense of phenomena. Taking a remix approach begins with the premises of a bricolage approach (Kincheloe, 2001, 2005) and then shifts to a level we might call "below method," where we engage in everyday practices of sense-making. The concept of remix highlights activities that are not often discussed as a part of method and may not be noticed, such as using serendipity, playing with different perspectives, generating partial renderings, moving through multiple variations, borrowing from disparate and perhaps disjunctive concepts, and so forth. Although methods texts offer extensive descriptions of how one might design research questions, collect data, manage and sort data, and apply analytical tools to this data, much of the actual process from data to conclusion remains a black box. Most often, especially in disciplines where interpretive reflexive inquiry is not taken for granted, these processes are not included in anything the audience might read. Instead, we see the tidied-up version of a long, messy, creative process of sense-making.

Adaptation and creative innovation is sorely needed to study the complexity of digital life. Internet research has been plagued by a constant reinvention of the wheel and a significant degree of trying to force fit methods that were invented for and function best in local face-to-face settings. I argue that by engaging in a greater level of attention to our everyday processes of sense-making within research projects, we can identify and then submit these practices to greater scrutiny. Remix is a metaphor that can help us get to this sort of reflexive attention to practice, product, and purpose and also is a fruitful mindset for engaging in highly responsive, ethically grounded, and context sensitive cultural interpretations.

In what follows, I discuss some of the complications associated with studying Internet-mediated contexts. I offer a research-centered definition of remix and then describe particular elements of remix that have proven to be valuable pedagogical tools for helping disrupt traditional frames for conducting qualitative research in digital contexts: generate, play, borrow, move, and interrogate.

As a brief caveat, remix is a generative tool for thinking creatively about methods, not a new method, or even a framework. It resides alongside other metaphors that seek to challenge how we envision research, such as dance (Janesick, 1994), jazz (Oldfather & West, 1994), crystallization (Richardson, 1994), bricolage (Kincheloe, 2001, 2005), or facets (Mason, 2011). These sorts of metaphors remind us that the process of research is, among other things, exploratory and creative, a mix of passion and curiosity. And that the product of our inquiry,

> whether an article, a graph, a poem, a story, a play, a dance, or a painting, is not something to be received, but something to be used; not a conclusion but a turn in a conversation; not a closed statement but an open question; not a way of declaring "this is how it is" but a means of inviting others to consider what it (or they) could become. (Bochner & Ellis, 2003, p. 507)

Social (Research) Contexts in the 21st Century

The past three decades mark tremendous growth in digital social interaction, from early experiments in virtual reality, text-based communities, and role-playing games to today's saturation in social media, where we are always on, tethered to mobile devices, enacting what Neilson in 2012 labeled "Generation C" (for connected). At the turn of the 21st century, technologies for communication became much more pervasive through mobility and convergence. The collaborative and distributive features of the web were more fully realized at this time with the rise of blogging. The capacity to easily connect—via commenting, tagging, and sharing—facilitated a huge growth in complex networks among people both locally and globally, across any media form imaginable. In both the blogosphere and commercial spheres, a system developed whereby value was linked to reputation and connectivity in these networks. This reputation and sharing economy has shifted our traditional understandings of authorship, blurring the boundaries between producer and consumer.

Throughout this time, frameworks for understanding and defining identity and social constructs have continued to shift away from the individual and toward networks and information flows. The performance of everyday life is seen as increasingly inseparable from the technologically mediated and mediatized confluences in which our information flows, with or without our attention or intention. Materiality in this mobile epoch is better understood as connection, process, and relationship.

Gergen (1991) discusses this as an inevitable but slow-incoming recognition of the relational self. Turkle (2011) describes it more in terms of fragmentation, or a cycling through of various virtual personae, each with sets of attributes to suit particular situations. Scholars such as Latour (2005; Latour et al., 2012) go further, emphasizing that in contemporary culture, we need to move beyond the notion and privileging of the individual to better understand the multiple agencies influencing any social situation. Characteristic of actor network theorists, the actor is not just embedded in networks but is "defined by its network … entirely defined by the open-ended lists in the databases" (Latour et al., 2012, p. 3). From this perspective, anything we might call an individual is simply a temporary constitution of attributes.

For social researchers, this means that many taken-for-granted techniques for identifying discrete situational boundaries, individuals, or other objects or for analysis are far less useful than they may have once seemed. As I have noted elsewhere (Markham, in press), at least four complications emerge when we consider the entanglements of the social contexts involving humans, Web 2.0 technologies, and smart mobile devices:

1. Boundaries between self and other are often unclear, particularly when information develops a social life of its own, beyond one's immediate circumstances.

2. Boundaries of situations and identification of contexts are often unclear as dramas play out in settings and times far removed from the origin of interaction.
3. Agency is not the sole property of individual entities, but a temporal performative element that emerges in the dynamic interplay of people and their technologies for communication.
4. Performativity can be linked not only to individuals but actions of the devices, interfaces, and networks of information through which dramas occur and meaning is negotiated.

To deal with the challenges of conducting qualitative research in mobile, global, and fragmented mediatized and mediated environments, do we cling to tradition, hoping for steady grounding? Or do we continually experiment? These questions are complicated by other axiological questions. Part of the difficulty of being innovative is linked closely to the persistence of positivist models and procedures. Whether discussed within the larger backlash against interpretivism or postmodernism, or within the economy-driven shifts toward evidence-based research models, it still feels like academia is battening down the hatches. This occurs in the midst of a cultural explosion—outside the walls of the academy—of collaborative, open source, reputation knowledge production.

This becomes an ethical concern on many levels, not the least of which relates to how and whether we are interrogating our methods adequately to protect people (our participants, their communities, and ourselves) from harm. With the automated scraping of data occurring on massive levels across all media platforms and by various agencies, individuals, and privatized interests, how can we ensure data privacy? How can we be sure our techniques for anonymizing sources will work? The simple answer to this question is we can't, unless we adjust our methods of representation. Or take the issue of privacy and informed consent. There are no easy answers, as was emphasized in the latest ethics guidelines of the Association of Internet Researchers (Markham & Buchanan, 2012). People engage in activities that would traditionally be considered highly sensitive, even when understanding that their actions are public and the potential audience is vast. It's not just that we have blurred the boundaries of what constitutes public and private spheres, it's that the concept itself is changing (see, e.g., boyd & Marwick, 2012; Markham, 2012; Nissenbaum, 2011).

To add to this dilemma, technological advances teach us that we cannot predict how our information will be used in the future. Now, more than ever, we have the obligation to try to proactively protect participants or to consider ways of doing inquiry that minimize the risk of future harms. My effort to invoke innovative metaphors for thinking about inquiry is embedded, then, in a larger argument that interpretive studies of digital experience would be not only stronger but probably more ethically grounded if we more radically disrupted—or revisited previous disruptions of—still taken-for-granted parameters for qualitative inquiry.

What Is Remix?

'Remix' is a term that came into usage in the late 20th century to refer to the practice and product of taking samples from audio tracks and putting them together in new and creative ways. The history of remix is most often linked to the music form of Jamaican Dub, represented well by artist King Tubby. King Tubby, whose work influenced generations of hip hop artists engaged in dub, scratch, rap, and DJ, began deconstructing and reconstructing musical tracks in the late '60s. We're now very familiar with the way songs are remixed in ways that extend or reinterpret them for different audiences. But remix goes well beyond music.

Remix has become a term that is used to describe the widespread practice of mashup videos, most evident on YouTube, or the phenomenon of Internet memes, which are typically composed of small units of cultural information (a phrase, an image, a short audio or video clip) that get mixed in different ways, generally for comedic effect. A meme is characterized by its evolution—in effect, it doesn't exist unless it morphs through reproduction and dissemination.

We could say remix is everywhere, or that "everything is a remix" (Ferguson, n.d.), as both a practice and outcome in all forms of cultural production. Navas (2006) notes that "cut/copy and paste, the fragmentation of material, is today part of everyday activities both at work and at home thanks to the computer" (para. 13), whereby easy-to-use software applications allow people to develop sophisticated mashups. Lessig (2008) and Ferguson (n.d.) offer extensive discussions of remix, offering many historical as well as contemporary artists and contexts to argue that it's the content of an idea, not the originator, that matters, and that borrowing, sampling, and creatively remixing ideas is an inherent aspect of any culture. Conceptualized broadly, remix is not something we do in addition to our everyday lives, it is the way we make sense of our world, by transforming the bombardment of stimuli into a seamless experience. If we take seriously the idea that everything we take to be real is a constant negotiation of relationships between people and things, and that culture is habit writ large, remix as a form of sense-making embraces this framework.

For purposes of talking about qualitative inquiry and the study of digital experience, I find two aspects of remix to be critical: First, remix relies on sampling, borrowing, and creatively reassembling units of cultural information to create something that is used to move or persuade others. The key to the power of remix is that it doesn't matter where the elements are drawn from as long as the resulting product has resonance for the audience. Remix is about working in the liminal space to create a particular way of connecting the familiar with the unfamiliar, or the original elements and the remixed.

Second, remix always occurs as part of a larger community of remix. It is a process of creating temporary assemblages that change almost immediately after initial production. The very power of remix relies on the participation of others as "produsers"[3] or collaborative remixers. Producers of any remix understand that once their product leaves their hands and is distributed, others will potentially remix it, again and again. The form of the remix will change over time. It might grow in quality and cohesion over time through various iterations. Or it might morph into something completely unrecognizable, with very few elements to trace it back to the origin points (or it might wither and die from neglect). A meme might appear to have a life of its own as it morphs and changes. But it is negotiated, interactive. It is transformed and it transforms its users and creators.

Remix is an inherent part of digital culture. As we surf, we create momentary meaning structures, mini-remixes that get remixed again and again, every time we surf similarly, with different outcomes. Our own actions yield these remixes at one level, yet these remixes are influenced by many other factors.

Indeed, remix undergirds the infrastructures of everything we understand to be part of the Internet. As Navas points out (2012), Google is an excellent example of a very different sort of remix, one that selectively presents us with results based on a complex (and often hidden) set of algorithms. Amazon.com recommendations, YouTube's "related content," and Facebook feeds are likewise remixed for us, based on proprietary algorithms that function beneath the surface of activity. Remix may not be the only lens for thinking about this, but it highlights the ways that meaning, contexts, and structures can be seen as temporary outcomes of interaction, emerging and fading, morphing into something slightly new every time we engage.

Thinking about digital culture through the lens of remix offers powerful means of resisting the focus on individuals and objects to get closer to the flows and connection points between various elements of the media ecology system, where meaning and assemblages and imaginaries are negotiated in relation and (inter)action. At the meta-level, thinking about qualitative research practice through the framework of remix offers a means of reconfiguring some of the practices associated with qualitative research. It allows us to embrace and grapple with complexity (rather than trying to simplify) by focusing less on methods (as templates to either apply to experiences and organize these experiences into particular categories and structures) and more on meaning as derived from a creative process of inquiry.

My application of remix as a concept embraces the essence of bricolage, as described by Kincheloe (2001, 2005). Extending the concept of bricolage, remix focuses on everyday practices of enacting method, as well as the way inquiry is—or can be—situated within a Web 2.0, social media-saturated, remix culture. Remix focuses our attention on the way temporally situated arguments are assembled and reassembled as they traverse various audiences. Each of these renderings has meaning and will be assessed by the reader/viewer/listener, but the quality and credibility of each is not predetermined by the way the data (cultural material) is collected, or the tools used to manage, sort, and categorize this data into something that can then be reorganized and edited by the remixer. Rather, quality is embedded in the extent to which the production (whether we call it argument, story, or finding) demonstrates resonance with the context, and also has resonance with the intended audience.

Instead of marginalizing the concepts of copy/cut & paste, collage, pastiche, and mashup, these practices become resonant and thus appropriate lenses for thinking about cultural formations as well as adaptive modes of inquiry. By letting go of the idea that our academic projects should provide answers, remix provides the researcher with a greater freedom to build creative and compelling arguments that enter larger conversations, both inside and outside the academy.[4]

This approach also tackles the difficulty of accomplishing the practices that Latour (2005) and others advocate through actor network theory. As Latour notes:

> Any given interaction seems to overflow with elements which are already in the situation coming from some other time, some other place, and generated by some other agency. This powerful intuition is as old as the social sciences. As I have said earlier, action is always dislocated, articulated, delegated, translated. Thus, if any observer is faithful to the direction suggested by this overflow, she will be led away from any given interaction to some other places, other times, and other agencies that appear to have molded them into shape. (2005, p. 166)

Remix is a way of following the overflow, being willing to flatten the social by considering all elements to be equal, without trying to identify individuals or contexts or distinguish the local from the global. The outcome of one's activities—if considered an act of making an argument—influences one's process in that it matters less where one begins or ends, because patterns and possibilities always emerge. It also shifts one from matters of fact to matters of concern.

Looking under Methods to Find Remix Practices: An Experiment in Play

A significant percentage of scholars who study digital culture, Internet-mediated contexts, or social media are new to qualitative inquiry. This is an important consideration when it comes to imagining the common models informing the definitional parameters for how qualitative inquiry gets done. Even when defined as a non-positivist process, procedures still retain linear and compartmentalized foundations. One begins with a phenomenon that informs one's research questions, which, in turn, inform particular strategies for data collection, analysis, and interpretation. Various stages are described as separate moments, and findings are written up at the end. Although the process can be displayed as iterative, the fundamental working metaphors are not nearly as innovative as those of us with extensive background or experience with innovative qualitative inquiry might imagine.

From the standpoint of researchers entrenched in positivist forms of inquiry, understanding the strength of interpretive qualitative inquiry requires going back to the basic question: What do we do when we engage in qualitative inquiry? These are the five elements of remix:

Generate
Move
Play
Borrow
Interrogate

These terms have proven very successful in cross-disciplinary workshops exploring innovative or creative approaches, as they help disconnect the practice of inquiry from methodological or epistemological baggage. These five activities of inquiry actually look a lot like what we might think people are doing when they are engaged in the practice of remix. Each of these terms will be conceptualized and operationalized in different ways for any researcher, depending on his or her perspective, discipline, project, and so forth. Likewise, the terms will take on different meaning at different stages of the project. Thus, the following brief descriptions of each term serve as only a starting point, illustrating how I might situate these terms in my own world of research.

Generate

When I think of this term, I immediately visualize the physical stacks of material that would collect on my desk over the course of a study. It was easier to understand what the term meant when the stuff of our research was more physically noticeable. The changing dimensions—in width and height—of the stack over time would indicate a state of progress. The more I investigated, the more stuff was generated: draft documents, field notes, concept maps, sketchbooks full of doodles, photos, and drawings, notes on literature I was reading, printed copies of theory and concept articles, untouched transcripts from interviews, the same transcripts coded the first time, the same transcripts coded a second time or in a different way, and on and on. I considered this teetering pile a treasure trove, full of data. Picking up random objects might trigger certain connections among ideas. Flipping open a research journal might spark a memory and open a floodgate of new information to consider. This wonderful chaos of inquiry is less visible when we work digitally. Much of this generative quality of inquiry is forgotten, never experienced, or lost.

We might think about the process of generating as one whereby we transform data according to different thematic classification schemes. Every iteration of this presents a new (in that it is different) data set, which represents the phenomenon in a new way. *The act of transformation is one of interpretation and remix.* Likewise, we generate a "new" participant every time we transform their raw activities into a different form, such as a written text, an edited version of their talk, a grammatically corrected version of their discourse, or a summary of themes emerging from their activities and interactions. Reflecting on these and other practices, we can see that inquiry is not only about simplifying and narrowing, but generating layers upon layers of informational units that influence our interpretations. Focusing only on the first layer of data (the original stuff we collected) doesn't allow us to fully appreciate what is actually at play when we engage in the long, involved, inductive, and explorative art and science of "writing culture."

When this inherent generative process is understood, it can enable fuller analysis of multiple layers of meaning. Simply put, more stuff is laid out on the table to be considered as data.

Play

Play is sometimes a guided or rule-driven activity, as when we play games. At other times, play is an open-ended leisure activity, as when we play with or play around. It's easy to see remix as a product of both types of play. As a process of inquiry, remix relies on experimenting with various combinations of elements to produce something meaningful. Successful remixes are inventive and often yield outcomes that seem quite new, despite the fact that the elements that are being combined are borrowed from other sources. So remix is a highly open-ended process. And, like most artistic endeavors, passion and innovation work in tandem with the skillful if not expert performance of one's art/craft. At the same time, most remix occurs in a larger community of remix, where certain goals and guidelines apply.

In academic contexts, we have been far less willing to characterize research as play, or playful (see Ellingson, this volume). Particularly if one's practices are closely directed or controlled by outside forces such as supervisors or funders, play may seem a disrespectful, lazy, or non-rigorous form of activity. In qualitative inquiry, this is a mistake, since what we do in the best moments of the interpretive process is just that. As any athlete or musician will say, getting in the zone of play or engaging in improvisation requires at least some element of skillful application of certain techniques and also functions as an important tool for honing one's skills. Curiosity and exploration mark a significant type of play. Experimentation without any particular purpose allows the researcher to move beyond what is already known to a point of learning, making new connections. Imaginative play allows one to let go of what ought to be done or thought and work in the realm of possibilities. As Marantz Henig (2008, para. 39) notes, "[f]or all its variety … there is something common to play in all its protean forms: variety itself. The essence of play is that the sequence of actions is fluid and scattered." Bekoff likewise describes play as "training for the unexpected. … Behavioral flexibility and variability is adaptive; in animals it's really important to be able to change your behavior in a changing environment" (in Marantz Henig, 2008, para. 39).

In terms of exploring complex social media contexts, play can actually become a critical turning point for research design that resonates better with contexts of flow, analysis that moves with or into these flows rather than abstracting and isolating objects arbitrarily and artificially, finding forms of representation that have contextual integrity and finding rather than simply applying conceptual models that help make sense of these phenomena.

Borrow

In the context of copyright, Lessig (2008) reminds us that a basic foundation of writing is quoting from other works. Referring to the writing of a particular individual, he says, "Were it music, we'd call it sampling. Were it painting, it would be called collage. Were it digital, we'd call it remix" (p. 51). In academic research, borrowing is essential, in this and other ways. To make sense of any phenomenon, we borrow all the time, whether or not we recognize it. We borrow ideas about sampling strategies, genres of writing, tools for analyzing data, and so forth.

As I take short-term engagements at various universities, I often end up sitting for days, weeks, or months in other scholars' offices. While I think or write, I wander around the offices of computer scientists, feminist technoscientists, linguists, postphenomenological theorists, or actor network theorists, gazing at the titles on their bookshelves. Flipping through books, gazing at art on walls, and reading articles left on desktops, it's no surprise I find a lot of useful concepts, theories, and phrases that I would never otherwise encounter. Through serendipity, I make new connections and find alternate perspectives. All of this broadens my perspectives, no matter the topic.

Of course, it's messy when I leave the comfort of my home discipline to struggle with new concepts. But it makes good sense when I consider the target of my inquiry. Most aspects of Internet-related phenomena occur across multiple platforms, media, and/or devices. Interactions that seem cohesive or complete are just partial traces of interactions, abstracted from lived experience, displaced in time and space. When we consider the way in which people use and relate to technologies for communication, the variation is endless. Borrowing approaches, perspectives, and techniques from not only outside one's discipline but from outside the academy seems not only natural but essential to figuring out creative ways to grapple with these contexts.

Move

Everything discussed above, whether applied to the activities of remix or the activities of qualitative inquiry, is about moving and being moved. Inquiry is always situated, but never motionless. This is an important thing to remember, particularly in globally entangled networks of cultural flow that comprise ever-shifting terrains of meaning. George Marcus (1998) uses the term "follow" to describe creative ways to engage in multi-sited ethnography: Follow the story, follow the people, follow the metaphors. We can add to this many other ways of thinking about following: shifting one's perspective, changing the questions, moving in and out of the flows of information, following the silences, gaps, and absences.

In many ways, what's most important is not how one moves but acknowledging that movement is inevitable, natural, and productive. It is also not necessarily forward, in that many movements will take us back to the beginning or will cause us to see the entire project in different ways, forcing us to mark our current point as a new beginning to move from.

Interrogate

Successful remix interrogates pieces of culture, torquing and integrating them into something unique so the audience can see each piece or the whole in a different way. This has happened throughout time, in literature, painting, architecture, design, film, music, and so forth. Now, we see it in fan fiction, mashup videos, street art, Internet memes—everywhere we see the production of culture, we know we are witnessing the outcome of a process of reflexive interrogation.

Perhaps interrogate seems too forceful to describe the act of reflexively questioning everything we're doing, seeing, feeling, or everything about the project and the phenomenon itself. I use this term to highlight that any close reading, detailed analysis, or inductive interpretation requires a steady stream of questioning. Sometimes we direct this interrogation at the object, to see how it is situated, to focus on what surrounds, embraces, encompasses, or encloses it, to wonder how it might look or be otherwise, to think about its existence in time and space. At other times, we direct this interrogation inward, to consider why we're interested in this and not another phenomenon, to ask how we are situated in relation to this stuff of our curiosity, to consider how we might think otherwise, by focusing critically on what surrounds, embraces, encompasses, or encloses us. This constant questioning may not be directly acknowledged as part of one's method, but it comprises a powerful everyday practice of all inquiry. Noticing it allows us to get better at doing it well, with purpose, and to incorporate the processes and products of our interrogations more clearly, or rigorously.

Searching for Resonance

These five elements of remix—generating, playing, borrowing, moving, and interrogating—usefully resist disciplining and can prompt more freedom to innovate when exploring contexts that defy easy encapsulation. As with bricolage or layered accounts (see Rambo Ronai, 1995), remix presumes that the resulting pastiche will never constitute a complete or whole picture. Rather, each outcome is an iterative rendering. Each is a work in progress. All are possibilities. Each builds on the others, informs the others, and influences the overall perspective one ends up with at the end. This is an unending process, one that invites conversation, collaboration, and further remixing. Remixes might show connections among elements or present a beautifully cohesive piece, as we see in Eric Whitacre's virtual choirs (http://ericwhitacre.com/the-virtual-choir). Or remixes can illustrate juxtaposition, disjuncture, or discontinuity. Rather than trying to resolve complexity in the research project, a remix might illustrate very clearly the irresolvable complexity of the phenomenon.

To be sure, questions of quality and credibility arise. There are many ways to think about criteria for quality,[5] but here I just mention one: The most successful remixes are those that have longevity and can be seen by many to hold a mark of quality. Whether this quality is closely analyzed by experts or simply felt by cultural members, and whether this quality is in the way something is made or in the story it tells, it likely has something to do with how much the product resonates. Successful remix reaches beyond the merely sufficient to the monumental. Ethical, context-sensitive, creative research does the same, if, in the end, it captures the attention of the reader, moves the reader to think differently, or causes the reader to want to engage, contribute further to the conversation, and continue the playful process of remix.

Notes

1 For more information and to view video, go to http://www.youtube.com/watch?v=ThvBJMzmSZI

2 Also inspired by the work of Lashua and Fox (2007), using remix as a method of action research.

3 "Produser" and "prosumer" are both terms that have come to represent the collapsed roles of producers and users and producers and consumers.

4 This sort of work has long been projects of Yvonna Lincoln and Norman Denzin (e.g., 1994, 2003), Art Bochner and Carolyn Ellis (e.g., 2003), Laurel Richardson (e.g., 1994), and many others who comprise the late 20th-century interpretive movement in the United States.

5 See, for example, various writers in Denzin and Lincoln's *Handbook of Qualitative Research* (all editions, published by Sage). Questions of criteria for quality are considered paramount and comprise a consistent theme throughout these volumes.

References

Bloggit, H. (2011). The world is changing—Tahrir Square revolution spreads (Jan. 27, NBC). http://www.youtube.com/watch?v=o-0Hm-n_LAM (accessed January 4, 2013).

Bochner, A., & Ellis, C. (2003). An introduction to the arts and narrative research: Art as inquiry. *Qualitative Inquiry, 9*, 506–514.

boyd, d. & Marwick, A. (2011). Social privacy in networked publics: Teens' attitudes, practices, and strategies. Unpublished manuscript. http://www.danah.org/papers/2011/SocialPrivacyPLSC-Draft.pdf (accessed August 11, 2011).

Deuze, M., Blank, P., & Speers, L. (2012). A life lived in media. *Digital Humanities Quarterly*, 6, para. 1–37.

Fergusen, K. (N.d.). Everything is a remix. (Four-part video series.) http://everythingisaremix.info (accessed January 4, 2013).

Gergen, K. (1991). *The saturated self: Dilemmas of identity in contemporary society.* New York: Basic Books.

Hayles, K. (2012). *How we think: Digital media and contemporary technogenesis.* Chicago: University of Chicago Press.

"Introducing Generation C: Americans 18-34 are the most connected." *Nielson.* (2012). http://blog.nielsen.com/nielsenwire/online_mobile/introducing-generation-c/ (accessed January 20, 2013).

Janesick, V. J. (1994). The dance of qualitative research design: Metaphor, methodolatry, and meaning. In N. K. Denzin & Y. S. Lincoln (Eds.), *Handbook of qualitative research* (pp. 209–219). Thousand Oaks, CA: Sage.

Kincheloe, J. (2001). Describing the bricolage: Conceptualizing a new rigor in qualitative research. *Qualitative Inquiry, 7*, 679–692.

Kincheloe, J. (2005). On to the next level: Continuing the conceptualization of the bricolage. *Qualitative Inquiry, 11*, 323–350.

Lashua, B. & Fox, K. (2007). Defining the groove: From remix to research in the beat of Boyle Street. *Leisure Sciences, 20*, 143–158.

Latour, B. (2005). *Reassembling the social. An introduction to actor network theory.* Oxford: Oxford University Press.

Latour, B., Jensen, P., Venturini, T., Grauwin, S., & Boullier, D. (2012). The whole is always smaller than its parts: A digital test of Gabriel Tarde's monads. *British Journal of Sociology, 63*, 590–615.

Lessig, L. (2008). *Remix: Making art and commerce thrive in the hybrid economy.* New York: Penguin Press.

Lincoln, Y. S. & Denzin, N. K. (1994). The fifth moment. In N. K. Denzin & Y. S. Lincoln (Eds.). *Handbook of qualitative research* (pp. 575–586). Thousand Oaks, CA: Sage.

Lincoln, Y. S. & Denzin, N. K. (2003). *Turning points in qualitative research: Tying knots in a handkerchief.* Thousand Oaks, CA: Sage.

Marantz Henig, R. (2008). Taking play seriously. *New York Times Magazine*, February 17. http://www.nytimes.com/2008/02/17/magazine/17play.html?pagewanted=all (accessed December 1, 2012).

Marcus, G. (1998). *Ethnography through thick and thin.* Princeton, NJ: Princeton University Press.

Markham, A. (2012). Fabrication as ethical practice: Qualitative inquiry in ambiguous Internet contexts. *Information, Communication, & Society, 15*, 334–353.

Markham, A. &. Buchanan, E. (2012). *Ethical decision-making and Internet research: Version 2.0. (Recommendations from the AoIR Ethics Committee.)* Chicago: Association of Internet Researchers.

Markham, A. (in press). Dramaturgy of digital experience. In C. Edgley (Ed.), *Handbook of dramatugry.* London: Ashgate Press.

Mason, J. (2011). Facet methodology: The case for an inventive research orientation. *Methodological Innovations Online, 6*, 75–92.

Navas, E. (2006). Remix: The bond of repetition and representation. http://remixtheory.net/?p=361 (accessed January 4, 2013).

Navas, E. (2012). *Remix theory: The aesthetics of sampling.* New York: Springer/Wein Press.

Nissenbaum, H. (2010). *Privacy in context: Technology, policy, and the integrity of social life.* Stanford, CA: Stanford Law Books.

Oldfather, P. & West, J. (1994). Qualitative research as jazz. *Educational Researcher, 23*, 22–26.

Rambo Ronai, C. (1995). Multiple reflections of child sex abuse: An argument for a layered account. *Journal of Contemporary Ethnography, 23*, 395–426.

Rheingold, H. (2002). *Smart mobs: The next social revolution.* New York: Basic Books.

Richardson, L. (1994). Writing: A form of inquiry. In N. K. Denzin & Y. S. Lincoln (Eds.), *Handbook of qualitative research* (pp. 516–529). Thousand Oaks, CA: Sage.

Shaaban, T. (2011). The Most AMAZING video on the internet #Egypt #jan25. YouTube video. http://www.youtube.com/watch?v=ThvBJMzmSZI (accessed January 4, 2013).

Turkle, S. (2011). *Alone together: Why we expect more from technology and less from each other.* New York: Basic Books.

Chapter 14

Dangerous Ethnography

D. Soyini Madison

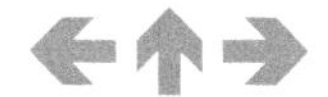

The Merriam-Webster pocket electronic dictionary describes "dangerous" as an adverb, defining it first as: (1) hazardous, perilous (a dangerous slope); and second as: (2) able or likely to inflict injury (a dangerous man)

—Madison

I. Three Vignettes

1. It was 1988, my first year teaching at the University of North Carolina (UNC) at Chapel Hill. My advisor, Dwight Conquergood, had flown in from Northwestern University in Evanston, Illinois, to give final approval of what I hoped would be the last draft of my dissertation. The dissertation needed to be completed within a few weeks for me to be awarded the Ph.D. that year and to be promoted from lecturer to assistant professor at UNC (this was the agreement UNC mandated on my hire). While Dwight was managing all-nighters proofing dissertation chapters at my kitchen table and I was running back and forth between my study and the kitchen giving him chapter

Originally published in *Qualitative Inquiry and Social Justice*, edited by Norman K. Denzin and Michael D. Giardina, pp.186–197. Republished in *Qualitative Inquiry—Past, Present, and Future: A Critical Reader*, edited by Norman K. Denzin and Michael D. Giardina, pp. 261–271. Left Coast Press, Inc.

after revised chapter, hot off the computer, one night we took a break from the intensity of dissertation deadline madness and started talking about the nature of fieldwork and the notion of a "dangerous ethnography."

Earlier that morning, Dwight went to campus with me to talk to a group of people who were interested in his fieldwork with Chicago street gangs. At the end of his presentation, the familiar question rose again: "Professor Conquergood, you are involved in very dangerous work with some very dangerous characters—are you safe?" Dwight, affectionately referred to in those days as the "Indiana Jones" of performance studies, was asked versions of this question time after time. At my kitchen table that night, he slowly shook his head and quietly said, "With these communities and entire families in peril, everyone is more worried about the lone white man."

2. Ten years later, in 1998, as an associate professor I was on my way to Ghana, West Africa, to conduct fieldwork with local human rights activists. Before I left for Ghana, the investigative television news magazine *60 Minutes* aired a feature on a traditional cultural practice in a particular region of Ghana where the reporter depicted innocent women and girls being forced and condemned to village shrines where they were placed in bondage as reparation for a crime committed by a family member, usually a male. After the *60 Minutes* program, when I mentioned to certain individuals that I was going to Ghana to research human rights in the rural areas, the response was "Be careful, Soyini, it is dangerous there. They steal women and put them in shrines." An entire country had been reduced to a unique location with no critical questions regarding the *60 Minutes* representation or concern for the women and girls reported.

3. Now, in 2008, as a full professor, I remember a transatlantic phone call from my student Hannah Blevins several years ago. I was in Ghana continuing my fieldwork on human rights and local activism and Hannah was in southern Appalachia in the last stages of her fieldwork to complete her dissertation on the cultural economy of the coal mining community and black lung disease. Hannah called from Tennessee to tell me she was going down

into one of the mines that had recently been closed. Her purpose was to see for herself where so many miners had worked and died. I was silent, but my immediate thought was, "No, you cannot, it is too dangerous." Sensing my fear through the phone, Hannah said it would be safe. She said experienced miners would guide her and protect her through the passageways of the mine. We talked for a bit. Hannah *did* go deep into the mine and completed a brilliant dissertation. But while she was thousands of feet below ground in a closed mine—to go where the miners had gone, to enter the risky knowledge of the body—I was on the other side of the Atlantic thinking of her and in fear of the danger.

II. Flipping the Script on Danger: Danger in Reverse

What if we stop for a moment and rethink the "dangerous"? What if we were to consider putting the dangerous in reverse? Instead of conventionally positioning the dangerous inside the field, what might happen if we think of *ourselves* as being dangerous? What if danger is no longer somewhere "out there" in the field? What if we carry danger with us, embody it, and carry it with us *into* the field? Consider the option that we, ourselves, could be dangerous. Consider what it might mean to be an *agent* of danger, what it might mean to become dangerous ethnographers doing dangerous ethnography. "Flip the script" and reposition the dangerous from individuals or communities that are and can be dangerous to some of us (i.e., a street gang member, a shrine in the Third World, a restricted coal mine) to now include the structures of power that generate and sustain what is systematically dangerous to *all* of us: systematic poverty, the machinery of imperialism, structures of homophobia, and phallocentric power. What if we were dangerous to the force of these dangers? What if we were dangerous to the systematic abuse of power? What if we were to be perpetrators of danger to that which is dangerous to our universal well-being?

The street gang member, a village shrine, and a restricted coal mine are dangers at the surface; structures of urban poverty, phallocentrism, imperialism, and homophobia are dangers at the root. An ethnography that labors to injure the foundation and the root cause of what is dangerous and that is not diverted by its symptoms or surfaces of danger might contemplate a new appropriation of danger. We can speak truth to power and we can also be dangerous to its perpetuation and continued abuse. Don't get me wrong: We must and should pay attention to the dangers at the tip and the surface, because they are no small matters. A troubled gang member, a shrine of slaves, and a restricted coal mine legitimately invoke fear and are dangerous at a number of levels. *Both* root and surface are forceful, significant, and scary. A dangerous ethnography seeks to enter surfaces, but, moreover, enters what is often hidden in plain sight—the convolutions and complications below the surface, the systems that generate and keep surfaces in place.

We will keep listening with our hearts and minds to the poignant ethnographic accounts of Darfur because the human horror is too great for us not to hear or care. A dangerous ethnography will carry those stories forth while not ignoring how oil money funds government weapons, how the militias are aligned with national and transnational exploitation, and how ignorance is warming the globe and drying up the land to spark one of the most vicious ethnic conflicts in recent history. Every story about the horror of Darfur is not only a story of human suffering that must be heard, it is also about oil and the warming of our planet. Another example of dangerous ethnography might include entering various urban dance communities to examine how everyday city life is identified, sustained, contested, and remade through the labor, imagination, and global connections of community dance dancers. A dangerous ethnography is reflected in the work of Judith Hamera, who unearthed the urban political infrastructures of dance to critique and complicate notions of difference, cosmopolitanism, the distributions of urban space, and the politics of globality and urban migration. Another example is the intimate ethnography of Della Pollock and her retelling of birth stories, documenting them as reperformances of how men and women recast the ritual of giving birth. Within the poetics of birth narratives, Pollock lends a penetrating analysis of U.S. medical discourse, reproductive technologies, and the tensive intersections of maternity, sexuality, and reproduction as well as how pain is constituted and represented.

My plea is for us not only to speak truth to power but also to put power in peril, in jeopardy, to endanger it. This all comes quite frankly from being weary of being angry. I have made up my mind in my golden years that I shall aim to be a danger to dangerous power, from the tip to the root, from the surface to the foundation.

III. The Body as Bearing Witness

I will argue that a *dangerous ethnography* does not begin with interventions on political economies or structures of the state or the nation, on global capitalism or corporate greed, or even on ideologies of neoliberalism or fundamentalism—these are the targets of a dangerous ethnography (with some complication) but they are not the starting point, not the inspiration. My inspiration for a dangerous ethnography begins with performance—that is, the body in performance.

In performance studies, we do a lot of talking about the body. For performance ethnographers, this means we must embrace the body not only as the feeling/sensing home of our being—the harbor of our breath—but the vulnerability of how our body must move through the space and time of another—transporting our very being and breath—for the purpose of knowledge, for the purpose of realization and discovery. Body knowledge, knowledge through the body, is evidence of the present. It is the truth that I exist with you—with myself—right here, right now. Further, it is evidence that I am not anywhere, I am not nowhere, I am not over yonder, I am not absent. I am not dead. I am alive here and now and I am vulnerable to this feeling/sensing present moment. My body breathes here unmediated and unprotected. The Other can reach across me and touch my wounds, can feel the beating of my heart, can hear my nervous breathing, can strike me down and make my blood flow.

This is intersubjective vulnerability in existential and ontological order, because bodies rub against one another flesh to flesh in a marked present and where we live on and between the extremes of life and death. Another can love me and another can kill me; I can love and kill in the corporeal present tense of another. I cannot live or die in my body's absence—I can only die and live in the present moment, in the presence of my body, and where my body is present. The immortality of the soul withstanding, we end when our bodies end and we begin when our bodies begin—body presence with another is fraught with intersubjective risks.

So what is my point? The point is that where my body is I am vulnerable to the radical extremes of life and death; the point is that where my body is I am vulnerable to the disgust and desire of all my senses; and finally, the point is that because my body is vulnerable to life and death in this particular ethnographic moment as well as the penetrating depths of its sensual meanings, I am living evidence that this moment, in this time and space, does exist and I am a surviving witness to its living realities of life and death and the infinite in-between. This is why, for better and for worse, we say: "Are you safe?" "Is it dangerous?" "I am afraid for you."

So how is the body specifically implicated in a dangerous ethnography? The body must testify, it must speak—it must provide a report—it must bear witness to the surfaces and the foundations, the symptoms and the causes.

"What should I do with what I have witnessed?" I have strong responses to what I witnessed during my fieldwork. These responses demanded that I be responsible for providing an opportunity for others to also gain the *ability* to respond in some form.[1] I bear witness and in bearing witness I do not have the singular response-ability for what I witness but the responsibility of invoking a response-ability in others to what was seen, heard, learned, felt, and done in the field and through performance. As Kelly Oliver states, "We have an obligation not only to respond but also to respond in a way that opens up rather than closes off the possibility to respond by others" (2001, pp. 18–19). Steven Durland says, "A person who bears witness to an injustice takes responsibility for that awareness. That person may then choose to do something or stand by, but he may not turn away in ignorance" (1987, p. 65).

Response, response-ability, and responsibility became aligned with advocacy and ethics. To be an advocate is to feel a responsibility to exhort and appeal on behalf of another or for another's cause with the hope that still more others will gain the ability to respond to your advocacy agenda. Being an advocate has a different intent than speaking in the manner of a ventriloquist, in the sense of muting Other voices to only amplify one's own. Being an advocate is to actively *assist* in the struggles of others, or (and) it is learning the tactics, symbols, and everyday forms of resistance of which the subaltern *enact* but "do not speak" (Spivak, 1988) so that they may provide platforms for which their struggles can be known and heard.[2] As advocates, we aim for a cycle of responses that will set loose a stream of response-abilities that will lead to something more, something of larger philosophical and material effects.

In addition, the position of advocate and the labor of advocacy are riddled with the pleasure and burden of representation that is always already so much about ethics. Advocates represent who and what they are advocating for: their names, narratives, histories, and their logics of persuasion as well as imagining what more is needed in the service of advocacy. All this requires labor that is entrenched in power relations and representations that are inextricable to ethics. Representation happens at different points along power's spectrum—we are all "vehicles and targets" of power's contagion and omnipresence.[3] As advocates, surrounded by the far and wide entanglements of power's disguises and infinite forms, we aim to invoke a response to its consequences—a response-ability—to its operations. In doing the work of advocacy, whether we consider ethics or not, it is always already present within the horizons of representation and the machinations of power. Because ethics requires responsibility (and the ability to respond), it is inherently antithetical to apathy.

If apathy cannot rest beside the ethical responsibility to respond and if ethics also includes providing opportunities for others to gain access to the ability to respond, then performance can form a vibrant and efficacious partnership with ethics. Ethics and advocacy now pave the way as we move from the field to the stage. Stage performance becomes a dynamic space where response-ability, advocacy, and ethnics are heightened and ultimately culminate.

The fieldwork data *travel* to the public stage with the hope that the performance will invoke a response (ability) among a group or spectators. It is said that theater and performance *show ourselves to ourselves* in ways that help us recognize our behavior and life worlds as well as the behavior and life worlds of others, for better or worse, as well as our/Others' unconscious needs and desires. Victor Turner said, "When we act in everyday life we do not merely re-act to indicative stimuli, we act in frames wrested from the genres of cultural performance" (1982, p. 122). He also said:

> It might be possible to regard the ensemble of performative and narrative genres, active and acting modalities of expressive culture as a hall of mirrors, or better magic mirrors. ... In this hall of mirrors the reflections are multiple, some magnifying, some diminishing, some distorting the faces peering into them, but in such a way as to provoke not merely thought, but also powerful feelings and the will to modify everyday matters in the minds of the gazers, for not one likes to see himself as ugly, ungainly, or dwarfish. Mirror distortions of reflection provoke reflexivity. (p. 105)

These performances not only reflect who we are, they shape and direct who we are and what we can become. The major work of performance ethnography is to make performances that do the labor of advocacy and do it ethically to inspire realms of reflection and responsibility. Bertolt Brecht reminds us that performance must also proceed beyond that of a mirror reflection to become the hammer that breaks the mirror, distorts the reflection, to build a new reality. Brecht's charge to "build a new reality" leads us closer to a methodology of *dangerous ethnography* and beckons the need for utopian performatives.

IV. Utopian Performatives

Performance scholar Jill Dolan reminds us that utopian performatives aim for "a different future, one full of hope and reanimated by a new, more radical humanism." She goes on to state that a Utopian Performative is capable of lifting us "above the present, into a hopeful feeling of what the world might be like" and that it is always already "a 'doing' in linguistic philosopher J. L. Austin's sense of the term, something that in its enunciation *acts*—that is, performs an action as tangible and effective as saying 'I do' in a wedding ceremony" (Dolan, 2005, pp. 5–6; emphasis in the original). Therefore we may understand Utopian Performance, in their "doings," as making palpable an affective vision of how the world might be better.

What is significant here is that Dolan is rearticulating the move from the ideal fantasy of Utopia in the Marxist sense by asserting that the utopian is "historical," it is "*this*-worldly" and involves human agency (Bamer, 1992, p. 6). That is, as Bamer states, we need to

> replace the idea of a Utopia as something fixed, a form to be fleshed out, with the idea of "the Utopian" as an *approach toward*, a movement beyond set limits into the realm of the not-yet-set. At the same time, I want to counter the notion of the utopian as unreal with the proposition that the utopian is powerfully real in the sense that hope and desire (and even fantasy) are real, never "merely" fantasy. It is a force that moves and shapes history. (Bamer, quoted in Dolan, 2005, pp. 5–6; emphasis added)

This notion of a utopian performative is articulated as a characteristic of the theater and stage performance but it is also appropriated by performance ethnographers and, I would argue, is the very motivation and inspiration leading us toward a dangerous ethnography. Adapting the philosophy of a utopian performative means that danger is not simply a threat to life but a praxis toward a better life and future that moves us from "as is" to "what if." I will now outline how a utopian performative, within critical performance ethnography, "flips the script" on danger through the ontology of performance.

First, performance invites us to understand the body as its own evidence. Our research is radically animating the intersubjective (corporeal) vulnerability of a particular present. We are not only participant-observers with Others, but flesh-to-flesh co-performative witnesses in the risky business of a contagious desire, passion, and urgency that affects us all, propelling back and forth between us/among us through our feeling/sensing vulnerable bodies. The utopian performative of a dangerous ethnography does not simply observe but bears the responsibility of witnessing, and it does not simply participate but embodies performance with a deeply felt sensing empathy.

Second, performance invites us to understand that "bearing witness" is a form of truth. The truth of not what precisely happened here but what profoundly and phenomenologically happened here to me, to us—to an/Other. It is a different measure than quantifying accuracy, because it constitutes the multiple makings of subjectivity and the emotional processes of witnessing, not for witnessing sake but for politics and praxis. Bearing witness to the culminating affects/effects of social live and symbol-making in action and the living narrative(s) that swirl within and against the creation and consequence of life and symbol are different encounters and challenges than the culminating answers, numbers, and checked boxes held as evidence, as more true.

Third, performance invites us to understand that the performative is always and already about a doing—a doing that transforms a reality. Again, "the performative is something that in its enunciation *acts*," makes action and makes action possible in its "affective dimensions" (Dolan, 2005, p. 5).

V. Coda

> *The current historical moment requires morally informed performance and arts-based disciplines that will help people recover meaning in the face of senseless, brutal violence, violence that produces voiceless screams of terror and insanity.*
>
> —N. K. Denzin, 2003

My hope is that we strive to be a danger to "the face of senseless, brutal violence" in the creation of its demise and that the "violence that produces voiceless screams of terror and insanity" (Denzin, 2003, p. 7), endangered by utopian performatives and our labors of love for the future, comes to an unalterable end, but, like a troubled memory and a regrettable history, inspires the words "ever again."

Notes

1 This concept draws from Kelly Oliver (2001).

2 This is a reference to Gayatri Chakravorty Spivak's classic essay, "Can the Subaltern Speak?" (1988). I am appropriating Spivak here to assert the temporalities of speaking within indigenous locations where the subaltern speaking subject escapes and/or transgresses the bounds of allowed speech constituted by Western epistemologies and venues.

3 I am drawing here from Michel Foucault's articulation of power as set forth primarily in *Discipline and Punish* (1991).

References

Bamer, A. (1992). *Partial visions: Feminism and utopianism in the 1970s*. London: Routledge.

Denzin, N. K. (2003). *Performance ethnography: Critical pedagogy and the politics of culture*. Thousand Oaks, CA: Sage.

Dolan, J. (2005). *Utopia in performance: Finding hope at the theater*. Ann Arbor: University of Michigan Press.

Durland, S. (1987). Witnessing: The guerrilla theater of Greenpeace. In J. Cohen-Cruz (Ed.), *Radical street performance*, p. 65. New York: Routledge.

Foucault, M. (1991). *Discipline and punish: The birth of the prison* (trans. A. Sheridan). London: Penguin.

Oliver, K. (2001). *Witnessing: Beyond recognition*. Minneapolis: University of Minnesota Press.

Spivak, G. C. (1988). Can the subaltern speak? In C. Nelson & L. Grossberg (Eds.), *Marxism and the interpretation of culture*, pp. 271–313. Champaign: University of Illinois Press.

Turner, V. (1982). *From ritual to theatre: The human seriousness of play*. New York: PAJ.

Chapter 15

Performative Writing

The Ethics of Representation in Form and Body

Ronald J. Pelias

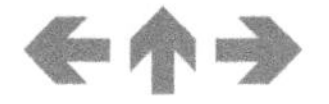

Performative writing, like other modes of qualitative inquiry, makes a bid as an alternative form of scholarly research. Such a bid often works by definitional opposition to positivist, objectivist logics that, as the argument goes, remain trapped in the Cartesian mind/body split. Work that is not qualitative is often called out as being cold and heartless, unreflective, unreadable and unread (boring), misguided, elitist, unethical, or simply wrong headed. Such name calling may seem a caricature when one remembers that objectivists operate from a desire to minimize, but not deny, the influence of researchers on those they study, to privilege others at the expense of themselves, and to predict so that they might take reasoned actions in the world. The "devil," dressed in such clothing, may not be as frightening a figure as qualitative researchers often suggest. Qualitative scholars feel that what is driving the uneasiness most likely comes from the devil's rejection of their claims to legitimacy. Earning legitimacy, however, does not have to come by constituting a devil and then calling for its demise. I would rather not make the case for qualitative inquiry in oppositional terms, although I have done so in the

Originally published in *Ethical Futures in Qualitative Inquiry*, edited by Norman K. Denzin and Michael D. Giardina, pp.181–196. Republished in *Qualitative Inquiry—Past, Present, and Future: A Critical Reader*, edited by Norman K. Denzin and Michael D. Giardina, pp. 272–287.

past (Pelias, 1999, 2004). Suffice it to say that I believe qualitative scholars proceed in a different way, a way that offers insights into human behavior and works on behalf of social justice. If I am correct, I am happy to be engaged in this line of scholarship. In particular, I have found performative writing a most appealing and productive research strategy.

This chapter, however, is not a celebration of performative writing, although I remain ready to toss the confetti at the performative writing dance. Instead of tossing confetti, I take this opportunity to tell a cautionary tale in the back corner of the performative writing festivities. My design is not to spoil the performative writing party, but to enhance its ethical practice. This cautionary tale, then, is an inquiry into the ethics of performative writing but without any desire to stop the celebration. It locates performative writing by outlining its definitional complexities before identifying a number of ethical issues about performative writing as a representational form. I end the chapter with a performative writing oath. I see it as a personal guide and as an invitational call for ethical practice. Much of what I have to offer can be applied equally well to a number of other associated forms. As I make my case, I quote researchers who speak directly to performative writing, those who would encompass performative writing under their own labeling, and those who may feel uncomfortable with my application of their ideas. To the last group, I apologize and hope that my borrowing is seen as a tribute to the productivity of their offerings.

Locating Performative Writing

Performative writing is a slippery term, in part because it resists its own containment. It is always writing and performing its way against satisfied representations. At its core, performative writing is an intervention in the crisis of representation. The intervention may stake its claim as a better, but never complete, form of representation, as an ongoing critique of representation's seduction, or as a continual, but never attainable, effort to escape language's hegemonic force. Despite this commonality, scholars, who have wed these two close, but at times squabbling, writing, and performing cousins, remain unsure of their own enunciation. "Performative" emerges as the contested cousin, even though "writing" carries its own troublesome history. Two differing, but not incompatible, conceptions of "performative" are prevalent, one that privileges "performative" as an adjective and the other that underlines it as a noun.

As an adjective, "performative" qualifies writing, telling what kind of writing is operative. In this usage, the page becomes a place where a performance can happen, where a writer can present for consideration a self speaking from the body, evocatively. The performance on the page parallels a performance on stage. It offers a bodily staging of a speaker—conceived variously—who engages personal, relational, cultural, historical, and political phenomena. Through monologue or dialogue, it makes present its topic, notes its investment, and is reflective and reflexive about its own workings. This ludic enterprise lives in the subjunctive, the "as if" (Turner, 1982, pp. 82–84), always holding itself up as a possibility. It "stands in" (Wilshire, 1982) for those who audience, offering language they may or may not claim as resonant. As it calls on the sensuous, the figurative, and the expressive, it is simultaneously confidant in and skeptical of language's abilities. Its speakers command, order, and trust in their linguistic constructions as well as mock, reject, and wrestle with their own efforts.

As a noun, "performative" is a speech act that accomplishes what it says (Austin, 1980). In this sense, language is a constitutive action, a productive mechanism that can reify and dismantle ongoing normative logics. Language, always repetitive and reiterative, is an obstinate discursive system, but it allows space for alternative possibilities, for disrupting the conventional and taken-for-granted, and for substantive change. As an utterance participating within or against performativity, a performative, then, is always partial and material. Its partiality speaks to its inadequacy; its materiality recognizes its force. When working to disturb and alter the normative, the performative labors in excess, engages in an ongoing play between presence and absence, and, in the doing, becomes a material intervention.

Thinking of "performative" as an adjective and a noun implies an emerging set of procedural precedents or stylistic conventions associated with performative writing. In this chapter, I rely on four organizing features of performative writing to begin the discussion of the ethical issues related to the form. I deploy the labels embodied, evocative, partial, and material as defining characteristics. Such a generic move may permit some organizational tidiness, but it obscures performative writing's power to perform against its own established boundaries. This reminder is in keeping with Pollock's (1998) caution before giving her own list (evocative, metonymic, subjective, nervous, citational, and consequential) of the "descriptive/prescriptive, practical/theoretical" characteristics of performative writing. She notes her intent is "to map directions/directives for performative writing without foreclosing on the possibility that performance may—at any moment—unhinge or override its claims" (Pollock, 1998, pp. 80–81). I use embodied, evocative, material, and partial in the same spirit, recognizing that the ethical issues discussed below are both prevalent and provisional.

The Ethics of Performative Writing's Form

Embodied

Performative writing's call for embodied speech is a bid to make the body relevant, a recovery gesture designed to intervene in the mind/body split. It asks the body to stand in for a number of perceived absences in traditional research practices. In general, the body is solicited to bring forth the researcher's presence. As Spry (2001) notes, "Performative writing composes the body into being. Such a praxis requires that I believe in language's representational abilities, thus putting my body at (the) stake" (p. viii). This interpellated presence takes four primary, and at times, combined forms, each carrying ethical pitfalls.

First, the body becomes a *troubling presence* by acknowledging that all claims are filtered, positioned, subjective, located in interaction, historical, cultural, and so on. The troubling presence is a nervous one, always questioning its own assertive rights, always reminding listeners to be leery of its claims, always turning back on itself to inquire: What, if anything, do I really know? What, if anything, can I claim without doing harm? The troubling presence emerges as humble, self-conscious, and self-effacing. In its reflexive move, however, it may take more space than it ethically requires or deserves. Those who encounter such accounts may wish researchers would simply get on with the claims they wish to make.

Second, the body is rendered as an *affective presence*. It is a container of our sensate and emotional beings. This affective presence speaks from and to the senses; it speaks of passions and feelings; it speaks from the heart. It offers a vulnerable self, exposed, presented bare for its personal and social curative value, for its articulation of a site for identification, and for its power as political intervention. The affective presence insists on its right to speak in its own register knowing that it may ridiculed, sacrificed, and dismissed. It finds comfort in Behar's (1996) claim that research "that doesn't break your heart isn't worth doing anymore" (p. 177). Such comfort, however, begs the ethical question of what should be told, of whose interests are privileged in the telling. It opens the door for those who would claim that the affective leads to self-indulgence, narcissism, and public therapy (Parks, 1998; Shields, 2000), to privileging self over others (Buzard, 2003; Hantzis, 1998; Madison, 2006), and to situating listeners into problematic stances (Terry, 2006). Such concerns, I believe, are misplaced. A more productive ethical question is what work is accomplished by an affective self.

Third, the body is brought forth as an *authentic presence*. As an authentic presence, it strives for an honest unfolding of self, a genuine display of the real, hidden self. The "true self" is there to be uncovered, probed, revealed. The authentic is what one deeply feels, what one seldom says. This construction carries the questionable assumptions that the authentic is found most fully in the hidden rather than in the typically shared, that the authentic is stable and unchanging, storied into coherence rather than always in flux and contingent, and that the authentic is something one possesses rather than something constituted in interaction. Regardless of how an authentic presence might be conceived, the ethical task reaches toward both self and other. As Guignon (2004) explains, "Authenticity is a personal undertaking insofar as it entails personal integrity and responsibility for self. But it also has a social dimension insofar as it brings with it a sense of belongingness and indebtedness to the wider social context that makes it possible" (p. 163). Embodied authenticity carries its greatest ethical force when it invites individual introspection as well as social deliberation and connection.

Fourth, the body emerges as a *political presence*. In doing so, it brings forward bodies that are marked differently, have been historically denied speech, and have been unrecognized and unacknowledged. The politically present body demands its rights in behalf of social justice, often placing itself at risk, often becoming a location where others can rally. It asserts its identity, claims its voice, refuses to back away. It also brings forward bodies that are familiar, normative, and privileged, in control of the legislative and material apparatus that makes their presence of little surprise. Such voices, if speaking on behalf of themselves, may seem selfish, unaware, calculating; if speaking on behalf of others, they may seem presumptuous, pedantic, and self-righteous. Making the body present is always a political act, raising the ethical questions of who gets to speak, who gets to speak for whom, and who should remain silent. Speaking for those who have been denied access can become an ethically silencing gesture. Failing to do so carries its own, more troubling, ethical risks.

These four presences articulate the body as a sensuous, originating center that situates speech in the felt, muscular, and somatic; as an identity marker, perhaps estranged, that requires personal and cultural negotiation; and as an authentic and truthful representation of self that can be deployed on behalf of oneself and others. When the body speaks as an originating center, it may assume that perception is direct, uncontaminated, untouched by historical and cultural circumstances. It may miss how the senses censor and contain. When it speaks as an identity marker, it stands in for others who may identify, but it places itself in danger. The self becomes vulnerable, subject to others' mercy and judgmental predilections, open to others' control and policing capabilities. The self emerges as "the person who …," a labeling that reduces the self into its identity claim. In some cases, the self is stigmatized, marked with suspect value and exposed to psychological and physical violence. As Ellis (2006) succinctly puts it, "You become the stories you write" (p. 20). Caught between the demand to tell and to be silent, the ethical choices weigh heavy on the body that performs its positionality. When the body speaks as an authentic representation of self, it reifies the mind/body spilt, exchanging the body for the mind. It forgets Gingrich-Philbrook's (2001) reminder that "cast[ing] 'the body' as performative writing's champion and 'language' as logic's, pitting them against one another … we jeopardize the mutuality of language and the body" (p. 1). It forgets, as Gingrich-Philbrook says, "My body makes language. It makes language like hair" (p. 3). When the body speaks as a political agent, its advocacy always comes at personal, cultural, and perhaps legislative cost. It is engaged in an exchange of power.

Evocative

Performative writing resides in the evocative, housed as an expressive and provocative form. As an expressive form, it summons the creative, the imaginative. It claims literary status. Its bid for the literary comes not only by reference to the various critical norms of poetry, prose, drama, and creative nonfiction, but also insists that the evocative be coupled with the embodied, partial, and material for its critical criteria. In other words, performative writing is its own form. To the extent, however, that it reaches for the literary it may be productive to ask if creative practices lead performative writers to compose with an affinity for, to use Lockford's (1998) distinction, "true *to* experience" rather than "true *in* experience" (p. 217; emphasis in the original). If so, performative writing confronts the same charges that fabricated memoirs such as James Frey's *A Million Little Pieces* and Binjamin Wilkomirski's *Fragments* face. To knowingly misrepresent when under the contract of truth telling is unethical. This principle carries significant weight for performative writing, a form of scholarly writing. To lie intentionally is the equivalent of falsifying data.

The notion of truth and lies, however, may become the target of performative writing, particularly when truth and lies are linked to power. The expressive task is to call into suspicion easy comfort in any narrative. Such work often takes away what it gives through an ongoing process of constant deferral and proliferating excess. Afraid of exchanging one system of power with another, performative writers may offer what Gunn (2006) calls a "shit-text," a text that stands as an endless generation of possibilities, but none sufficient, except, I would argue, its own implicit assumption of its own value. Although such writing celebrates the possible in its often witty and playful uncovering, it is hard to know where ethically to land, to decide what ethical action should be taken. Even so, such expressive displays are often provocative.

As a provocation, it is critical and rhetorical, challenging the status quo and calling for action. It is a speech act, a performative with the potential to stir, dismantle, and proliferate discursive systems. Prodding, always trying to change the direction of the herd, it persuades by bringing forward alternative pastures for our consumptive needs. Its efficacy depends on the evocative power of language to present imaginative visions against performativity's ongoing reiterations. The ethical burden, particularly given its playful textuality in constituting possibilities, is to become a counter-force, an animating center for social intervention. It runs the risk of never pointing beyond itself.

Partial

Performative writing recognizes that regardless of the number of possibilities one might generate, all accounts are partial, incomplete. There will always be slippages, gaps, and hauntings in any claim one might wish to make. Performative writing attempts to speak to those slippages, gaps, and hauntings by offering selves who, following a concentrated consideration of who they story themselves to be, are willing to stand by and question their commitments in the social world. As they do so, they write themselves and others.

Writing themselves, they construct speakers who, in their best renderings, are open, inquisitive, empathic, cautious, dialogic, and committed to social justice. In their worst articulations, they may appear disgruntled (nothing is right with the world), arrogant (my position is the only correct position), and saintly (see the good I do in the world). Equally problematic, a speaker will seldom appear who is unlikable, insincere, or unsympathetic, even when the speaker tells about his or her own social or moral inadequacies. Such limiting representations miss the potential, as Hoagland (2003) suggests, that "there is truth-telling, and more, in meanness" (p. 13). Hoagland desires a space where "the decency of the speaker" (p. 13) is not a predetermined or mandatory compositional strategy.

Writing others, like writing oneself, is always an exercise in partiality and always ethically inflected. Doty (2005), in discussing the memoir, offers an instructive summary of what is at stake:

> My picturing will distort its subject. ... This particular form of distortion—the inevitable rewriting of those we love we do in the mere act of describing them—is the betrayal build into memoir, into the telling of memories. ...The lives of other people are unknowable. Period. I wouldn't go so far as a poet colleague of mine who says that "representation is murder," but I would acknowledge that to represent is to maim. [p. 17]

He then adds, "But the alternative, of course, is worse: are we willing to lose the past, to allow it to be erased, because it can only be partially known?" (p. 17). Performative writing is caught in the same negotiation: how does one negotiate the rights of others with the rights of the individual to formulate his or her story, particularly when the self is understood, not as autonomous, but as a relational being? The writer, possessing the power of the pen, may be at less ethical risk than others but should not be neglected in our ethical considerations. We might ask: with what rights do writers write? Having raised that question, I want to turn to four ethical issues in the representation of others.

First, informed consent, the standard requirement of institutional review boards, is an essential but insufficient step. As Denzin (2003) rightly remarks, "Obtaining a person's signature on an informed consent form is not the same as demonstrating true respect" (p. 252). Participants, after giving their initial approval, may have recognize that they have agreed to more than they bargained for, may feel trapped by the emergent interpersonal relationship that at times develops between participants and researchers, or may decide that their participation requires disclosures they are uncomfortable making. Whatever the reason, following Ellis's (2006) counsel to engage in ongoing participant checks or even to consider co-constructed narratives is ethically sound. But even when researchers operate with such careful consideration, participants are unlikely to be aware of how they might feel once a piece receives response from an external audience. Anticipating the consequences of being rendered a particular way is at best difficult. Such was the case, for example, for the South Carolina students who appeared in the mock-documentary film, *Borat: Cultural Learnings of America for Make Benefit Glorious Nation of Kazakhstan*. Initially, they gave their consent and accepted payment for their participation, but after seeing how they were perceived, they filed a lawsuit. The lawsuit reads that the film "made plaintiffs the object of ridicule, humiliation, mental anguish and emotional and physical distress, loss of reputation, goodwill and standing in the community" (CNN.com, 2006). Such responses typically come, not in negotiation with researchers, but from viewing reception. Helping participants understand how their renderings might be seen becomes a researcher's obligation.

Second, negotiating facts when representing others is tricky business. As Eakin (2004) notes, criticism comes to writers "for not telling the truth" as well as "for telling too much truth" (p. 3). "Not telling the truth" and "telling too much" have a number of permutations. Intentional deception, as noted above, is a problematic stance for researchers. But the principle is not always easy to follow. Sometimes, researchers fail to tell the truth by omission. Such lies are often motivated by good reason—denied consent, fear of harming others, ideological sensitivity. Such reasons are no small matters but do not escape the problem of representing others in less than full light. Noting what cannot be told may at least make the light a bit brighter. Other times, researchers hide behind the production of truth (i.e., since "X" really happened, I am not responsible for the consequences of sharing it). Because a tale may be true, however, does not mean it serves a productive purpose in the world. It begs the question of how researchers should write with or against, partial though it may be, the discursive systems they confront.

Third, representations invite identification. This invitation may allow others to find their own voice and to take political action, but it may also permit false associations and lessened obligations. Constructing texts that essentialize attributes may encourage false associations by suggesting that the target audience shares the same position as the speaker. Duped into believing that the speaker is one of them, they allow the speaker to do their work, to become their surrogate, to shoulder their responsibilities.

Their identification is too easily claimed. Just as easily, identification may be too quickly dismissed. The reluctance or refusal to associate, to claim alliances, diminishes membership in the human community and weakens political will. Given such potential responses, performative writers should both establish commonality and demonstrate individuality. This charge is not only ethical but also fosters good writing. Representations also invite "disidentification" (Muñoz, 1999). Such is the case when writers offer a portrayal that audiences see enough similarities to recognize themselves but reject the depiction as fully resonant. Again, the ethical burden is to write toward marking commonality and specifying individuality.

Fourth, the failure to portray and the frequency of representation of others also lead performative writers to additional ethical considerations. People who are not rendered in a given account may feel slighted, surprised, or suspicious that the writer did not see their presence as essential to the tale. Some may wonder why a writer has not considered their relationship worthy of written commentary, particularly in situations in which they understand their relationship as close. Others may believe that they are occupying more space in a writer's work than they desire or merit. In extreme cases, they may feel that they are being stalked by the pen. Who to include and to what degree and who to omit in a given account requires relational and ethical consideration.

Do no harm, the common ethical adage offered to those who represent others, is not an easy task and begs the question of how harm might emerge. Partial renderings cannot be escaped but solipsism is not the corrective. Representation demands, more than anything else, an empathic sensibility, a move toward others that is relationally figured and practiced with compassion. As Doty (2005) suggests, writing "becomes, unexpectedly, an empathic adventure, a quest for trying to see into the lives of others. Even if such a 'seeing into' is by nature partial, an interpretive fiction, it's what we have" (p. 20). The simple but insufficient advice—don't share anything about a person you wouldn't share if that person were present—assumes an ethical desire and insists that empathy is the first mandate for ethical responsibility.

Material

Performative writing has consequences. It is taken in, processed, used. It carries a material force. Calling on the performative to pull against performativity's weight, it is both a material substance that locates its presence and an action in the world that articulates the unsaid, unnoticed, and unquestioned. It languages potential, by promising alternatives and propagating prospects. In this way, it is a "mobilizing praxis" that intervenes in language's endless deferral by "materializing possibility" (Pollock, 1998, p. 96). It pushes the unseen into the real, offering utopian visions and pedagogical exemplars. As a pedagogical practice, it turns "the performative into the political ... allow[ing] us to dream our way into a militant democratic utopian space" (Denzin, 2003, p. xiii). Such a critical performative pedagogy is, as Alexander (2005) explains, "radical and risky—radical in the sense that they [performative methods] strip away notions of a given human condition, and risky in that our sense of comfort in knowing the world is made bare" (p. 425). Performative writing embraces this risk in the name of social justice.

The desire for social justice, however, may require more than articulating possibilities. Opening possibilities may allow for action but may not be of much help to the transvestite who walks down the wrong street, the person of color who wants a quality school for his or her children, or the Sudanese people who daily confront genocide. Possibilities, in such situations, are a weak helping hand; they are necessary and productive but, in many cases, insufficient to alter material circumstances. Short of fostering legislative change, writing, no matter how provocative, may seem empty. Writer D. W. Fenza (2006) offers a chilling reminder:

> While intellectuals of the right engineered the conservative control of the House, Senate, White House, federal budget, tax codes, state courts, federal courts, news media, public opinion, and a few foreign nations, intellectuals of the left seized control of the Norton anthologies. Never before in the history of liberalism have so many words been spilled to accomplish so little. [p. 32]

Perhaps performative writers have settled for their own righteousness, finding too much comfort in the utopian language of social justice, care, and hope. Such abstractions, unless made concrete, may be good rallying calls but transform little.

I complete this discussion of the ethical issues surrounding performative writing without explicitly describing the ethical principles guiding my concerns. These concerns take their roots in Denzin's (2003), Alexander's (2005), Conquergood's (1991), Madison's (2005), Ellis's (2006), and others' calls for ethical practice. Based on their foundations, my desire has been to write in their spirit. I end this chapter with a performative writing exercise designed to make evident my ethical convictions implied throughout by my questioning and demanding claims.

A Performative Writing Oath for Ethical Performative Writing

I must write.

I must write naming and unnaming and, then, name again. Language is my most telling friend, my most fierce foe. I must write knowing that categories collapse without details and details contaminate containment. I must write with promises I cannot keep. I must write with hope in my failure.

I must accept that with every utterance I am guilty. Power lurks, will grab me at every turn. I must stare it down, write it down.

I must write a body, mine. I must write from my bruises and scars, from my skin that once was touched, from my demanding mouth.

I must trouble my body until its language tells more than it should.

I must identify myself so that I might turn on myself. I am implicated, always under suspicion, accused. The privilege of position offers no protection—neither a majority nor minority posture pulls a free pass. I must remember others deserve their turn.

I must let my body speak with its heart exposed. I must be raw, raucous, rabid. I must rage, razor sharp. I must cry out, cry in. Then, I must ask the reason. I must be sure I can deal with the mess after I spill my guts.

I must body myself next to others so that we move together, muscle together. I must feel the ache, the joy. I must speak while holding another's hand. I must let others tell me if I am sincere.

I must put my body where it needs to be, must know when it should be removed, ridiculed, revoked.

I must demand literature's presence; cheer and fear its seductions. I must figure the fictive for what it is. There is no telling the truth. There is only knowing the lie.

I must allow myself to enter, to see the possible. I must imagine what is not there, what seems to haunt, what needs a creative tug on language's sleeve.

I must provoke by pointing to power and must stand with authority. Then, I must question my power by pointing. I must consider defending my territory by inviting my enemies in, by offering what I can.

I must display myself, pants up or down, without arrogance. Even if I am right today, tomorrow I will be wrong. I must display myself without doing damage to myself, to others. I must display myself without delicacy, disguise, or delusion. I must disrobe the personal.

I must protect those I write as I protect the truth of my writing. If anyone must be sacrificed, I must sacrifice myself. I must do no harm, unless I must, and I must as I manage my motives, maneuver my methods, and market my ideas.

I must invite identification, empathy. I must call for the utopian us. I must beware of its dangers—slippery alliances sliding by substance, imposition of dominant positions, a tear substituting for social action. I must not let its dangers stifle me. It is my only chance for connection.

I must be responsible for my words—they break bones. I must sentence my way until my words might heal.

I must perform to accomplish what I believe, even if my belief is momentary, even if belief is all I have. I must perform feeling, for the sake of the felt. I must perform for the heart's reasons. I must perform to make a difference.

I must act. I must act without delay. Each word declares my death. I must act as if this were my last chance. I must build my legacy in sweat, in the street. I must make haste. I am falling away.

I must be suspicious of this oath.

References

Alexander, B. K. (2005). Performance ethnography: The reenacting and inciting of culture. In N. K. Denzin & Y. S. Lincoln, (Eds.), *Handbook of qualitative research*, 3rd ed. (pp. 411–442). Thousand Oaks, CA: Sage.

Austin. J. L. (1980). *How to do things with words*. New York: Oxford University Press.

Behar, R. (1996). *The vulnerable observer: Anthropology that breaks your heart*. Boston: Beacon Press.

Buzard, J. (2003). On auto-ethnographic authority. *The Yale Journal of Criticism*, *16*(1), 61–91.

CNN.com. (2006). Humiliated frat boys sue over "Borat" portrayal. Available online at http://www.cnn.com/2006/SHOWBIZ/Movies/11/10/film.boratlawsuit.ap/index.html. Accessed November 25, 2006.

Conquergood, D. (1991). Rethinking ethnography. *Communication Monographs*, *52*(1), 179–194.

Denzin, N. K. (2003). *Performance ethnography: Critical pedagogy and the politics of culture*. Thousand Oaks, CA: Sage.

Doty, M. (2005). Return to sender: memory, betrayal, and memoir. *The Writer's Chronicle*, *38*(October/November), 15–21.

Eakin, P. J. (Ed.). (2004). *The ethics of life writing*. Ithaca, NY: Cornell University Press.

Ellis, C. (2006). Telling secrets, revealing lives: Relational ethics in research with intimate others. *Qualitative Inquiry*, *12*(1), 1–27.

Fenza, D. W. (2006). Advice for graduating MFA students in writing: The words and the bees. *The Writer's Chronicle*, *38*(May/Summer), 30–35.

Gingrich-Philbrook, C. (2001). Bite your tongue: Four songs of body and language. In L. C. Miller &. R. J. Pelias (Eds.), *The green window: Proceeding of the Giant City Conference on Performative Writing* (pp. 1–7). Carbondale: Southern Illinois University.

Guignon, C. (2004). *On being authentic*. New York: Routledge.

Gunn, J. (2006). Shittext: Toward a new coprophilic style. *Text and Performance Quarterly*, *26*(1), 79–97.

Hantzis, D. (1998). Reflecting on "a dialogue with friends": Performing the "other/self" OJA 1995. In S. Dailey (Ed.), *The future of performance studies: Visions and revisions* (pp. 203–206). Annadale, VA: National Communication Association.

Hoagland, T. (2003). Negative capability: How to talk mean and influence people. *American Poetry Review*, *32*(March/April), 13–15.

Lockford, L. (1998). Emergent issues in the performance of a border-transgressive narrative. In S. Dailey (Ed.), *The future of performance studies: Visions and revisions* (pp. 214–220). Annadale, VA: National Communication Association.

Madison, D. S. (2005). *Critical ethnography: method, ethics, and performance.* Thousand Oaks, CA: Sage.

Madison, D. S. (2006). The dialogic performative in critical ethnography. *Text and Performance Quarterly, 26*(4), 320–324.

Muñoz, J. E. (1999). *Disidentifications: Queers of color and the performance of politics.* Minneapolis: University of Minnesota Press.

Parks, M. (1998). Where does scholarship begin? *American Communication Journal, 1.* Available online at http://acjournal.org/holdings/vol1/Iss2/special/parks.htm. Accessed October 1, 2002.

Pelias, R. J. (1999). *Writing performance: Poeticizing the researcher's body.* Carbondale: Southern Illinois University Press.

Pelias, R. J. (2004). *A methodology of the heart: Evoking academic and daily life.* Walnut Creek, CA: AltaMira.

Pollock, D. (1998). Performative writing. In P. Phelan & J. Lane (Eds.), *The ends of performance* (pp. 73–103). New York: New York University Press.

Shields, D. C. (2000). Symbolic convergence and speech communication theories: Sensing and examining dis/enchantment with theoretical robustness of critical autoethnography. *Communication Monographs, 67*(4), 392–421.

Spry, T. (2001). Preface. In L. C. Miller &. R. J. Pelias (Eds.), *The green window: Proceeding of the Giant City Conference on Performative Writing.* Carbondale: Southern Illinois University.

Terry, D. P. (2006). Once blind, now seeing: Problematics of confessional performance. *Text and Performance Quarterly, 26*(3), 209–228.

Turner, V. (1982). *From ritual to theatre: The human seriousness of play.* New York: Performing Arts Journal Publications.

Wilshire, B. (1982). *Role playing and identity: The limits of theatre as metaphor.* Bloomington: Indiana University Press.

Chapter 16

Learning to Remember the Things We've Learned to Forget

Endarkened Feminisms and the Sacred Nature of Research

Cynthia B. Dillard
(Nana Mansa II of Mpeasem, Ghana)

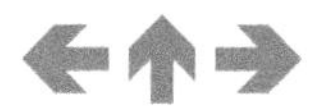

The Question of Memory

I can remember the day as if it were yesterday. … Ma Vic, with whom I stayed during my time in the village, was not only my dear friend, but my guide in the maze of the market. She had her favorite sellers: the woman from whom she bought baskets of plump red tomatoes; another woman her plantain, another yam; still another, her spices and food staples. And as a regular customer, her loyalty was rewarded with the expected "dash" of a few extra onions or an additional handful of rice. As Vic very confidently maneuvered her way through the market, I warily negotiated the open sewers, the sharp corners of the metal roofs, and the young market women who, without a stall, carried their store—big trays of fish or mango or other goods—on their heads. So my eyes faced downward most of the time, tenuously watching every step. My observations of the market were primarily at the places where we stopped to make a purchase, the places where my eyes could focus on what was around me and not on my feet.

We stopped at the plantain woman's stall. "My sister!" the woman exclaimed, greeting Vic with the enthusiasm of someone

Originally published in *Qualitative Inquiry and Global Crises*, edited by Norman K. Denzin and Michael D. Giardina, pp. 226–243. Republished in *Qualitative Inquiry—Past, Present, and Future: A Critical Reader*, edited by Norman K. Denzin and Michael D. Giardina, pp. 288–305. Left Coast Press, Inc.

who knows she's going to make a big sale. "You are welcome," she said to me, the customary greeting in Ghana when you haven't seen someone for a while. Her smile was warm, seeming to remember my presence on previous visits to her stall. Exchanging more small talk in Twi, Vic and the woman began their search for the biggest and the best plantains in the pile. And that's when our eyes met. About 70 years old, this woman (possibly the aunt or mother of the seller) was sitting in the shadows of the stall. She stared at me, a clear combination of curiosity and suspicion in her eyes, yellowed with age. She looked me up and down. I smiled at her, very uncomfortable with her unwavering gaze. As Vic and the seller were finishing their transaction, the old woman reached over and touched Vic's arm, her face now absolutely perplexed, nodding in my direction: "What *is* she (me)? Is she a white woman?" I nearly fell over, a rush of emotions running through me, from absolute horror to disgust to disbelief to sadness. Vic giggled and explained to the woman (who had still not quit staring at me) that I was not a white woman but a black American.

That evening in my researcher's journal (and through confused, angry, and sad tears that could've filled a river), I wondered aloud as I wrote: "How could she see *me* as a white woman?" "Couldn't she see the African woman I could see in myself?" "Didn't she know what had happened to millions of Africans who'd been forcibly taken from the shores of Ghana and other West African countries?" "Where did she think we had gone?" "Had she never imagined that some of us would return?" "How can this sister/mother see me this way?" On reflection, what frightened me most about her question was that, at that very moment, I couldn't answer it myself:

> What had been the rather solid taken-for-granted nature of my African American identity—an identity that I'd used to make sense of myself—melted down like butter on a hot summer's day in that moment in Ghana. Something very rich that I loved dearly had become useless fat on the sidewalk, no help whatsoever in explaining and understanding what she saw, or who I was. But I know there is wisdom in her question or it wouldn't have come to teach me a lesson. If I'm to "be" a researcher in this space, I will have to struggle with the butter on the sidewalk,

> the shifting ground of African identity through Ghanaian eyes. Neither here nor there (Ghana or the US), neither African nor American, neither recognizably Black nor white. Maybe it's not either/or: Maybe it's both/and? Somehow, it feels like it's beyond these dualities. They seem too simple. Regardless, it hurts to do this work. (Journal, 1/22/98)

And this pain stayed with me until the following week, when market day came again:

> Today is market day again. Honestly, I'm dreading it. But I don't think there's an acceptable excuse not to go and help. … As we approached the plantain seller's stall, my stomach churned and my nerves were shattered, afraid of what "insult" (however innocent) would come from the old lady. Vic, oblivious to my inner turmoil, again greeted the plantain woman and went about her business. But before I could properly greet the seller, I glanced to my right and caught the eye—and the smile—of the old lady. "Morning Black American lady! How are you?" she says happily, clearly concentrating hard to speak to me in her heavily accented English. I replied in my equally faltering Twi: "Me ho ye," ("I'm fine.") And she reached over and grabbed my wrist. "Black American. Yea." (Journal, 1/29/98)

This story is from my book *On Spiritual Strivings* (Dillard, 2006a). In the book, I sought to examine the ways that centering spirituality in an academic life transforms its very foundations, creating the site for spiritual healing and service to the world. And I chose to begin this talk with that story because it is still on my mind and in my heart, gnawing in the pit of my gut. "*What is she?* Is she a white woman? A black American—yea!" Both the question and the way the old lady asked it threw my entire sense of who I was into confusion. Yet, in retrospect, it is in the answer to that question that I have come to better understand my self, my life's purpose and a new direction for my work.

What I would like to do in this chapter is to try to reflexively read and remember this story and so many others created and lived by black women everywhere, to make visible the spiritual, cultural, and ritual memories that are necessary to appreciate the complex and contested spaces and places of black women's lives in our fullness. What I am also suggesting here is that you too must travel with me/with us in this journey, in the same engaged process of re-membering and seeing what Busia (1989) calls our "icons of significance" as well. This is our re-search *together*, in community, the goal being to develop a better sense of reading the Diaspora, of truly being able to see Africa's children at home and in the New World. And although this may seem like a very private and singular her/story of travel, journey, awakening, and cultural memory, it might also be read/considered as a metaphor of the history/herstory of African people as we traverse and settle, move, and create homeplace in the New World and Africa as well.

These memories are about the concrete aspects of our lives, where meaning—within our memories—"becomes what we can read and what we can no longer or could never read about ourselves and our lives" (Busia, p. 198). Busia goes on to say: "This act of reading becomes an exercise in identifications—to recognize life experiences and historic transformations that point the way toward a celebration, a coming together attainable only through an understanding and acceptance of the demands of the past, which are transformed into a gift of the future" (p. 198).

And as researchers, we will read and hear differently, and at varying depths, depending on our ability to read productively, to read the signs along the way.

Central to my thinking about the meanings of culture and race in research and other decolonizing projects is an often unnamed element of identity, one that is inherent in the acts of research and teaching. And both are *deeply embedded in the act of memory and of re-membering*. Often in research by scholars of color and others, we see that racial/cultural memory is at least part of what is raised up in our on-going quest to be "seen" and "heard" and "unlimited" in the myriad ways we approach our questions, our scholarship (see Alexander, 2005; Coloma, 2008; Daza, 2008; Strong-Wilson, 2008; Subedi, 2008; and Subreendeth, 2008 for examples). In common, memory can be thought of as a thing, person, or event that brings to mind and heart a past experience—and with it, the ability to "re"-member, to recall and think of *again*. The *American Heritage Dictionary* (2000) goes so far as to say that to remember is "to bear in mind, as deserving a gift or reward" (p. 597). And the very intimate nature of research narratives like the story from Ghana suggests that memory is also about an *awakening*, an opening to the spirit of something that has, until that moment, been asleep within us.

For many researchers of color, embracing an ethic that opens to spirit is fundamental to the nature of learning, teaching, and by extension, research. We seem to inherently recognize that such spaces and acts—and our memories and ways of being with/in them—are always and in all ways also political, cultural, situated, embodied, spiritual: They are alive and present within us. However, all too often, we have been seduced into forgetting (or have chosen to do so), given the weight and power of our memories and the often radical act of re-membering in our present lives and work, that is remembering as a decolonizing project. And if we assume, as I do, that the knowledge, wisdom, and ways of our ancestors are a central and present part of everything that has existed, is existing, and will exist in the future, then teaching and research must also undertake an often unnamed, unrecognized, unarticulated, and forgotten task that is important for individuals who yearn to understand ways of being and knowing that have been marginalized in the world and in formal education. Simply put, *we must learn to re-member the things that we've learned to forget*. Whether through wandering into unfamiliar/always familiar contexts, making conscious choices to use/not use languages and cultural wisdom, or strategically choosing to cover or uncover, in returning to and re-membering, an awakening in research and teaching is possible and powerful. And there are several lessons we must learn to remember, to answer the question asked by the old lady: *What is she?* The first lesson we must recognize and remember is embedded in this very story, a lesson that many African-ascendent people already know:

> Being scattered in diaspora is an act of dispossession from our past, from our original homeland, from our languages and from each other. We must re-member, "to see again the fragments that make up the whole, not as isolated individual and even redundant fragments, but as part of a creative and sustaining whole." (Busia, 1989, p. 197)

So part of the old lady's questions is about remembering as an act of piece-gathering. But the bigger part of this lesson is about seeing ourselves in the gaze of another and not looking away, but looking deeper. It is fundamentally to answer the question: Who are we in relation to others—and staying long enough to find out.

A Memory in Time: Praisesong for the Queen Mother[1]

You woke me this morning
And I became part of Your divine plan
Chosen on this day
To be among the living.
You dressed me in a purple kaba[2]
And I became the color of royalty,
Traveling to the village in a dirty old van
That felt like my royal carriage,
The curtains drawn for the privacy
Of the new Queen Mother.
You introduced "Professor Cynthia Dillard"
To the Chiefs of the kingdom,
And I became my own desire
To know as I am known,
You honored my family name
On the front of the community center and preschool,
And I became my parents, their parents, parents, parents,
Those who, by virtue of the Blackness of Africa
Were considered by some
Not to be fully human,
But whose depth of humanity shone like the sun in this
moment.
You brought my sister-mothers to bathe me in the soothing
waters of life,
And I once again became the child of all my mothers
Marion Lucille Cook Dillard
Wanda Amaker Williams

Florence Mary Miller
Nana Mansa, the first,
And those unknown to me.
You wrapped me in the swath of traditional kente,
And I became the weavers of that cloth,
The men who learned from their fathers and their fathers' fathers,
An art so special that had taken months and months
Of skill, patience, and love in its creation.
You sat me on my Queen's stool
And I became Nana Mansa II, Nkosua Ohemaa[3]
The spirit of Nana Mansa, the first, now residing
not in my head,
But in the stool,
She speaks centuries of cultural memories
directly to my heart, as an African American,
"I had many children, but you are the only one who has returned."
You lovingly dress me in beads old and new,
Adorning my fingers with gold rings, my Queen's chain around my neck,
And I became the precious riches and treasures of the Universe
Now and then.
You fanned me with cloth and palms and bare hands,
And I became the wind
Carrying Your voice:
"Don't be afraid, Nana.
Trust me.
You have all that you need.
I will show you what you already know."
You poured libation
And called me into the sacred ritual of remembering,
And I became my own full circle as a researcher,

A searcher again, honoring the knowledge of
Who and what is here and there
Of what's been and is to be,
Inseparable realities, united by Your gift of breath,
A committed teacher and student of my own becoming.
You drummed and we danced
And with each beat,
I became the rhythms of my passed on ancestors,
Who gathered with us on that day
Brothers and sisters of the village, the community, the diaspora,
A holy encounter indeed!
You gave food to feed the whole village,
And I became my own full belly,
And the too often empty bellies of the village children and families,
For that moment, we were all satisfied.
Full.
Happy.
Joyful in Your bounty.
You've blessed me with life,
A chance to manifest extraordinary works
Through You.
By becoming all of myself
I can live not into the smallness of the world's expectations
But into the greatness of the true names
You've given to me.

Praisesongs are traditional types of poems, sung in various places all over the continent of Africa. They are ceremonial and social poems, recited or sung in public at celebrations such as outdoorings (in Ghana, a christening or naming ceremony) or anniverseries or funerals. Embracing the history, legends, and traditions of a community of people, praisesongs can be used to celebrate triumph over adversity, bravery and courage, both in life and death. They can also mark social transition, upward movement culturally, socially, or spiritually. While the meditation above is a praisesong to my ascent as a queen mother in Ghana, here's the question: How might our memories, our encounters and representations of those, act as praisesongs in the world? As we teach, conduct research, and examine and create texts—whether the research narrative, the lesson plan, the interview transcript, the representational text in publication—our sense of who we are, our identity, our very selves and spirits are seen/understood/recognized/grounded in our past: They make sense to us based on something that has happened (in memory) versus simply as a present moment or a future not yet come. I am arguing here that it is from our memories that we can recognize and answer the question: "Who am I?" and collectively "Who are we?" This isn't just about being able to recognize times past on a calendar or datebook. This is fundamentally to see that our known and unknown and yet-to-be-known lives as human being are deeply imbued with meaning that is based in our memory. Booth (2006) suggests that to answer the question of who we are, we have to go deep into the well of memory:

> to draw a boundary between group members and others; to provide a basis for collective action; and to call attention to life-in-common, a shared history and future. … All of these involve claims about identity across time and change, and about identity and responsibility as well. … Statement[s] of identity turn out to involve a strong *temporal* dimension. (p. 3; emphasis added)

This is also fundamental to an African cosmology, one that is based on understanding one's place, space, and purpose in time through recognition of a common destiny: I am because we are. And for those of us who think and feel ourselves into our scholarship through frameworks and paradigms that are African in nature and that just "*feels* right" to us[4] (Lorde, 1984, p. 37; emphasis added), we also recognize that we cannot feel or engage our scholarship without seeing that, as singer Dianne Reeves (1999) suggests in her song "Testify": "God and time are synonymous/and in time God reveals all things/Be still/Stand in love/and pay attention." Within African spaces, time is not thought of in the abstract, but in relation to Spirit. Time is what has happened here, what continues to happen here, and the honoring of "the relationships that linger [here]" (Bargna, 2000, p. 25). This is one of the major ways that African cosmology challenges Western conceptions of time, space, and location: It is circular, based in past, present, and future as intricate connective, and collective webs of meaning making:

> You honored my family name
> On the front of the community center and preschool,
> And I became my parents, their parents, parents, parents,
> Those who, by virtue of the Blackness of Africa
> Were considered by some
> Not to be fully human...

That brings us to the second lesson: Our memories are based in a sense of connective and collective time, from which we both re-cognize our identities and from which we can transform those identities.

For example, any research of the African American might need to explicitly acknowledge the importance of the transatlantic slave trade and the Middle Passage as relevant experiences in the collective memory of African-ascendent personhood. The Middle Passage was the forced enslavement and forced journey of millions of Africans from Africa to the New World. Spaces associated with this trade in human beings—the slave dungeons that dot the western coast of Africa, the routes and rivers that were used for the inland walk to the coastal forts and dungeons, sites in the United States that commemorate the places where enslaved African people resisted and created new homes, new communities—are ripe with memory and with meaning for African-ascendent peoples who *chose* to remember, who *choose* to make pilgrimage to these spaces to feel, see, and better understand the place of such memories in the formations of our identities, our personhood.[5]

And although the events of the Middle Passage and slavery in the New World are now centuries old (and often unrecognized in the memories of many both on the continent of Africa and in the Diaspora), for those who choose to remember, these engagements have the profound ability to transform us, to bring us back to places (both literally and spiritually) that we hear in the praiseong: *"I had many children, but you were the one who returned."* How do we see these recognitions in our scholarship? "*Everything* about the placing of the questions of research is important here, as our lives and those of the participants we study are full of 'icons of significance'" (Busia, 1989, p. 201; emphasis in the original). With every question we ask, don't ask, answer, don't answer, it is crucial for us to recognize and remember that our participants are being forced to ask central questions of their lives as well. As we are "studying" literacy practices, or teacher education or the ways that African American culture shapes mathematics instruction, what does it really mean to say: "Tell me about yourself." Where is the place of racial/cultural memory of the Middle Passage there, both for the researched and the researcher? This is key, as so many "study" with/in/about African-ascendent communities. How do we—or might we—re-cognize the child you are observing as an *African* American, as connected to and collectively a part of the circle of African time? How is our entire enterprise shaped by the lack of memory of an event so very traumatic that it forever changed the very time, space, and spirit of humanity, that there would be no African American without it?

Irwin-Zarecka (1994) states that "personal relevance of the traumatic memory and not personal witness to the trauma [is what] defines community" (p. 49). But the power and relevance of the memory endures. It matters. An African cosmology requires that we see and better understand this persistence across time (it's enduringness, as described by Booth, 2006), as its presence describes one of the ways that the African community is bounded and has borders and cultural understandings that bind and define its members. Such boundedness within community when conscious and connected transforms one's identity such that the question "Who am I?" is no longer a total and bewildering mystery for African Americans and others in Diaspora. It may become, as we see in my praisesong imbued with meaning and with response-ability, both at the core of claims to membership from an endarkened feminist epistemology (see Dillard,

2000; Dillard & Bell, 2011; Dillard & Okpalaoka, in press). It is the time where we find ourselves a part of something bigger than what we already are.

One of the many ways that African feminist scholars working from/through endarkened frameworks are re-membering, or putting back together notions of time that honor and lift up "the relationships that linger there," is to attempt to ask a different set of questions, starting first with ourselves. These are the echoes that you heard in the praisesong, an interrogation of the ways that memory is always already there. It is the way that the sacred also shapes memory and is inseparable in memory. Within the temporal and physical movement that Africans in Diaspora have undergone, it is also what gives the memory shape within Western epistemological frameworks, including frameworks of feminism.[6] It is embedded in the ways that a researcher like myself can re-member, put it back together again:

> By becoming all of myself
>
> I can live not into the smallness of the world's expectations
>
> But into the greatness of the true names
>
> You've given to me.

What is needed are models of inquiry that truly honor the complexities of memories. Of indigenous and the "modern" time, experienced not just in our minds, but in our bodies and spirits as well. Frameworks that approach research as sacred practice, worthy of reverence. A way of thinking and feeling and doing research that honors the fluidity of time and space, of the material world and the spiritual one. Mostly, as we point out in recent work located in the slave dungeons in Ghana (Dillard & Bell, 2011), we need a way to inquire that acknowledges both the joy and pain of location/dislocation and the transformation of both in our stories: African women are not stories of a singular self, but are stories of *we*, collective stories deeply embedded in African women's wisdom and indigenous knowledges. In his discussion of the Middle Passage, Tom Feelings (1995) further and eloquently states:

> I began to see how important the telling of this particular story could be for Africans all over the world, many who consciously or unconsciously share this race memory, this painful experience of

> the Middle Passage. … But if this part of history could be told in such a way that those chains of the past … could, in the telling, become spiritual links that willingly bind us together now and into the future, then that painful Middle Passage could become, ironically, a positive connecting line to all of us, whether living inside or outside the continent of Africa. (p. ii)

Formed as a question, what do such memories mean for the teacher/scholar of color (and conscience), and how might we more explicitly and systematically engage them, re-member what we have forgotten as a way toward healing not just ourselves but those with whom we teach and research? Turning back to Feelings (1995) above, he suggests first that such memories, from a spiritual framework, have the potential to connect those on the continent of Africa to those in the Diaspora, the result of the traumatic acts of the trans-Atlantic slave trade. This is a central characteristic of racial/cultural memories for all who live with/in Diaspora. So, first, *these are memories acknowledge an ever present thread between the Diaspora and the continent, a heritage "homeplace."*

It is not accidental that many scholars of color take up the exploration and research into/about connections to or with/in some version of an ancestral, heritage, or cultural homeplace and that our representations—in art, in inquiry, in personhood and identity—represent those cultural spaces and places. Second, *racial/cultural memories are intimate*: They are memories that, good or bad, make you ache with desire "to find the marriage of meaning and matter in our lives, in the world" (Mountain Dreamer, 2005, p. 42). I believe this may be true for Whites and others who have not carried or been politically or culturally marked or "racialized"—and it is worthy of being explored by all researchers, regardless of race. Such intimacy is inextricably linked to racial and cultural identities; that is, memories are part and parcel of the meanings of identity, of the meaning of who we are and how we are in the world. Husband (2007), in his work on African American male teacher identity, suggests that cultural memories are those memories of experiences and/or events related to collective and or individual racial/cultural identity "that are either too significant to easily forget or so salient that one strives to forget"

(p. 10). He goes on to describe the fundamental nature and character of racial/cultural memories:

> In the case of the former, cultural memories can be thought of as memories of events as racial/cultural beings that are/were so remarkable that we consider them to be defining moments in our life histories. … Pertaining to the latter, race/cultural memories are those related to our racial/cultural identities that are so potent [often painful] that we tend to suppress [them] in order to function as human beings. (p. 10)

What we see here is that the intimate nature of racial/cultural memories and their work in identity creation is inseparable from what it means to be vulnerable in our work, from reaching down inside of one's self and across toward others to places that may "break your heart" (Behar, 1996)—but, like many courageous researchers, choosing to go there anyhow.

That brings us to the final part of a definition of racial/cultural memories: *They are memories that change our ways of being (ontology) and knowing (epistemology) in what we call the present.* They are inspirational, breathing new life into the work of teaching, research, and living. They are the roots we must first grow in order to have our leaves. They are memories that *transform* us, a place within and without that feeds our ability to engage new metaphors and practices in our work (Dillard, 2000).

The Claim of Memory

Here's lesson #3:

> *While remembering is about claiming, it is also about being claimed in a space of recognition that has "[held] your people to this earth"* (McElroy, 1997, p. 2; emphasis added).

> It's been lights off (no electricity) since about 7 pm. Around 7:30 pm, the seamstress arrives with my dresses. They are both really beautiful. But so was what happened with the purple kaba. The seamstress asked me to go and try it on so she could make any adjustments that might be needed. Given my experience with the old lady in the market, I was a little leery about what she might say once I put the dress on. I carefully tied my head wrap

> and tentatively came out of the side room. "Mmmmmm," she exclaimed, looking at me in my kaba, clearly in admiration. "Who tied it for you?' she said, pointing to my head wrap. "I did it," I said, realizing that I had done so in a manner that surprised her. "Turn around," she said sternly. And as her hand brushed down the back side of my body, I knew that, like the brothers earlier in the day, she too recognized [another] one of the many carry-overs of African womanhood that could not be oppressed or suppressed, even through the violence of the slave trade: The African woman's ass [as she wears the slit skirt]. She turned to Vic: "She **is** an African woman." So, however weak were our identifications of these links between us, as African women, they were clear and apparent to her and to me in that moment. And her look of recognition is one I will never, ever forget. (Journal, 1/22/98)

Irwin-Zarecka (1994) speaks brilliantly of how people make sense of the past, particularly relevant to this discussion of memories and personhood of African people. That is that, in a wholly racialized society, our collective memories are less about an intellectual "truth" about what we are referencing, what we are working to construct, what we desire to put back together again. That is spiritual and sacred work, the "rules" of which will be different for different groups of people. Mostly, these memories bear weight on the experiences being remembered for these different groups shape our claims to "mine," "theirs," "ours." I'm arguing here that this memory-work is critical for marginalized peoples, to be able to see ourselves more clearly in order to see how we are mutually recognized, mutually remembered, mutually mediated. Such memories are reference to the place that holds us to this Earth, the ways we are because we have been. And as researchers, while our claims to knowing are always subjective,

> it is the definition shared by people we study that matters. In many cases there is a rather radical difference between the observer's and the participants realities. ... But whether the past as we understand it and the part as understood by our subjects are closer or further apart, we ought to consider both in our analysis. Our baseline is a needed standard for critical judgment and their baseline

is what informs remembrance [and hence, the answers]. (Irwin-Zarecka, 1994, p. 19)

In many ways, this positions the qualitative researcher as a narrator and creator of memory, both her and his own and the collective memory of, the hearts and soul of humanity, in all its variations. However, for the black or endarkened feminist researcher, whose work is often deliberately situated in indigenous spaces and places, and focused on knowledge and cultural production, this is not simply the narration of a story: It is the *deliberate* work of engaging and *preserving* these stories, both of the "thing" itself and our engagements and experiences with it. But mostly, it is also our *duty*—our responsibility—to *remember*: We are those who can bear witness to our African "past," diasporic "present," and future as a full circle: That is, after all, what it means to be in community, to be in the spirit collectively. Let it be so.

Notes

1 Becoming a Queen Mother is part of a collection of meditations from an unpublished manuscript entitled *Living Africa: A Book of Meditations*. This is also in honor of Paule Marshall's *Praisesong for the Widow* (1984), a book that has had a profound influence on my thoughts on the endarkened nature of memory.

2 Kaba is a style of dress worn by Ghanaian women made from batik/wax print cloth. It consists of a fitted top, often embellished with very elaborate necklines, sleeves, and waist and a form-fitting skirt with a slit and a head wrap.

3 Queen Mother of Development

4 See Dillard (2006b) for a full discussion of paradigms and endarkened feminist thought.

5 For further explorations of these memories, see Dillard & Bell (2011). See also Dillard (2008).

6 See Dillard & Okpalaoka (in press) for an in-depth look at the sacred and the spiritual in endarkened transnational feminist praxis and research.

References

Alexander, M. J. (2005). *Pedagogies of crossing: Meditations of feminism, sexual politics, memory, and the sacred.* Durham, NC: Duke University Press.

American Heritage Dictionary of the English Language. (2000). Boston: Delta Books.

Bargna, I. (2000). *African art.* Milan, Italy: Jaca Books.

Behar, R. (1996). *The vulnerable observer: Anthropology that breaks your heart.* Boston: Beacon.

Booth, W. J. (2006). *Communities of memory: On witness, identity, and justice.* Ithaca, NY: Cornell University Press.

Busia, A. (1989). What is your nation? Reconnecting Africa and her diaspora through Paule Marshall's *Praisesong for the widow.* In C. Wall (Ed.), *Changing our own words: Essays on criticism, theory, and writing by black women* (pp. 116–129). New Bruswick, NJ: Rutgers University Press.

Coloma, R. (2008). Border crossing subjectivities and research: Through the prism of feminists of color. *Race, Ethnicity and Education, 11*, 1, 11–28.

Daza, S. (2008). Decolonizing researcher authenticity. *Race, Ethnicity and Education, 11*, 1, 71–86.

Dillard, C. B. (2000). The substance of things hoped for, the evidence of things not seen: Examining an endarkened feminist epistemology in educational research and leadership. *International Journal of Qualitative Studies in Education, 13*, 6, 661–681.

Dillard, C. B. (2006a). *On spiritual strivings: Transforming an African American woman's academic life.* Albany: State University of New York Press.

Dillard, C. B. (2006b). When the music changes, so should the dance: Cultural and spiritual considerations in paradigm "proliferation." *International Journal of Qualitative Studies in Education, 19*, 1, 59–76.

Dillard, C. B. (2008). When the ground is black, the ground is fertile: Exploring endarkened feminst epistemology and healing methodologies of the spirit. In N. K. Denzin, Y. S. Lincoln, & L. Tuhiwai-Smith (Eds.), *Handbook of critical and indigenous methodologies* (pp. 277–292). Thousand Oaks, CA: Sage.

Dillard, C. B., & Bell, C. (2011). Endarkened feminism and sacred praxis: Troubling (auto)ethnography through critical engagements with African indigenous knowledges. In G. Dei (Ed.), *Indigenous philosophies and critical education* (pp. 337–349). New York: Peter Lang.

Dillard, C. B., & Okpalaoka, C. L. (in press). The sacred and spirtual nature of endarkened transnational feminist praxis in qualitative research. In N. K. Denzin & Y. S. Lincoln (Eds.), *Handbook of qualitative research* (4th ed.). Thousand Oaks, CA: Sage.

Feelings, T. (1995). *The middle passage.* New York: Dial Books.

Husband, T. (2007). Always black, always male: Race/cultural recollections and the qualitative researcher. Unpublished paper presented at The Congress of Qualitative Inquiry, May 3–6, University of Illinois, Champaign-Urbana.

Irwin-Zarecka, I. (1994). *Frames of remembrance: The dynamics of collective memory.* New Brunswick, NJ: Transaction Publishers.

Lorde, A. (1984). *Sister outsider: Essays and speeches by Audre Lorde.* Freedom, CA: The Crossing Press.

Marshall, P. (1984). *Praisesong for the widow.* New York: Dutton.

McElroy, C. J. (1997). *A long way from St. Louie: Travel memoirs.* Minneapolis: Coffee House Press.

Mountain Dreamer, O. (2005). *What we ache for: Creativity and the unfolding of the soul.* San Francisco: Harper Collins.

Reeves, D. (singer). (1999). Testify (audio recording). On album "Bridges." New York: Blue Note Records.

Strong-Wilson, T. (2008). *Bringing memory forward: Storied remembrance in social justice education with teachers.* New York: Peter Lang.

Subedi, B. (2008). Contesting racialization: Asian immigrant teachers' critiques and claims of teacher authenticity. *Race, Ethnicity and Education, 11*, 1, 57–70.

Chapter 17

The Exquisite Corpse of Art-Based Research

Charles R. Garoian

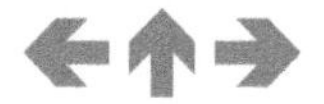

There was a lot of multi versions of all kinds of things, we were always pulling things apart, I had like a big junk yard of stuff, as the year went by, if something wasn't complete, I just pulled out the parts I liked, it was like pullin' the parts you need from one car, put 'em in the other car so that car runs[1]

— Bruce Springsteen (2010) on writing "Darkness on the Edge of Town"

twenty, twenty acres, empty land, twenty acres of empty land, nothing, absolutely nothing could grow on it, nothing but sand, tumble weeds and Johnson grass that is … gopher holes everywhere, jack rabbits all over the place, but otherwise empty God-forsaken land where Chester Alexanian[2] *lived, collected, and installed rusted, broken, cannibalized tractor parts, worn out farm implements, some animal powered, others powered by machines … corroded cultivators, plows, thrashers, buggy parts, dilapidated cars, junked pick ups, delivery trucks, forklifts, tractors, you name it, he had it, spread across that barren twenty acres of land, a veritable outdoor museum of agricultural implements, historical artifacts, material culture from the late nineteenth century*

Originally published in *Qualitative Inquiry and Global Crises,* edited by Norman K. Denzin and Michael D. Giardina, pp. 155–177. Republished in *Qualitative Inquiry—Past, Present, and Future: A Critical Reader,* edited by Norman K. Denzin and Michael D. Giardina, pp. 306–327. Left Coast Press, Inc.

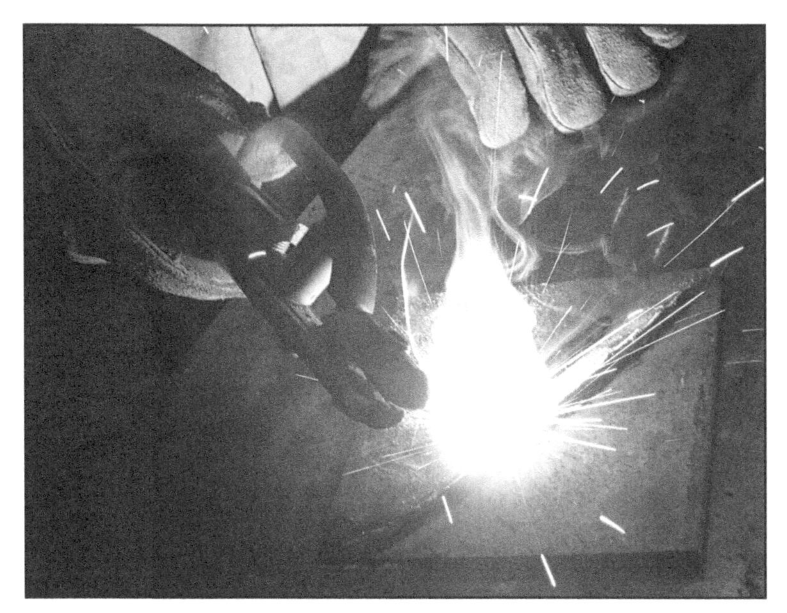

Figure 17.1: Z-Z-Z-Z-Z-Z-Z-Z-Zuht. *Photograph courtesy Charles Garoian.*

to the present, he had one of everything it seemed ... others' throw-aways, he was collector, curator, conservator, and docent, all in one, Chester's eccentricity was conspicuous, not a hoarder, but close to it. ... I didn't relate even though I was studying to become an artist, I didn't understand the logic of his eclectic impulse even though I was amassing my own load, I didn't get it even though, even though my stuff was being exhibited in galleries and museums ... it was only afterwards, after Chester constructed his rickety forklift that my burden of assumptions lifted ... the forklift that he composed from parts, fragments of a rundown '32 Ford Model A, '52 Chevy flatbed, and a '55 Yale forklift, all of which were appropriated from his junk heap, the anthology that he had archived on that empty patch of land, the twenty acres where he stockpiled his stuff ... where he was played by play, the tinkering play that anthropologist Victor Turner[3] refers to as the "supreme bricoleur of frail transient constructions," ... Z-Z-Z-Z-Z-Zuht, Z-Z-Z-Z-Z-Z-Z-Z-Zuht, Z-Z-Z-Z-Z-Z-Z-Z-Z-Z-Z-Zuht, Chester cut here and there, then he welded there and here (see Figure 17.1), Z-Z-Z-Z-Z-Zhut, he cut and welded, welded and cut and welded again to assemble an elaborate Frankenstein algo-rhythm,

Z-Z-Z-Z-Z-Z-Z-Z-Z-Zhut, a monstrous forklift with its linkages and sutures readily apparent like the folds of Exquisite Corpse... cannibalized Ford, Chevy, and Yale body parts whose differences were easily discernable, there was no attempt, none at all to conceal the radical juxtaposition of junk, rusted yellow contours adjoining a dented black frame adjoining scarred yellow-orange forks, Chevy, Ford, Yale, all three absent yet present, their surfaces and parts grimy and pitted from years of use and oxidation, their three-in-one differences and particularities exposed, yet, yet like those incongruous constructions of the Dadaists and Surrealists, the crazy thing actually worked on many levels, visually, conceptually, materially, but most of all mechanically ... notwithstanding its raw aesthetic, what pleased him most about his resurrected Corpse was its ability to do the heavy lifting, the hard work of hauling fresh and dried fruit, and wine grapes to the market, Chester's objective was always steadfastly modest ... it was only then, then, after my assumptions had blurred, that I associated and understood his assemblage work and those that I was ironically constructing in my studio by affixing cultural fragments and detritus to my canvas ... was mine fine art and his simply junk? There was a beauty in the way his forklift monstrosity looked and worked, while lacking pretension its differential forms and functions overwhelmed, restored and renewed my way of seeing and understanding the world.

I offer the story that you have just read as a prelude to my exploration and characterization of the "Exquisite Corpse of Art-Based Research," the topic of this chapter. My objective in complicating its narrative is to draw attention to *what* my story is about, the precarious construction of Chester's forklift, and *how* my collaged, stammering prose is constructed to expose in-between spaces where you, as readers, can linger on its juxtapositions, and fold your own stories among its contiguous, disjunctive associations, correspondences and complementarities. About such lingering philosopher John Dewey (1938) writes: "The crucial educational problem is that of procuring the *postponement of immediate action* upon desire until observation and judgment have intervened" (pp. 64, 69; emphasis added). Such postponement affords the contemplation, seeing, and transformational becoming of subjectivity through art research and practice.

Indeed, in exposing the *how* of my writing about Chester's forklift, I am responding to the call of arts-based researchers and educators like Graeme Sullivan (2005), Cahnmann-Taylor and Siegesmund (2008), and Dónal O'Donoghue (2009) who advocate for educational research that more closely follows the imaginary and improvisational processes and practices of artists, poets, and musicians as compared with inquiry that is commonly associated with the logical-rational approaches in the sciences and social sciences. My premise is that the Exquisite Corpse folding of complex and contradictory narratives into and through each other offers significant possibilities for engaging in democratic discourse, understanding alterity, and respect for cultural differences and peculiarities.[4] Respect for alterity is possible, according to philosopher Emmanuel Levinas, by virtue of a nonreciprocal relationship with the other, where the self remains open and susceptible to difference, to not knowing, and to indeterminacy. Such "unknowable and unassimilable alterity" is possible insofar as the relationship with the other is only ever as strangers (Todd, 2001, p. 69).

In complementing my narrative about Chester's forklift, in what follows I briefly discuss the historical positioning of Exquisite Corpse in twentieth-century art, and I invoke artists' and scholars' research and creative works that correspond with the creative strategies proposed by the Exquisite Corpse process. In doing so, I address the following questions: What is Exquisite Corpse and how was it historically situated? How does it function visually and conceptually? How are subjectivity and otherness constituted by its incongruous discourse? How does its fragmented research and practice enable creative and political agency? And, how does its abstruse, heterogeneous criticality differ from the ideological discourses of academic, institutional, and corporate power?

Like Chester's forklift, the surrealists' Exquisite Corpse parlor game consisted of three or more individual sections, each rendered by a single player and joined together into a single, collaborative visual or written artwork. In the visual example of the game, a sheet of paper was folded horizontally into its sections (Figure 17.2) and assigned a vertical, corporeal order beginning with the head in the top section of the paper, the torso in its middle section, then the feet in the bottom section.[5] Important to preserving the chance element

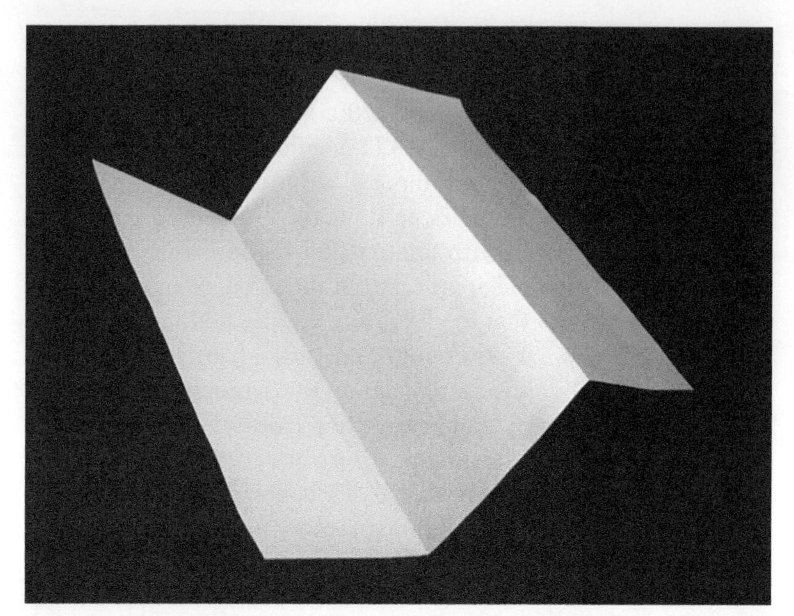

Figure17.2: Folded paper for Exquisite Corpse.
Photograph courtesy Charles Garoian.

of the game, each section was made in secret, then folded and concealed under the previous sections until all were completed and the sheet was unfolded at the end of the game to reveal the juxtaposing of an Exquisite Corpse. For a sectional drawing to remain hidden, a player completed his or her part of the body out of sight from the other players, then continued its ending lines to the bottom edge of the section and just over the top edge of the next section to provide the next player clues as to where to start drawing their part of the body. While this collaborative procedure among the players seems constrained and regimented, any such limitations were dispelled when the adjoining and disjoining play between its sections were revealed at the unfolding of the sheet.

This oscillating movement between congruity and incongruity conjoins game theorist James Carse's (1986) differentiations of *finite* and *infinite* games, in which the prescribed structure and rules of the former are contrasted with the ambiguity, indeterminacy, and contingent improvisational structures of the latter. Given this to and fro movement of Exquisite Corpse, it is at its

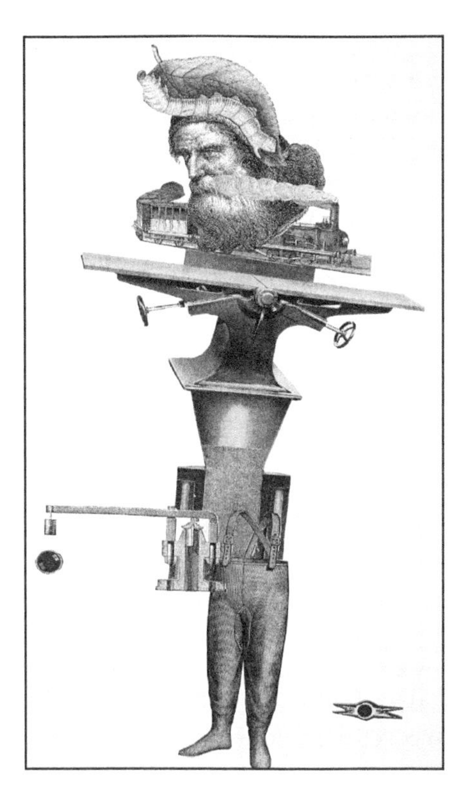

Figure 17.3: André Breton, Jacqueline Lamba, Yves Tanguy, *Cadavre exquis* [Exquisite Corpse] February 9, 1938. Collage on paper, 31.00 x 21.20 cm (unfolded 31.00 x 42.20 cm).
Collection of National Galleries of Scotland. © 2010 Artists Rights Society (ARS), New York/ADAGP, Paris. © 2010 Estate of Yves Tanguy/Artists Rights Society (ARS), New York.

unfolding when the incongruities of the sections are revealed and when viewers are left with an interminable conundrum in fusing the disjunctions of its heterogeneous body; a monstrous body whose excessive figurations and reconfigurations resist normalization, homogenization, and what critical theorist Donna Haraway (1992) calls the hegemony of "artifactualism,"[6] within the singular frame of the paper sheet upon which it has been rendered.

The paradoxical and heterogeneous characteristics of Exquisite Corpse are evident in the 1938 playing of the game (Figure 17.3) by surrealists André Breton, Jacqueline Lamba, and Yves Tanguy.[7] The head section contains a large leaf with a caterpillar attached atop a bearded old man's head, like the adorned headdresses of military leaders in antiquity; a steam locomotive pulls a train of cars around the old man's right side, tunnels under his beard across his neck, and out the other side demarcating the area of his shoulders; while the juxtaposed beard, caterpillar, leaf, train, and its smoke seem incongruous, they have in common a biomorphic, serpentine configuration as compared with the geometric, machinic forms of the following sections.

In the torso section, what appears to be a machinist's or cabinet maker's industrial lathe stretches across what would be considered the man's chest area with the lathe's adjustment wheels and their extended rods stretching one to the left and the other to the right suggesting short, outstretched arms; the lathe is positioned at an angle on a teetering conical stand that rests on a round, drum-like form whose sides appear like pistons tightly contained in cylinders; in the foreground of the table a long pipe-like form extends at a slight angle but horizontally along the bottom fold of the paper and toward its outer edge.

In the third, the feet section, the pipe-like form in the previous section elbows downward at one end and into this section; together with a similar form nearby, and what appears to be a dangling counterweight at the opposite end, the apparatus suggests fittings among other components in an ambiguous hydraulic mechanism that is adjoined to the left hip of a workman's insulated underpants, leggings that also cover the feet, with suspenders that are strapped, buckled, and hooped adjacent to the section's fold like a garment hanging from a clothes line.

The effect of each individual section in relation to the composite is a collaged stacking of disparate images and ideas representing artifacts, detritus, and mechanical production processes of industrial culture. When unfolded, the consolidation of Breton, Lamba, and Tanguy's three sections transforms into a whole yet disjunctive body, an anthropomorphic machine; a machine-man; a monstrous man-machine suggested by the image of the bearded old man's head and accompanying adornments in the top section, and supplemented by the placements and configurations of machine components in the other two sections; hence, the body is constituted as a mutable, indeterminate assemblage.[8]

Like Breton, Lamba, and Tanguy's assemblage, the adjoining words "exquisite" and "corpse" befit and confirm the incongruent folds of the game's process. According to the *Oxford English Dictionary* (OED), "exquisite" is defined as follows: "A. *adj.*1.

Sought out, 'recherché'. a. Of an expedient, explanation, reason: Sought out, ingeniously devised, far-fetched. Of studies: Abstruse" (OED, 2011). Although the definition of corpse seems uncomplicated, specifically a dead body, its dormancy nevertheless serves as an important counterpoint to the differential possibilities suggested by exquisite. For example, two of the defining terms for exquisite, "*recherché*" and "abstruse," are pertinent to my argument in this chapter. While *recherché* is the French word for research, abstruse is defined as something concealed, hidden, or latent. Hence, searching, and searching again, and again ... for knowledge that is latent yet incipient and emergent is at the heart of art research and practice that resists concrescence, and exemplifies the characteristic ambiguities and incompleteness of Exquisite Corpse.[9]

In terms of its corporeality, Exquisite Corpse affirms the embodiment of art research and practice as a processual, dialectical "algorhythm,"[10] which mutates between what is known and unknown, seen and unseen, familiar and strange, self and other, in fueling the body's imagination, improvisation, and creativity. Accordingly, art theorists Kochhar-Lindgren et al. (2009) use the neologism "algorhythm" to describe Exquisite Corpse as a process of art, theory, and pedagogy that "endlessly reinvents itself and reappears in a number of different contexts" (p. xviv). As such, the neologism corresponds with critical theorist Theodor Adorno's (1997) characterization of the dialectical movement of art as a "processual enactment of antagonisms (p. 176), and philosopher Brian Massumi's (2002) concept of art embodiment as a "processual rhythm of continuity and discontinuity" in and across contexts (p. 217). Exquisite Corpse similarly constitutes eccentric, ecstatic, and eclectic embodiment; an imminent dynamic of folding and unfolding, revealing and concealing knowledge that is capable of rupturing sedimented, normalizing ideologies and practices of hegemonic power; in doing so, its antinomies offer irreducible possibilities for the body's creative and political agency.[11]

Understanding that "exquisite" constitutes "research," its conjoining with "corpse" brings to mind the seeking of knowledge that is yet to be discovered and learned; and presumably an "exhumation" and "re-habitation" of ossified understandings; the transformation of socially and historically determined assumptions and ideologies; those that inscribe, choreograph, and regulate the body and the body politic. The restoration and renewal of lived experience that lays dormant within dead and frozen metaphors is possible within the diverse and dynamic, interstitial conditions, "the *bursting at the seams* of "Exquisite [*and*] Corpse [*and*]" (Sapier, 2009, p. 197), where cultural differences and peculiarities are contiguous and fluid; where labile understandings in-between private and public knowledge are exposed and enable examining and critiquing academic, institutional, and corporate structures; a differential space where originary lived experiences are restored, renewed, and the newness of lived experience sustained interminably.[12] Hence, in resisting intellectual closure and ideological sedimentations, Exquisite Corpse research and practice, "does not dismiss all knowledge, but rather activates it [differently] as a performance" (Sapier, 2009, p. 197).[13] In doing so, it serves as public pedagogy that exposes, examines, and critiques sedimented, ideological assumptions of the body and the body politic (Denzin, 2003, p. 9).

Concerned with the exhumation of immutable metaphors, my aim in this chapter is to revisit *cadavre exquis*, one of several free associative parlor games with which the surrealists responded to Sigmund Freud's conception of dream cognition,[14] and to reconsider its mutable and indeterminate narrative as enabling the body's critical intervention within academic, institutional, and corporate culture. Within the context of modernist art, and the avant-garde's utopian ambitions, the disjunctive, mutable operations of Exquisite Corpse mirrored and mimicked the technological and production efficiencies of machine culture as evidenced by Breton, Lamba, and Tanguy's collaborative collage process. The dadaists' engineering of component fragments and parts of visual and material culture in collage, montage, and assemblage narratives, for example, is one parallel with industrial and mechanized construction, and the uncanny machinations of dreams, humor, and play in the mind as theorized and expounded by Freud and performed by the surrealists in games like the Exquisite Corpse, is another.

Art historian Susan Laxton (2009) describes the discrete yet significant differences between the disjunctive narratives of dada montage and surrealist Exquisite Corpse. She explains that the "tension of juxtaposition" of disparate fragments in montage represent "unambivalent 'difference,'" whereas that tension in Exquisite Corpse "is ameliorated by the way that drawing is regulated in the game, specifically by requiring each player to take up the contours of the image exactly where another player left off, effectively extending the previous contribution long enough to smooth the transition" (p. 32). In other words, while the fragments of montage remain disparate and disjunctive, the conjunctions of Exquisite Corpse oscillate between its disjunctive sections and its consolidated, figural structure, and in doing so they expose an interminable process of forming and becoming a figure.[15]

The radical procedure of Exquisite Corpse notwithstanding, the transgressive operations and contraventions of the surrealists' games were driven by a desire to break from and escape the codes and canons of historical art and culture. With progress as its imperative, the movement's dialectical critique of history fell short of its ambition to transform society. Relegated to the margins of art and culture by the procession of avant-gardism, the movement had little effect on "art's critical engagement with social praxis" as it had hoped for (Bürger, pp. 78–79; Laxton, 2009, p. 30). With minimal impact on society at large, its forceful critique remained bound to the art world as yet another ideological manifestation within the spectrum of modernist art, and its strategies and attempts at transforming social and historical regimes and ideologies of power were subsequently absorbed by the consumptive impulses and inducements of industrial capitalism in its endless thirst for novelty.[16]

Naive about the false consciousness of modernism, the differential critiques and strategies of the artistic avant-garde were easily co-opted by academic, institutional, and corporate systems of production and distribution in order to reinvent and expand their imperious positioning and power. Examples where the avant-garde's radical strategies have been appropriated by corporate capitalism are found in mass mediated advertisements that seduce and manufacture the body's desire for consumption by way of montage innuendos, parodies, and narratives on sex, health, and environmental issues. With consciousness raising as their purported aim, such spectacle entertainments and inducements deploy clever, fashionable juxtapositions of images and ideas whose interstitial contingencies are immediately claimed, tamed, and branded with corporate logos, and often endorsed by celebrities to ensure that consumers associate the advertisement's ingenuity and smartness with the commodities being advertised. In doing so, the impact of corporate capitalism on the body's creative and political agency is lost in the daze and dazzle of spectacle (Mirzoeff, 2002).

The profit motives of corporate capitalism are far reaching and have impacted institutions of higher education. Colleges and universities, for example, are experiencing rapid corporatization as the educational values of debt-burdened families are shifting from arts and liberal arts study toward academic disciplines that will ensure job security. Indeed, the high cost of tuition and accompanying expenses has resulted in a commodification of learning where students insist on high grades as an entitlement for merely showing up in class, and their helicopter-parents hover over them and their teachers to get the biggest bang for their tuition bucks. Political scientist Wendy Brown warns: "The danger [of liberal arts erosion] … is that the public will give up the idea of educating people for democratic citizenship. Instead, all of public higher education will be essentially vocational in nature, oriented entirely around the market logic of job preparation … [as such] universities will be expected to build human capital" (quoted in Glenn, 2010).

As capital, the body's desire for creative and political agency, which is constituted by indeterminate, individual, and differential processes like those of Exquisite Corpse and others in arts and liberal arts study, is usurped, rearticulated, and colonized as commodity fetishism by the spectacle of corporate culture. Critical educator Paulo Freire (1998) opposes the wholeness and wholesomeness that educational capitalism offers: "It is in our incompleteness, of which we are aware, that education is grounded. … Education does not make us educable. It is our awareness of being unfinished that makes us educable" (p. 58). Accordingly, the body's incompleteness, its "unfinished" awareness and desire for learning and creative agency, stands in stark contrast with the manufactured desire for and false promises of knowledge as power, which purport educational grounding and completeness by way of consumption rather than production. Like the proverbial emperor with new clothes, spectacle veils its control over the body by manufacturing a false sense of desire and agency (Debord, 1994, p. 23). By choreographing its choices and compulsion to consume through schooling and the mass mediated organs of newspapers, television, movies, magazines, advertising, and the Internet, the indifference of power toward the body continues to homogenize difference within the body politic.

Hence, my purpose in exhuming the spectacle of Exquisite Corpse from the confines of modernist art history is to reinhabit and reconstitute its originary abstruse research without underestimating, circumventing, or deserting the pitfalls of academic, institutional, and corporate power, but to ensure the "possibility of disarticulating their constitutive elements, with the aim of establishing a different power configuration" that challenges power's indifference toward the body's agency (Mouffe, 2010). It is my contention that situating the differential research and practice of art, like Exquisite Corpse, within regimes of power, be they classrooms, museums, or boardrooms, constitutes an interminable process of exposure, examination, and critique that counters ideological representations and sedimentations and facilitates latent power configurations that respect and allow for the differences and peculiarities of the body and the body politic.

Since its inception in the 1920s, visual artists have re-inhabited the dadaists' and surrealists' processes of radical juxtaposition in new and differing ways to disarticulate and reconfigure the sedimented and fetishized codes and practices of art and culture that stultify the body's creative and political agency. In the remaining portion of this chapter, I will describe and discuss two works of art as examples of how the generative research and practice of Exquisite Corpse has accrued since the surrealists. Before proceeding, however, I want to elaborate on the process of collaboration, which is usually identified with the surrealists' renderings of Exquisite Corpse. My purpose in doing so is to extend and expand the understanding of collaboration to include the contextual shifts and folds of experience with which viewers interact with works of art. Hence, contrary to the assumption that defines viewers as disembodied spectators, their embodiment of an artwork's movements, affects, and sensations constitute them as collaborators, which is consistent with the dynamic relational engagement of Exquisite Corpse. An expansive understanding of collaboration is a case in point in my discussion of the following works of art considering that solo artists created them.

In *One and Three Chairs*[17] (1965), conceptual artist Joseph Kosuth juxtaposed three representations of "chair" (Figure 17.4) to engage viewers' critical contemplation and participation. To the left of his installation, a large format photograph is pinned on a wall that contains an image of a life-sized wooden folding chair positioned on a white floor and against a white wall. The wall and floor in the photograph, it turns out, are those of the gallery where Kosuth has installed the actual folding chair positioned against the actual wall in the photograph, both of which are situated adjacent to a text panel tacked to the wall that contains

chair (châr), n. [OF. chaiere (F. chaire), < L. cathedra: see cathedra.] A seat with a back, and often arms, usually for one person; a seat of office or authority, or the office itself; the person occupying the seat or office, esp. the chairman of a meeting; a sedan-chair; a chaise†; a metal block or clutch to support and secure a rail in a railroad.

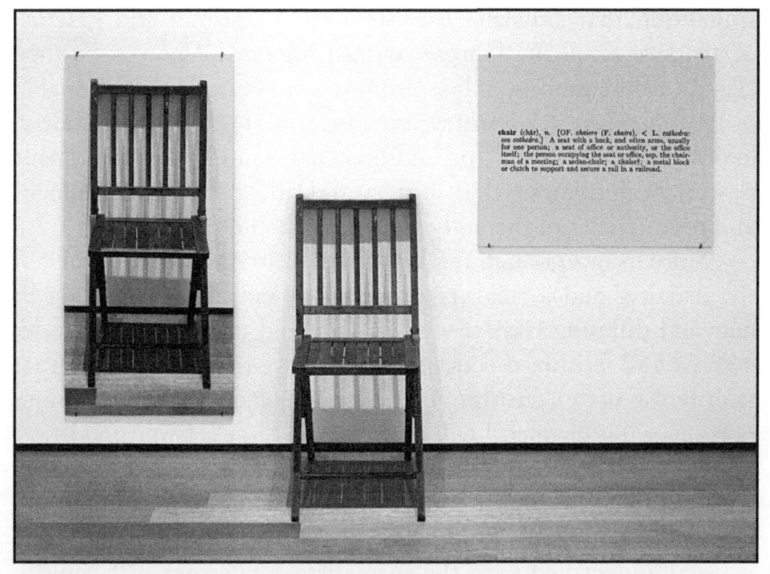

Figure 17.4: Joseph Kosuth (1945–). © 2015 Joseph Kosuth / Artists Rights Society (ARS), New York. *One and Three Chairs*, 1965. Wooden folding chair, photographic copy of a chair, and photographic enlargement of a dictionary definition of a chair; chair 32 3/8" x 14 7/8" x 20 7/8z"; photo panel, 36" x 24 1/8"; text panel 24" x 24 1/8". *Larry Aldrich Foundation Fund. Digital Image. © The Museum of Modern Art/Licensed by SCALA/ Art Resource, The Museum of Modern Art, New York.*

the dictionary definition of chair; hence "one and three chairs." Kosuth has created a visual and conceptual conundrum with this installation, which exposes differences between actual and virtual representations of cultural artifacts, and differences between textual representations and those of images. Like Exquisite Corpse, it is at the "unfolding" of Kosuth's three representations of the "folding" chair where viewers are invited to intervene, collaborate, and respond with questions, and to explore, experiment, and improvise possible associations and understandings that challenge socially and historically constructed assumptions of art and culture. Functionality, for example, is one issue that viewers may reflect upon and question in their response to the installation's disjunctive mode of address. While chair is socially and historically understood as an artifact for the body's sitting comfort, the understanding of that function is disturbed, brought into question, and rendered mutable by virtue of its placement in an art exhibit where touching is prohibited by security guards. As such, the gallery context unfolds and raises additional questions about *One and Three Chairs*.

Although it might seem an exaggeration and eccentric to suggest that art galleries *are* chairs, considering that artworks are exhibited and essentialized in galleries suggests that that is where they "sit" or come to rest. According to philosopher Ludwig Wittgenstein's language-games,[18] a chair's significance would depend on any number of contexts in which it would be placed. In other words, although we may assume that a chair is only a chair based on its familiar use and meaning, its placement within an art installation represents a shift in context that throws its function and significance into question and attaches it with other, unexpected ones. Questions about language use, such as those raised by Kosuth's compelling chair installation *One and Three Chairs*, correspond with the generative, folding-unfolding discourse of Exquisite Corpse research and practice.

While a folded structure is not readily apparent in artist Joel Kyack's *Superclogger: "Rush Hour–210 East-Pasadena"*[19] (2010), his live public artwork (Figure 17.5) during rush hour on a congested Los Angeles freeway does constitute movement across different contexts similar to Exquisite Corpse and

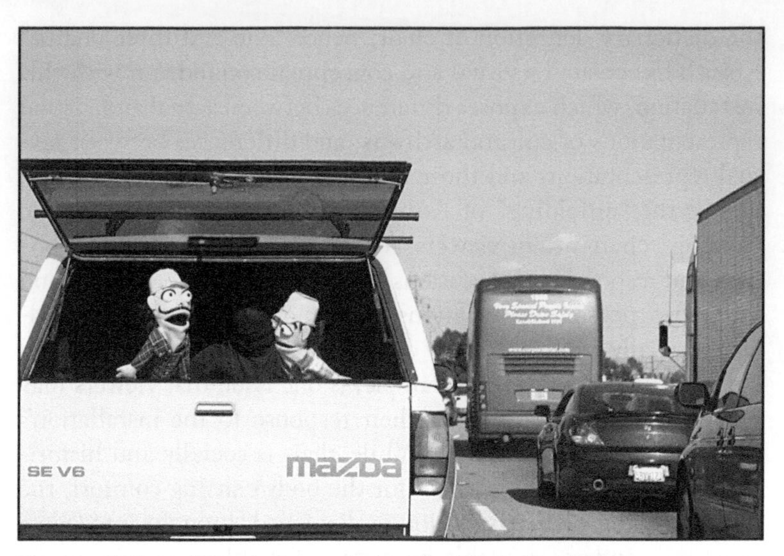

Figures 17.5. Joel Kyack, Superclogger (public art initiative documentation photograph), 2010, Rush hour-210 East-Pasadena. *Courtesy of the artist and LA><ART, Los Angeles.*

Kosuth's *One and Three Chairs*. *Superclogger* consisted of puppet shows that were co-conceived with artist Peter Fuller and performed by Kyack from the tailgate of an ordinary white Mazda pickup truck with the rear hatch of its shell opened for viewing by commuters jammed in traffic. The show's cast consisted of "a group of funky, grimy, homemade Muppets, acting out short vignettes on themes that might speak to people stuck in traffic. Coping with uncertain conditions, for instance, or the state of being controlled" (Ulaby, 2010). Using FM broadcasting equipment like that found in drive-in theaters, Kyack transmitted the soundtracks of his puppet performances by way of radio waves to commuters' cars that were stalled bumper-to-bumper in traffic within 200 feet of his pickup.

Assuming puppet theater as a unifying, figural structure like Exquisite Corpse, the disjunctive folds of *Superclogger* are suggested by the pickup truck as performance stage complete with its tailgate proscenium; the highway an open air stage where commuter traffic is performed; and, cars, a lot of cars, stopping and starting, weaving and inching forward, controlled by the unpredictable ebb and flow of rush hour traffic constituting drivers' performances of driving as puppetry—a staging that is further controlled and regulated according to the script of state traffic laws.[20] ArtDaily.org, a Los Angeles–based Internet art newspaper, described the impact of Kyack's puppet performances on traffic madness as follows:

> *Superclogger* engages the traffic jam as a formal materialization of the principles of chaos, providing a direct experience with the evolving conditions that can effect a system and help to predict outcomes—in this instance, a person breaking [*sic*] a millisecond earlier than expected because of the puppet show would, over time, drastically change traffic patterns. Intervening in the commute experience of people driving behind the truck, *Superclogger* aims to *briefly halt* the progression of chaos by temporarily drawing the audience out of the commute experience and placing them within an intimate space of engagement that highlights their own individual presence within the broader structure of the traffic jam. (ArtDaily.org, 2010; emphasis added)

ArtDaily.org's characterization of *braking* cars affecting traffic patterns on the highway as a formal materialization of chaos[21] during the traffic jam corresponds with the disjunctive sectional folds of Exquisite Corpse, which *break with,* and extend our patterns of perception and thought and interconnect with others. Like Exquisite Corpse, the complex and contradictory research of *Superclogger* opened liminal, contingent spaces of experience where drivers' escalations of aggression over the chaos in which they were situated were delayed; in-between spaces where drivers were able to linger on the abstruse juxtapositions as the highway/performance unfolded and where they experienced its dynamic, intimate space of engagement. In doing so, the liveness of the performance transformed drivers' assumptions and expectations about sitting in their cars waiting for traffic to abate; about how a pickup truck constitutes a stage and the highway a theatre; and the use of their car radios speaker systems that receive the sounds and narratives of a live performance. In other words, *Superclogger* created a differential space where drivers were able to renew and restore their understanding of traffic from across multiple contexts of experience.[22]

Based on the unfolding of Exquisite Corpse research and practice in Breton, Lamba, and Tanguy's *Cadavre Exquis,* Kosuth's *One and Three Chairs*, Kyack's *Superclogger,* and including Chester's forklift, let us now consider each of these four works as folds in the Exquisite Corpse unfolding of this chapter. Although each work differs from the others, there exist *generative, figural correspondences* in-between their *generative, figural structures*, a folding-unfolding movement across the various bewildering contexts of Exquisite Corpse research. Such deterritorializing and reterritorializing machinations constitute the work of art as a body without organs (BwO) according to Deleuze and Guattari (1987); that is, a cultural body that resists sedimented *organ*izational assumptions, significations and representations through its dynamic movements, affects and sensations. Accordingly, "the BwO is not at all the opposite of the organs. The organs are not its enemies. The enemy is the organism [sedimented body of organs]" (p. 158).

Such resistance to concrescence (those dead and frozen metaphors mentioned previously) in-between and among the formations of Exquisite Corpse constitutes embodiment as a "plane of consistency" (p. 251), where disparate and disjunctive folds of experience temporarily consolidate, and where interminable affinities generate via multiple lines of flight across various unfolding contexts. Hence, in resisting sedimentation, or intellectual closure, the four aforementioned works enable figural rhythms and associations to emerge between and among them, as their plane of consistency is unfolded.

Accordingly, let us consider the disparate discontinuities of Chester's welded assemblage in processual rhythm with the continuities of its forklift form; *and* consider the discontinuities of Breton, Lamba, and Tanguy's machinic folds in processual rhythm with the continuities of its unfolded machine body; *and* consider the discontinuities in Kosuth's installation in processual rhythm with continuities that consolidate as *one* in three chairs; *and* consider the discontinuities of controlled movement during rush hour traffic in processual rhythm with the continuities that consolidate a formal materialization of highway chaos as puppetry through Kyack's pick-up truck performance ... *and, and,* then consider the continues and discontinuities of Chester's forklift assemblage in processual rhythm with the continues and discontinuities of Breton, Lamba, and Tanguy's *Cadavre Exquis* in processual rhythm with the continues and discontinuities of Kosuth's *One and Three Chairs* in processual rhythm with the continues and discontinuities of Kyach's *Supperclogger* ... and consider ... in processual rhythm with the continues and discontinuities of ... *and, and, and.* ...[23]

Hence, like *Superclogger*, the agonistic associative movements of Exquisite Corpse destabilize the gridlock of sedimented cultural organs that traffic and stultify our bodies' creative and political agency by unfolding and materializing a chaotic field of excess and possibility that Grosz (2008) ascribes to the emancipatory affects of art: "the generation of vibratory waves, rhythms, that traverse the body and make of the body a link with forces it cannot otherwise perceive and act upon" (p. 23). Therein lies the paradox of contemporary cultural life: While this *excessiveness*, the sensate body's becoming other through art, is frequently misunderstood and misrepresented as *frivolous* by academic, institutional and corporate organs of power, it is by virtue of its destabilizing frivolities—the very mis-understandings, misrepresentations, and mis-firings of art research and practice like Exquisite Corpse—that our ways of seeing, understanding, and creating the world are transformed.

Notes

1 Rock musician Bruce Springsteen describing his song writing process for his 1978 album "Darkness on the Edge of Town" during an interview with actor Edward Norton in 2010.

2 Chester Alexanian (1924–1991), my father-in-law, owned and operated Chester Alexanian Trucking and Tractoring (CATT) beginning in the early 1950s until his death in 1991. He and his wife Ruby raised two daughters, Sherrie and Cindy, in the small agricultural community of Fowler, California, where they lived on 20 acres of land and Chester ran his business.

3 See Turner (1983, p. 234).

4 The Exquisite Corpse folding process of inquiry that is referred to in this chapter corresponds with the "braided metaphor" with which Sullivan

(2005, pp. 103–109) theorizes the complex movements and interconnections that are enabled through visual arts research and practice.

5 Laxton (2009) writes that in the written version of Exquisite Corpse, subject/verb/object corresponded with the head/torso/feet structure of the visual version (p. 30).

6 Haraway (1992) characterizes "artifactualism" as postmodernism's reductive hyper-production, reproduction, replication, and globalization of denatured images and ideas that permeate, homogenize, and dominate the body's creative and political agency. The principle of artifactualism is that "the whole world is remade in the image of commodity production" (p. 297).

7 See a color reproduction of Cadavre Exquis [Exquisite Corpse], 1938, by Breton, Lamba, and Tanguy in the collection of the National Galleries of Scotland at http://www.nationalgalleries.org/collection/online_search/4:324/result/0/31332

8 Breton, Lamba, and Tanguy's machinic construction corresponds with Deleuze and Guattari's (1987) concept of assemblage—a gathering of disparate elements in a single context that resist concrescence and interpretation. In doing so, its affect is one of extension and expansion across multiple contexts, a rhizomatic "deterritorializing machine" that releases an interminable web of associations and understandings (pp. 4, 333).

9 Critical theorist Adorno (1997) characterizes artworks' resistance to intellectual closure, like Exquisite Corpse, as the antithetical procedure of montage: "Artworks … that negate meaning must also necessarily be disrupted in their unity; this is the function of montage, which disavows unity through the emerging disparateness of the parts at the same time that, as a principle of form, it reaffirms unity" (p. 154).

10 The neologism "algorhythm" plays on the word "algorithm," which the OED defines as "a step-by-step procedure for reaching a clinical decision or diagnosis, often set out in the form of a flow chart, in which the answer to each question determines the next question to be asked" (OED, 2011).

11 Kochhar-Lindgren et al. (2009) argue that: "The Exquisite Corpse exemplifies one manner in which difference is produced as a means of disrupting the normalizing of the hegemonic power of current cultural regime" (p. xxii).

12 The restoral and renewal capacities of Exquisite Corpse correspond with philosopher Michel de Certeau's (1988) differentiation of *spaces* and *places.* He describes the characteristics of space as contingent, performative, and differential, which oppose the stability and singularity of place (p. 117). Also, philosopher Henri Lefebvre (1991) characterizes the differences and peculiarities of differential space as resisting the abstract space of corporate capitalism (pp. 52–53).

13 Literary theorist Craig Sapier describes correspondences between the folds of Exquisite Corpse and Roland Barthes's *punctum* (1981).

14 See film theorist Anne M. Kern's (2009) characterization of surrealism's "crucial and consistent" relationship with Freud's theories (p. 4).

15 Following philosopher Gilles Deleuze's conception of the *figural* as the "abandonment of art as representation," cultural theorist Elizabeth Grosz (2008) writes: "The figural is the deformation of the sensational and the submission [of the] figurative to sensation. It is the development of art as an 'analogical language,' a non-representational 'language' of colors, forms, bodily shapes, screams" (p. 88).

16 Adorno (1997) describes the institutionalization and subsequent neutralization of the social impact of surrealist art as a "false afterlife" considering that it "began as a protest against the fetishization of art as an isolated realm, yet as art, which after all surrealism was, it was forced beyond the pure form of protest" (p. 229).

17 See a color reproduction of Kosuth's *One and Three Chairs* (1965) in the collection of the Museum of Modern Art at http://www.moma.org/collection/browse_results.php?criteria=O%3AAD%3AE%3A3228&page_number=1&template_id=1&sort_order=1

18 Similar to Wittgenstein's language-games, in which the significance of a word or object is dependent on the context in which it is found, and its use determines its meaning.

19 See a color reproduction of and listen to the National Public Radio story about Kyack's *Superclogger*, 2010 at http://www.npr.org/templates/story/story.php?storyId=129128690

20 Such a multiplicity corresponds with Deleuze and Guattari's (1987) analogy of the untying of *puppet strings* [author's emphasis] from the will of the artist-puppeteer, which in this case is Kyack, and extends as multiple lines of flight to form an expansive web of connections between and among other "puppet[s] in other dimensions connected to the first" (p. 8).

21 ArtDaily.org's use of "chaos" to describe *Superclogger's* materialization of form is the inverse of absolute order; rather what Grosz (2008) argues "as a plethora of orders, forms, wills—forces that cannot be distinguished or differentiated from each other, both matter and its conditions for being otherwise, both the actual and the virtual indistinguishably (p. 5).

22 For additional information about *Superclogger* see report on National Public Radio website at http://www.npr.org/templates/story/story.php?storyId=129128690

23 My use of the ellipsis [...] is to suggest an affinity between Exquisite Corpse and the rhizomatic alliances that Deleuze and Guattari (1987) characterize as having "no beginning or end." Contrary to the genealogical and ontological filiations of a tap root-tree that "imposes the verb 'to be'... the fabric of the rhizome is the conjunction, 'and ... and ... and ...'" (p. 25).

References

Adorno, T. W. (1997). *Aesthetic theory: Theory and history of literature.* G. Adorno & R. Tiedemann (Eds.). Minneapolis: University of Minnesota Press.

ArtDaily.org. (2010). Public art project presents various puppet shows to drivers caught in traffic. file:///Users/crg2/Desktop/Superclogger.webarchive (accessed July 12, 2010).

Barthes, R. (1981). *Camera lucida.* New York: Hill and Wang.

Bürger, P. (1984). *Theory of the avant-garde.* M. Shaw (Trans.). Minneapolis: University of Minnesota Press.

Cahnmann-Taylor, M., & Siegesmund, R. (2008). Challenges to the definition and acceptance of arts-based inquiry as research. In M. Cahnmann-Taylor & R. Siegesmund (Eds.), *Arts-based research in education: Foundations for practice*, pp. 1–2. New York: Routledge.

Carse, J. P. (1986). *Finite and infinite games.* New York: Ballantine Books.

Debord, G. (1994). *The society of the spectacle* (D. Nicholson-Smith, Trans.). New York: Zone Books.

De Certeau, M. (1988). *The practice of everyday life.* Berkeley: University of California Press.

Deleuze, G., & Guattari, F. (1987). *A thousand plateaus: Capitalism and schizophrenia.* B. Massumi (Trans.). Minneapolis: University of Minnesota Press.

Denzin, N. K. (2003). *Performance ethnography: Critical pedagogy and the politics of culture.* Thousand Oaks, CA: Sage.

Dewey, J. (1938). *Experience and education.* New York: Macmillan.

Freire, P. (1998). *Pedagogy of freedom: Ethics, democracy, and civic courage.* Lanham, MD: Rowman & Littlefield.

Glenn, D. (2010). Public higher education is "eroding from all sides" warn political scientists. *The Chronicle of Higher Education.* http:/chronicle.com/article/Public-Higher-Education-Is/124292/ (accessed September 2, 2010).

Grosz, E. (2008). *Chaos, territory, art: Deleuze and the framing of the earth.* New York: Columbia University Press.

Haraway, D. (1992). The promises of monsters: A regenerative politics for inappropriate/d others. In L. Grossberg, C. Nelson, & P.A. Treichler (Eds.), *Cultural studies*, pp. 295–337. New York: Routledge.

Kern, A. M. (2009). From one exquisite corpse (in)to another. In K. Kochhar-Lindgren, D. Schneiderman, & T. Denlinger (Eds.), *The exquisite corpse: Chance and collaboration in Surrealism's parlor game*, pp. 3–28. Lincoln: University of Nebraska Press.

Kochhar-Lindgren, K., Schneiderman, D., & Denlinger, T. (2009). Introduction. In K. Kochhar-Lindgren, D. Schneiderman, & T. Denlinger (Eds.), *The exquisite corpse: Chance and collaboration in Surrealism's parlor game*, pp. xx–xxix. Lincoln: University of Nebraska Press.

Laxton, S. (2009). This is not a drawing. In K. Kochhar-Lindgren, D. Schneiderman, & T. Denlinger (Eds.), *The exquisite corpse: Chance and collaboration in Surrealism's parlor game*, pp. 29–48. Lincoln: University of Nebraska Press.

Lefebvre, H. (1991). *The production of space*. D. Nicholson-Smith (Trans.). Malden, MA: Blackwell.

Massumi, B. (2002). *Parables for the virtual: Movement, affect, sensation*. Durham, NC: Duke University.

Mirzoeff, N. (2002). *An introduction to visual culture*. London: Routledge.

Mouffe, C. (2010). The museum revisited. *Kostis Velonis*. http://kostisvelonis.blogspot.com/2010/06/museum-revisited.html (accessed January 16, 2011).

Oxford English Dctionary. 2011. http://www.oed.com/view/Entry/66815 (accessed January 15, 2011).

O'Donoghue, D. (2009). Are we asking the wrong questions in arts-based research? *Studies in Art Education: A Journal of Issues and Research in Art Education, 50*, 4, 352–367.

Sapier, C. (2009). Academia's exquiste corpse: An ethnography of the application process. In K. Kochhar-Lindgren, D. Schneiderman, & T. Denlinger (Eds.), *The exquisite corpse: Chance and collaboration in Surrealism's parlor game*, pp. 189–205. Lincoln: University of Nebraska Press.

Springsteen, B. (2010). Ed Norton interviews Bruce Springsteen on "Darkness." National Public Radio. http://www.npr.org/2010/11/12/131272103/ed-norton-interviews-bruce-springsteen-on-darkness (accessed November 15, 2010).

Sullivan, G. (2005). *Art practice as research: Inquiry in the visual arts*. Thousand Oaks, CA: Sage.

Todd, S. (2001). On not knowing the other, or learning from Levinas. *Philosophy of education archive*. http://ojs.ed.uiuc.edu/index.php/pes/issue/view/17 (accessed January 16, 2011) and http://ojs.ed.uiuc.edu/index.php/pes/article/viewFile/1871/582 (accessed January 16, 2011).

Turner, V.W. (1983). Body, brain, and culture. *Zygon, 18*, 3, 221–245.

Ulaby, N. (2010). 'Superclogger': Free theater on L.A.'s freeways. National Public Radio. http://www.npr.org/templates/story/story.php?storyId=129128690 (accessed August 11, 2010).

Chapter 18

The Death of a Cow

Jean Halley

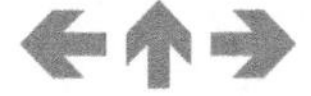

In this chapter, I explore the death of beef cows. I contrast these deaths with the death of my beloved childhood cat and with the sadness—a kind of dying—in my childhood. I look at the violence of these deaths, but also simply at the ways the deaths are a movement from one state to another, not only for the dying, but for all those involved in and surrounding the death. I try to capture the feel, atmosphere, and experience of these changes. And I use the data or evidence of my life experience along with the lives of cows to tell this story. This chapter is part of a larger project, a book in which I juxtapose the social history of beef ranching with the story of my childhood family, one side of whom were cattle ranchers.

The experience of living is the experience of change. Dying is perhaps a more significant change than many, but it is still only one change in the midst of an infinity of tiny and large changes making up our days. I contrast this movement, this change, with the ways in which we—cow, cat, all of us—are also momentarily caught, contained in emotional, physical, and body spaces. In other words, we are held in life, in our bodies and in our life

Originally published in *Qualitative Inquiry and Social Justice*, edited by Norman K. Denzin and Michael D. Giardina, pp. 229–247. Republished in *Qualitative Inquiry—Past, Present, and Future: A Critical Reader*, edited by Norman K. Denzin and Michael D. Giardina, pp. 328–346.

situations. There is no getting away from my own physicalness or my own life story, or my own emotional pain and joy. Even so, each of these things constantly changes, moves and transforms to something else. In its new form, the matter—be it me or a cow or a cut of meat—is both different and still the same. For even death does not stay still. Everything moves, everything changes.

Death as Production

Historically in the United States, the slaughterhouses have made most of the money to be made in beef. This is true even though the slaughterhouses were merely one stage in the production of meat. Some people bred and raised the cows; others slaughtered them and packed their meat to be sold; at the final stage, the consumer bought and ate the flesh. Jimmy M. Skaggs (1986) writes that the process was like an hourglass with lots of people in the beginning raising cows—the ranchers—and lots of people at the end eating cows—the consumers—but not many slaughtering them. The slaughterhouses had and continue to have a stranglehold on the industry. A small number of people have made and continue to make an immense amount of money off the backs of cows, literally, and less literally off ranchers. Indeed, Karen Olsson writes, "Four giant competitors—IBP, ConAgra, Excel (owned by Cargill) and Farmland National Beef—dominate the beef industry, together controlling over 85 percent of the US market" (2002, p. 12).

Similar to their counterparts in other industries, ranchers who supply the cows to these four companies, need to produce as much of their product—cow-to-be-meat—as possible with as little lost labor or other resources as possible in as short a time as is possible. To survive as a profitable business, they must raise their cows to make as much desirable meat as possible in as short a time as possible. The bigger the cow and the faster growing the cow the better. Yet there are other factors. American meat eaters want meat of a certain flavor and look. So cattle ranchers have slowly bred and raised bigger cows faster over the past century. This has a number of implications for the cow. Cows' lives have become significantly shorter. And they have slowly been ballooning out into larger and larger animals. Remarkably, this is the case even though they have less time to grow before slaughter.

When it comes time to be slaughtered, cows are either sold from their most recent owners, probably the people who own the feedlot or the slaughterhouse itself fattens the cows before slaughter. The cows need to be at a certain standard of health before the federal government allows them to be slaughtered. My grandfather owned a sale-barn. So he was a conduit from the people raising the cows to the people slaughtering the cows. Of course, he also raised cows himself. He made money by selling his own cattle as well as by auctioning other ranchers' cattle.

I remember walking above the cows on raised wooden pathways at my grandfather's sale-barn. I saw the cows from above. I walked up above these enormous pens filled with manure and mud and mooing animals, I walked and looked down on cow. But when you are around cows, you do not just see them. Perhaps the most dramatic experience of being with cows is the smelling of them. They have a very strong and very particular odor. The kind of odor—like breastfed baby poop or wet dog—that is definitively cow. Of course, like the poop of babies fed formula versus breastmilk, the odor changes depending on what you feed the cow. And our cows in the United States eat corn, lots of corn.

In killing cows, transforming this living, breathing, eating life into meat, the process has been routinized, much like the making of most other products in our postindustrialized world. Each step of a cow's death has been broken into its smallest component and done over and over again to thousands of cows. For instance, in the 1990s the John Morrell plant in Sioux Falls, South Dakota, then the only remaining tri-species plant, slaughtered "several thousand cattle, hogs, and sheep each day on three separate killing floors" (Eisnitz, 1997, p. 117). At the time of her research, journalist Gail A. Eisnitz found that

> one hundred and one million pigs are slaughtered each year in the United States. Thirty seven million cattle and calves. More than four million horses, goats, and sheep. And over eight billion chickens and turkeys. In all, annually in the United States farmers produce 65 billion pounds of cattle and pigs … 46 billion pounds of chickens and turkeys. (p. 61)

That is a lot of killing.

Federal law mandates that the killing happen at slaughterhouses in the following manner. First, the cow is herded and probed through a chute in a "knocking box," or they are herded one by one into a restrainer on a conveyor belt. The conveyor belt carries the animal to a person whose job it is to stun the cow, the aptly titled "stun operator" or "knocker." This person has a compressed-air gun with which he or she shoots the animal in the forehead. The gun "drives a steel bolt into the cow's skull and then retracts it. If the gun is sufficiently powered, well maintained, and properly used by the operator, it knocks the cow unconscious or kills the animal on the spot" (Eisnitz, 1997, p. 20). The also aptly named "shackler" shackles the animal. This person's job is to put a chain around one of the cow's hind legs for cow after cow after cow. The chain is attached to a powerful machine that lifts the cow by its leg up into the air, then carries the cow, hanging upside down, through the next stages of the slaughtering process.

Next a person called the "sticker" cuts the cow's throat; "more precisely, the carotid arteries and a jugular vein in the neck" (Eisnitz, 1997, p. 20). The sticker makes a vertical, not horizontal, incision in the animal's throat, near where the major vessels issue from the heart, to cut off the flow of blood to the animal's brain. "Next the cow travels along the 'bleed rail' and is given several minutes to bleed out. The carcass then proceeds to the head-skinners, the leggers, and on down the line where it is completely skinned, eviscerated, and split in half" (p. 20).

The federal government passed the first version of this killing process into law with the Humane Slaughter Act (HSA) in 1958. Congress expanded the HSA in 1978. "Among the HSA's most important provisions is the requirement that all animals be rendered unconscious with just one application of an effective stunning device by a trained person before being shackled and hoisted up on the line" (Eisnitz, 1997, p. 24).

The Jungle

The story of what actually happens to cows at the kill is another story. But that story requires yet another story before its telling.

In 1906, Upton Sinclair published his famous novel about an immigrant family new to Chicago and carrying the "American

Dream." As we watch this family struggle to survive, the "American Dream" is unraveled, and the American reality for new immigrants and the working poor is revealed. Sinclair wrote *The Jungle* out of his profound political commitments. Sinclair was a lifelong radical and activist, and a "significant presence within early socialist groups in American: In 1905, he cofounded the Intercollegiate Socialist Society with Jack London, Florence Kelley, and Clarence Darrow; in 1906 he established a socialist community, the Helicon Home Colony, in Englewood, New Jersey" (Spiegel, introduction to Sinclair 2003 [1906], p. v). Writing was one important venue for the expression of Sinclair's politics. "His work is identified with that of the writers Theodore Roosevelt dubbed 'muckrakers.' In all, he published more than ninety books and pamphlets and countless articles" (Spiegel, introduction to Sinclair, 2003 [1906], p. vi).

Through his perhaps most famous work, *The Jungle*, Sinclair revealed the underbelly of U.S. capitalism. Sinclair lived in

> an age of capitalist Titans, of magnates whose wealth, power, and hubris seemed unlimited: A single man owned a million acres of the Texas Panhandle, an American coal tycoon attempted to buy the Great Wall of China, and in the Midwest a combination known as the Beef Trust tightly controlled the production and sale of meat through pervasive wage and price fixing and the unrelenting exploitation of the stockyard workforce. (Spiegel, introduction to Sinclair, 2003 [1906], p. xv)

Sinclair intended to expose the terrible treatment of workers in the meat industry, particularly after the meatpacker's strike that failed to change the conditions of these workers in 1904. But the American public responded to the *conditions* under which their meat was processed from living animal to the product they bought and ate:

> *The Jungle* revealed slaughterhouse conditions so shocking and meat so filthy that meat sales plummeted more than fifty percent and President Theodore Roosevelt personally crusaded for enactment of the Federal Meat Inspection Act of 1906. That law and subsequent legislation established standards for plant sanitation and required federal inspection of all meat shipped interstate or out of the country. (Eisnitz, 1997, p. 21)

Although the American public *did* respond to the filth in their meat, they did not respond to the abuse of workers who produced their meat or to the violence against the animals that became their meat. As Sinclair himself said, "I aimed at the public's heart, and by accident I hit it in the stomach" (Spiegel, introduction to Sinclair, 2003 [1906], p. vi). Indeed, reading *The Jungle*, one often feels sick to one's stomach. For example, Sinclair describes the deceptive and unsafe practices of the Chicago meat industry and its complete lack of concern for the public's health. Every part of every animal was used to make some product to sell to the unsuspecting consumer. Even sick animals were used. Sinclair wrote:

> It seemed that they must have agencies all over the country, to hunt out old and crippled and diseased cattle to be canned. There were cattle which had been fed on "whiskey-malt," the refuse of the breweries, and had become what the men called "steerly"—which means covered with boils. It was a nasty job killing these, for when you plunged your knife into them they would burst and splash foul-smelling stuff into your face; and when a man's sleeves were smeared with blood, and his hands steeped in it, how was he ever to wipe his face, or to clear his eyes so that he could see? It was stuff such as this that made the "embalmed beef" that had killed several times as many United States soldiers as all the bullets of the Spaniards; only the army beef, besides, was not fresh canned, it was old stuff that had been lying for years in the cellars. (Sinclair 2003 [1906], p. 110)

These, along with Sinclair's other assertions, were all but one independently verified when his book was published.[1] Understandably, when discovering the real origins of their dinner, the public was outraged. However, Sinclair made vivid more than just the health hazards birthed by the industry. Nonetheless, in contrast to the rapid enactment of the Meat Inspection Act and the federal Food and Drug Act passed the same year the book came out, no legal or other formal changes were made on behalf of meat industry workers. And the HSA did not come about until 1958.

The HSA addresses, of course, the death of cows and other animals. Yet there is more to their lives than dying. Death is only one among other changes in the life of a beef cow. Another important change is that of calf to adult cow. In a capitalist economy, the most important part of this change is that of small cow to large cow, less cow to more cow. And maybe caught in pressing, pressing of more life into life, pressing of more cow into cow, more meat into the skin wrapping and bone rack of animal, there is only one way out, only one way, and that is back to the place from which we came, back to sadness, back to dying. Maybe it is silly to dwell any longer on cows, stupid creatures. But they are gentle and alive. And they do offer themselves to us, unknowing. They make the sacrifice of dying. And then they live again, allowing their flesh to become ours. It is a kind of passion, a fully giving of one's self.

Somewhere around fourteen to sixteen months old, fattened cows are loaded into cattle trailers and carried to their last stop, the slaughterhouses. Cows must walk the last few steps of this journey. In fact, in this walk, they have always taken part in their own dying. The distance they walked decreased significantly over the past two hundred years. They used to walk for miles, for days, even months to the place of their slaughter. Albeit a shorter walk, cows still walk to the site of their death. Indeed, there is a law requiring that the animal do so. This is not, of course, meant to benefit the cow. Humans have devised this test to be sure the cow is healthy before transforming its flesh into food. A cow that cannot walk, a "downed cow," could be a sick cow whose flesh is unfit for human consumption. Healthy cows tend to spend a lot of time on their feet. And obviously, almost all healthy cows can walk.

Given our profit-driven society, that cows must walk to their own slaughter has made things pretty rough for the cows. The Humane Society of the United States (2008) offers video footage at their website from numerous undercover investigations involving their "Factory Farming Campaign: Working to Reduce the Suffering of Animals Raised for Meat, Eggs, and Milk." Among its investigations, in 2008, the Humane Society looked into the sale and slaughter of dairy cows that were no longer producing enough milk to make them profitable.

Typically, dairy farmers sell unproductive cows for slaughter. The Humane Society secretly inspected numerous auctions and slaughterhouses where they find that downed dairy cows "too frail to walk may be dragged to their death or left suffering for hours" (2008). In the video footage, one views downed animals being beaten until they drag themselves on broken limbs to their own slaughter. And in the end, potential profit carries more weight than the law that the animals must walk. Machines drag animals, seemingly too sick to be forced to move. Workers attach a chain to the leg of one dairy cow. In the footage, they proceed to drag the cow's full body weight by her overextended leg to the slaughterhouse. One witnesses other animals being kicked, beaten, and shocked as workers attempt to force the downed animals up. One worker repeatedly and forcefully probes a downed cow in her eye. Another worker rolls a downed cow bellowing and crying in front of a farm vehicle. Before stopping this rolling, the worker drives over her head. After beating another downed cow to no avail, a worker tries to force her to her feet by spraying water down her nose so that she feels that she is about to drown.

Along with the issue of cruelty to these animals, as the Humane Society points out, if downed and sick animals are being slaughtered and processed for meat, consumers are probably (unknowingly) eating diseased meat from such sick animals (2008). Indeed, children at school seem to be the consumers of some of this meat. One of the slaughterhouses found to abuse and slaughter downed cows, the Hallmark Slaughterhouse, provided meat for the Westland Meat Company, itself a top supplier to the National School Lunch Program. The Humane Society believes that the National School Lunch Program has received and served a significant amount of meat from downed, and potentially sick, cattle.

At the slaughterhouse, all the cows' efforts bear fruit. And they become meat. They are stunned, bled, and eviscerated. Then they are graded, checked for disease, and broken down into cuts. And, given that at some beef plants, 390 animals are killed every hour, that is a lot of killing. And a lot of meat.

And so the cows offer themselves to be eaten. They become us. The body and the blood. It is a kind of passion, a kind of giving. And maybe no one, not cows, not us, maybe no one really owes anyone their passion. But they give it anyhow. I am one of those who gives passionately. The catch is that passion, given or received, brings something with it, some weight of its past it carried into new form. Passion is not freedom. It is a heavy kind of love.

I know about this. I love, at least a few people, with everything. They are my everything. But if this loving is giving, it is a funny kind of giving. Really, in it, in giving this love, I try to leave myself. I try to step away from the unbearable place that is me. I try to enter into them, and become anew. Passion can be dying. But passion can also act to kill, to press into, to push aside and away, bloating, exploding the walls of another.

But Here

My sadness leaves me no choice. It pushes all else aside. It is the hardest thing to name and yet demands naming. It is a dry, dusty washed-out-by-too-much-sun place. It is a place that swallows all else, all other desires, all color, all beauty. All gone to this still quiet.

We all risk returning to this emptiness that makes one long for dying because at least in dying there is a strength. Color and presence live on in dying. But here, but here, how can I tell it? I am again my horse before a storm, rushing along fence lines, frenzy whirling in the air, gripping me from inside out. I rush, seeking words to release me.

And yet, somewhere I know there is no release. My horse, too, lived forever in-between fences. His escapes were momentary. He was always caught, always brought home, always, to that place between wires. That is where I too live. It is no place and yet it fills everywhere, inside of me.

This. This is the ghost of my family. Somehow, of that, I feel a kind of sureness, even as the sureness slips away. This is the ghost. My grandfather, my father's father, whoever he was, was a man willing violence, willing rupture of another. And there lived the ghost. He was a man who got rich. A man who hated "niggers," who pulled my hair, who touched my breasts before breasts pushed forward. He voted Republican, drove crazy-like, beat his sons with a belt or worse when they misbehaved, and supposedly loved my grandmother, whatever that means. Or at least, that is the story as I now know it. They say my grandfather was sane. He was the wire fence line, dividing this from that, cutting through, controlling all things.

My father, like my mother's father, was out of control. He was insane. He was the waste left behind my grandfather's life. He was the violence ricocheting here and there, controlling nothing, moving wildly. But that, too, of course, is a kind of control. And so if my grandfather held the gun, steady and shot, my father, the bullet, ran until it found me. And I live with it, embedded inside. It will not let me go. Nor I, it.

Yet there is no quick way out, anyhow. The fences go to infinity. They live on with or without me. And I cannot leave, anyhow. My grandfather, dead fifteen years, is still here, of course. Everything stays.

And me too, just when I think I have turned away to somewhere else, no fence no land no frenzied horse no sun-bleached colorless sky no boy scarecrow hanging on a fence no girl wet with his release no story clinging to her no toilet whirling cat gut away no more, no more, just then I turn, and there it is again. Just then I turn and find the fence to meet me.

Barbed Wire

My grandfather worked among cows. His life was made of power and violence and a certain kind of success. And among other things, his spent his days containing cows, growing more cows and bigger cows, selling cows and starting over, containing more cows. As with most things growing and becoming, becoming cow, becoming meat entailed containing. Beef growing is contained most closely by skin stretched tight. Beyond skin, containing cows entails fence and fence entails wire. In its beginning, cow meat is often held by wire, barbed wire. And as with most everything, what holds us, what presses in on us, is as much us as we are who press out against our walls.

Barbed wire was invented in 1874 after Joseph F. Glidden was struck by a device on sale at an agricultural fair—nails stuck into a wooden board to be attached to the head of wandering livestock (Netz, 2002, p. 17). Whenever the animal tried to press herself into a limited area, she would cause herself intense pain. The board with its nails replaced the presence of human beings.

It was a punishing, portable wall. Through the pain it caused, the board demanded obedience. Glidden, recognizing its potential, developed this innovation. He took the nails off of the animal and put them on an actual wall, or really a fence (Netz, 2002, p. 18). The fascinating part of this invention was its frailty. The fence, made of strands of wire with nails or barbs attached, barbed wire, is insubstantial. The fence is frail. For strength, when it comes to pain, is often unnecessary. This is not because animals will not fight. We all fight. We all fight for our freedom in one way, or another. And, oddly, for some, the tighter we are held, the closer the walls, the more we desire freedom, the more we desire that which is far away. The more we desire.

The Walls in My Dream

And the basement went on and on and on, walls moving into halls and rooms, tunnels curving here, winding there, it unfolded back and again back in time, through years, then more years. And all the while, menace pressed in on us like a hand, reaching. It was always almost there, always almost grabbing hold, lurking panting pushing in on us, like a bad horror movie. Danger pressed against the windows that kept appearing in my mind. I was afraid. How many ways are there to say it. I was afraid. I tried to find a place where we could rest, the we that we were, always changing. Yet most important, my child, my son, my love kept slipping out of my reach. And then, I became the hand, only frantic, edging against panic, stretching to find him again, stretching to enclose him against, in, within me. In the dream, I tried to find a place where we could rest. I made resting places on the way as we ran on through time and basements of my past woven together, reaching across spaces, places too large to ever really cross. Finally, in the end, I made a bed in a cement unfinished basement room, a bed on the floor from sofa mattress pads and old blankets and memories and things. I tucked my child in. To sleep, my child, to sleep amid my fear. As the basement ran on, around us.

Maybe no one really owes anyone their passion. Even so, I am one of those who gives it. And in my life, no one ever loved me with passion except perhaps my cat, Thomasina. Thomasina was the only one that gave me her full allegiance. She loved me. It was final, forever and always. She, really, loved me. She gave me her body, warm and soft, small, gray, wrapped around my neck at night, gently, loudly purring. She gave me her full presence. And when I was away, she cried, for hours and through the night, loud calling, calling outside my mother's bedroom door. She insisted I be returned to her.

And now, she is gone. It was only her small cat body that kept me from the vastness of being totally alone. And I wonder how I can spend a lifetime this way. No matter what, unwanted. No matter what. How can I live a whole life this way. It will always be too long, too many days, too much hurt.

Thomasina died. But I know, I know it wasn't really because she was old. Her arthritis was making her ache in the freezing, bitterness of winter in Montana, at least nine months of cold, maybe more. By then, by the time Thomasina's arthritis chilled her limbs to stiff and aching, I was away. Her last winter was my semester abroad in Alicante, Spain. Even being in Spain, even being in college, that time when they say everything is good, even so, I longed to come home. And it was then that my mother said that Thomasina could not fully move her body. Instead she dragged her stiff back legs through the house to a resting place where she would stay until her hurting body's needs made her move again.

So that's when, that was when we decided to kill her. We decided that we would leave her to living for one more summer, one more summer in Montana with its gentle, sweet warmth, long days, free of suffering. Summer in Montana is a romance that the world has with itself. We decided that we would kill her at the end of summer.

And yet I know that she was really the only one that loved me more than anything; she loved me with intensity and faithfulness, focus. She really loved me. And so I decided to have her killed. It was because, really because, her love was unbearable. That's why. It was unbearable in the threat of its leaving. Because the leaving always comes. And in its passing, there is left behind, only the brilliant raw pain of myself. I could not bear for her to leave. I just couldn't.

It is ironic. Vegetarian, pacifist that I am. I am adamantly against killing. And yet I consciously decided to kill the one that loved me most.

So we chose a day for her dying. And even so, even being the one who decided, I could not endure her. The night before her death I spent with a man I hardly knew. My time with Thomasina was perfunctory. It was time I had to spend. And then I stroked her. And then I left. And the next day I got my brother to make photographs of her and me together one last time. Odd that there was no film in the camera, a mistake that made sure there were no traces left behind. She was really gone. And then we, my brother and sister and I, drove her to the veterinarian. My mother could not be there. And so we drove her, the three of us who knew so much about leavings from the place of being left. And then I held her on the veterinarian's shiny steel table. I held her down and still.

She died crying. And we laughed because she had done so much crying. We laughed, and she died. Maybe she knew that her leaving was really my leaving. I was gone again. It merited long cries, as many as she could manage before we each were gone. I had to do it. I had to go. I could not bear for her to leave. It was one more leaving I could not allow.

← ↑ →

Yet, you know that nothing ends. And dying is not always what it looks like. We often tell each other that dying is the end. But it's not. Even death is funny that way. Nothing really ends. There is always a resurrection. Life always pushes for life, again. We all do. We all push, for life, in one way or another. Even in the placidity of cow-being, life pushes for life. Some animals fight in a way that is wild. Some animals fight in a way that is breathless. But that is not the only way. Cows fight, too; cows fight by waiting.

From the perspective of the meat industry, there are a number of problems with the HSA. Ultimately, all the problems result in a loss of profit. And we must remember that the meat industry is not in the business to feed the hungry masses or to hearken back to a safer, saner time when we all lived on farms, or even to supply good work to those in need of it. The meat industry is, of course, all about profit. Not the animals, not the food made from their flesh, not the human beings who kill the animals and pack their meat, or the ones who eat it. It is, pure and simple, about profit. Following the HSA's mandated procedure for killing animals takes too much time. There is time involved in properly stunning an animal. There is time involved in correcting an improper stun. And there is time involved in keeping the line slow enough to protect the workers. Indeed, often in an attempt to speed up production, animals simply do not get stunned properly, if they get stunned at all.

With stunning, lost time is a central issue but not the only issue. There is a common belief in the meat industry that stunning an animal to the point of stopping its heart will make the meat less valuable. "It's an industry myth that an animal's heart has to keep beating in order to pump all the blood from its muscles. When the blood is retained in the meat, it provides a good medium for bacteria to grow, and that reduces the meat's shelf life" (Eisnitz, 1997, p. 122). Eisnitz interviewed Bucky White, a meatpacker at the John Morrell plant in Sioux Falls, South Dakota. About stunning cattle, Bucky White said, "We got a superintendent who claims the big bolt kills the cattle 'too dead' and they don't bleed properly … I've headed [skinned the heads of] and stuck cattle for twenty-one years, and I've never heard of cattle being too dead" (p. 122). Here Bucky White's spouse, Margie White added, "They're climbing up the walls and kicking you … but they're too dead" (p. 122).

Fully stunning animals, of course, is good for the animal about to be slaughtered and good for the workers processing its meat. The animal is then processed with minimal suffering. And workers stay safer, sticking, skinning, and cutting large animals that are dead rather than fighting the meatpackers as they work. In the early 1980s, many studies demonstrated that "killing an animal by stopping the heart instead of just stunning it has no effect on the amount of blood retained in the meat" (Eisnitz, 1997, p. 123). Nonetheless, the meat industry clings to the idea that animals should not be stunned to the extent that their hearts stop. Because of this worry over "too dead" cows, management often keeps the stun gun current turned down. Bucky White explained to Eisnitz "that the captive bolt knocking guns they used have two sizes of bolts. Plant management requires that the smaller, less effective bolt be used" (p. 122).

Eisnitz asked Bucky White how often alive and conscious cattle come through the stunning process: "The way I look at it," White said, "out of the 1,228 beef I stuck today it would have been okay if a few were still alive. But it's all day. Constantly, all day, I get live cattle" (Eisnitz, 1997, p. 121). In response to Eisnitz asking him how he can tell that the cattle are alive and conscious, White said, "The live ones you could tell 'cause they're bellowing, blinking, looking around" (p. 121). Because the animals are alive, they fight and this is dangerous for the workers attempting to process the animal's flesh:

"A month ago Bucky got kicked in the mouth," Margie said.

White pointed to his lip. "Right here, just about drove my tooth right through. Then I got kicked behind the ear."

"Two weeks ago he got it right above the eye," Margie said.

"So in the last month," [Eisnitz] asked, "how many times did you get nailed?"

"Got kicked in the mouth, the eye ..."

"Under the arm," Margie said, "And just yesterday, underneath the other arm, it's black and blue." (Eisnitz, 1997, p. 122)

Eisnitz also met with then United States Department of Agriculture (USDA) meat inspector, Kevin Walker, about his experience at a slaughterhouse in Bartow, Florida, Kaplan Industries. Before their meeting he had contacted her by mail with his concerns. He claimed that cattle were being skinned alive at Kaplan Industries.

"This is not only extremely cruel," he wrote, "but also very dangerous for the plant personnel who have to skin these kicking animals." Plant management knew about the problem, he said, but didn't want to correct it because that would mean slowing down the production line. "I have contacted a number of federal agencies but have been told there is nothing they can do. They also told me that the problems I described exist all over the country, that they are just a little worse at Kaplan's." (Eisnitz, 1997, p. 18)

Eisnitz, the chief investigator for the Human Farming Association, was initially skeptical about Walker's claims.

> Who in their right mind would attempt to skin conscious cows, particularly right under the nose of United States Department of Agriculture (USDA) meat inspectors? Sometimes involuntary reflexes in stunned or dead animals can look like conscious kicking. (Eisnitz, 1997, p. 18)

Eisnitz decided to look into the matter.

Clearly, animals alive and conscious violates the HSA. However, oddly enough, the very group who is supposed to enforce the HSA, the USDA, opposes the act. Indeed, the USDA is itself allied with the meat industry. Further, there are no penalties—no fines or possible prison time—for violating the HSA. USDA meat inspectors are merely supposed to shut down the kill line until the slaughterhouse remedies the violations. Of course, shutting down the kill line, even momentarily, cuts into company profits. The danger of even a brief loss of time in production is meant to keep the meat industry complying with the law.

Unfortunately, Eisnitz found that rather than forcing a shut down, the USDA simply ignores nearly all violations of the HSA. Eisnitz interviewed numerous workers at various levels of work inside U.S. meat-packing businesses and found that the slaughterhouses are consistently violating the HSA. Again and again, different people involved in meat packing with different companies reiterated similar stories. Cows are being skinned alive and conscious. Conscious pigs are regularly immersed in scalding water and boiled alive. Awake and aware chicken are normally bled out and scalded in boiling water (to loosen their feathers). And because the HSA does not protect poultry in the United States, the USDA does not have to bother ignoring the brutal poultry slaughtering process. Scalding live chickens in boiling water is completely legal.

Eisnitz found that the Kaplan company was killing around six hundred cows every day. "Not as many as some of the nation's newer high-speed mega-operations, but still high enough to make it the largest beef slaughterhouse in Florida" (Eisnitz, 1997, p. 19). Yet, according to Walker, the facility was in poor repair and simply could not even handle the slower line times such as when they slaughtered only fifty to seventy cows an hour. "As a result, when the line speed was increased—particularly when the foreman was trying to push through as many cattle as possible at the end of the work day—plant employees just couldn't keep up" (p. 28). Rushing at their work, stun operators would sometimes miss and knock the animal at the side of its head instead of straight on. Some of the improperly stunned cows respond by breaking free and running wildly through the plant. Most however, "regained consciousness after they'd been shackled and hoisted onto the overhead rail" (p. 28). These animals, hanging by one leg, fight, twist and turn, trying to break free. Walker told Eisnitz that in "addition to kicking and thrashing as they hung upside down … they'd be blinking and stretching their necks from side to side, looking around, really frantic" (p. 28).

Conscious animal or not, the overhead moving rail continues either way, and with it the cow moves to the next stage in the process, to the sticker. When the cow is conscious and fighting, and particularly when the line is moving fast, the sticker sometimes does not manage to cut the cow's throat in such a way that it bleeds out fast. Nonetheless, within seconds after being cut, the cow arrives at the head-skinners who skin the hide off of the animal's head. Eisnitz quotes Walker as saying, "A lot of times the skinner finds out an animal is still conscious when he slices the side of its head and it starts kicking wildly. If that happens, or if a cow is already kicking when it arrives at their station, the skinners show a knife into the back of its head to cut the spinal cord" (Eisnitz, 1997, p. 29). Eisnitz writes, "This practice paralyzes the cow from the neck down but doesn't deaden the pain of head skinning or render the animal unconscious; it simply allows workers to skin or dismember the animal without getting kicked" (p. 29).

It is an understatement to say that skinning the hide off of a conscious animal is cruel. Even so, cruelty to the animal is not the only issue. Live cattle struggling and fighting as they are being processed into meat present an extremely dangerous situation for the workers, the meat packers, processing them. The workers are themselves crowded together and unprotected, many carrying knives. It is a perfect set-up for accidents. Walker told Eisnitz,

> Sometimes animals would break free of their shackles and come crashing down headfirst to the floor fifteen feet below, where

other men worked. … It's a miracle that nobody's been killed. There were three in one day, one right after another. One hit a worker, just a glancing blow, broke his leg. I almost got crushed by a falling bull. (Eisnitz, 1997, p. 29)

At the National Beef plant, almost four hundred animals die every hour. They are set free, to become something else. They become us. You know, everything passes. Everything passes away, leaving a shadow of itself behind, transformed into something else.

And cows become us. Of course, in the food chain, we aren't the only ones eating cow. In fact until August 1997, even the cows ate cows. And they still eat meat, just meat from more distant relatives. "When a cow is slaughtered, about half of it by weight is not eaten by humans: the intestines and their contents, the head, hooves, and horns, as well as bones and blood. These are dumped into giant grinders at rendering plants, as are the entire bodies of cows and other farm animals known to be diseased" (Lyman, 1998, p. 12). Yet not only farm animals are "rendered." Euthanized pets such as the six or seven million cats and dogs put down in animal shelters each year and road kill are all transformed, rendered into something else. The whole mix, forty billion pounds of dead animals each year, is ground up and steam-cooked. Then the lighter fatty material floats to the top of the mix and is separated out to be used for making candles, waxes, cosmetics, soaps, lubricants, and whatnot. The renderers dry and pulverized the heavier protein material into a powder. This "protein concentrate" is used as an additive in almost all pet food as well as to livestock feed.

So. We eat cows. And the cows used to eat cows. They eat other meat now in the form of protein concentrate. Who cares really? Well, the problem is not just the meat eating meat before we eat the meat. There are a number of problems with meat. But not only problems; meat is not only laden with problems. Meat is also food. It is a gift of sorts from the cows, and the labor and the land. And those who eat meat devour it and are, at least a little bit, renewed. And the cows die unto us, and eventually we to the land, and the land feeds. And we begin again.

Note

1 The only assertion in his book that could not be verified involved Sinclair's report of workers who accidentally fell into open vats of hot water in the tank rooms. He wrote, "When they were fished out, there was never enough of them left to be worth exhibiting, sometimes they would be over-looked for days, till all but the bones of them had gone out to the world as Durham's Pure Leaf Lard!" (Sinclair 2003 [1906], p. 113).

References

Eisnitz, G. A. (1997). *Slaughterhouse: The shocking story of greed, neglect, and inhumane treatment inside of the U.S. meat industry.* Amherst, NY: Prometheus Books.

Humane Society of the United States. (2008). Factory farming campaign: Working to reduce the suffering of animals raised for meat, eggs, and milk. Available online at http://video.hsus.org/ (accessed July 16, 2008).

Lyman, H. (1998). *Mad cowboy: Plain truth from the cattle rancher who won't eat meat.* New York: Simon & Schuster.

Netz, R. (2002). Collections of confinement: Thoughts on barbed wire. *Connect: Art, Politics, Theory, Practice, 12*(1), 15–22.

Olsson, K. (2002). The shame of meatpacking. *The Nation*, September 16, p. 12.

Sinclair, U. (2003 [1906]). *The jungle, with an introduction and notes by Maura Spiegel.* New York: Barnes & Noble Classic.

Skaggs, J. M. (1986). *Prime cut: Livestock raising and meatpacking in the United States, 1607–1983.* College Station: Texas A&M University Press.

Section IV

Indigenous & Decolonizing Interventions

Chapter 19

Choosing the Margins

The Role of Research in Indigenous Struggles for Social Justice

Linda Tuhiwai Smith

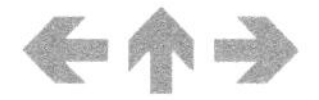

Introduction

Ka whawhai tonu matou, ake, ake, ake—
We will fight on for ever and ever.
—Rewi Maniapoto, 1864

A nineteenth-century prophecy by a Māori leader predicted that the struggle of Māori people against colonialism would go on forever and therefore the need to resist will be without end. This may appear to be a message without hope, but it has become an exhortation to Māori people that our survival, our humanity, our world-view and language, our imagination and spirit, our very place in the world depends on our capacity to act for ourselves, to speak for ourselves, to engage in the world and the actions of our colonizers, to face them head on. Māori struggles for social justice in New Zealand are messy, noisy, simultaneously celebratory and demoralizing, hopeful and desperate. Although there have been incremental gains, they have often been made from the depths of despair, accepted reluctantly as the crumbs of compromise.

Originally published in *Qualitative Inquiry and the Conservative Challenge*, edited by Norman K. Denzin and Michael D. Giardina, pp. 151–173. Republished in *Qualitative Inquiry—Past, Present, and Future: A Critical Reader*, edited by Norman K. Denzin and Michael D. Giardina, pp. 349–371.

The demands on scholars and intellectuals in similar contexts have been discussed in the revolutionary texts by writers such as Gramsci and Fanon, in feminist and indigenist literature, and in research texts. In the research literature, the issues are often discussed in terms of the methodologies, ethics, theoretical and discursive representations, emancipatory possibilities, and power relations associated with studying marginalized and vulnerable communities, the outsider Other, or within specific populations and communities such as urban youth.

Qualitative researchers are trained to "see things." Researchers working in the field of social injustice witness or see things that may impact directly on their own relationships, identities, safety, and freedom. Speaking for, and speaking out, can land a researcher in considerable trouble; being "named" as a leftist researcher or native sympathizer is likewise a risk that is carried even in societies that value freedom of speech and of academic discovery. In these conservative times, the role of an indigenous researcher and of other researchers committed to producing research knowledge that documents social injustice, recovers subjugated knowledges, helps create spaces for the voices of the silenced to be expressed and "listened to," and challenges racism, colonialism, and oppression is a risky business.

This chapter is written from that messy intersection, from the borders of the vast and expanding territory that is the margin, that exists "outside" the security zone, outside the gated and fortified community. The first part of the chapter revisits Chandra Mohanty's (1991) cartography of struggles, as faced by indigenous and marginalized communities. The purpose is to provide a sense of the landscape that researchers negotiate and seek to understand. In this first part, the chapter emphasizes the notion of struggle and what it means to live a life in struggle. The second part examines some of the implications for indigenous researchers who choose to work in indigenous and marginalized communities, communities that are in engaged struggle. These researchers work the borders, betwixt and between institutions and communities, systems of power and systemic injustice, cultures of dominance and cultures in survival mode, politics and theory, theory and practice.

Revisiting the Concept of Struggle

Struggle, as many social activists have identified, is an important tool in the overthrow of oppression and colonialism. Struggle is a dynamic, powerful, and important tool that is embedded in what at first glance often seems to be just part of the apparatus of Marxist rhetoric and radical discourse. In its Marxist revolutionary sense, the concept of struggle can also be associated with forms of psychological torture and political haranguing, as individuals are coerced into losing their memories of a past regime or into informing on their family and friends.

In its broader sense, struggle is simply what life feels like when people are trying to survive in the margins, to seek freedom and better conditions, to seek social justice. Struggle is a tool of both social activism and theory. It has the potential to enable oppressed groups to embrace and mobilize agency and to turn the consciousness of injustice into strategies for change. Struggle can be mobilized as resistance and as transformation. It can provide the means for working things out "on the ground," for identifying and solving problems of practice, for identifying strengths and weaknesses, for refining tactics and uncovering deeper challenges.

But struggle can also be a blunt tool. As a blunt tool, it has often privileged patriarchy and sexism in indigenous activist groups or been used to commit groups to modes of operation that undermine the very values they espouse and expect of others. As a blunt instrument, struggle can also promote actions that simply reinforce hegemony and that have no chance of delivering significant social change.

Paolo Freire's model of change argues that conscientization leads to action or struggle; when people learn to read the word (of injustice) and read the world (of injustice) they will act against injustice. However, Graham Smith (2004) has argued that in the Māori context, participation in struggle can, and often does, come before a raised consciousness. Smith's research has shown that people often participated in struggles more to show solidarity with friends and family, or some other pragmatic motivation, than as a personal commitment to or knowledge about historical oppression, colonialism, and the survival of Māori people. Along the way, many of those people become more conscious of the politics of struggle in which they are engaged. As Smith points out "Māori experience tends to suggest that these elements [conscientisation, resistance, transformative action] may occur in any order and indeed may occur simultaneously" (p. 51).

Struggle, then, can be viewed as group or collective agency rather than as individual consciousness. The political leaders of struggle need some form of collective consent or mandate to act and to sustain action over time. The story of struggle is also a story about activist leadership and collective consent and the tension between these two processes (leading and consenting). It is in this area that much revolutionary literature tends to focus on the hegemonic role of intellectuals who occupy the establishment and their power to influence others and command over what counts as legitimate knowledge.

Struggle is also a theoretical tool for understanding agency and social change, for making sense of power relations, and for interpreting the tension between academic views of political actions and activist views of the academy. Theorizing the politics, psychology, and pedagogy of struggle is the role of activist scholars and the organic intellectuals who work in that intersection between the community and the academy. It often presents itself as a phenomenon that researchers "see" when they see communities living on the edge and in crisis; when they attempt to interpret or make ethnographic sense of life in the margin; when they attempt to account for behaviors, attitudes, value systems; and when they attempt comparisons with their own communities and social class. People, families, and organizations in marginalized communities struggle every day; it is a way of life that is necessary for survival and, when theorized and mobilized, can become a powerful strategy for transformation.

Multiple Layers of Struggle

The Māori struggle for decolonization is multilayered and multidimensional and has occurred across multiple sites simultaneously. Graham Smith (2004) has argued that theorizing this struggle from a Māori framework of Kaupapa Māori has provided important insights about transformation, about how transformation works and can be made to work for indigenous communities. Similarly, Leonie Pihama (2005) writes that "Kaupapa Māori is a transformative power. To think and act in terms of Kaupapa Māori while experiencing colonisation is to resist dominance." In this section, I focus more on the conditions that intersect or are external to this transformative process and that, at times, can work for or against change, can destabilize the struggle or can present opportunities to be exploited, can provide creative resources, or can unleash a counterhegemonic and narrow agenda of change.

I conceptualize five conditions or dimensions that have framed the struggle for decolonization. I define the first as a critical consciousness, an awakening from the slumber of hegemony and the realization that action has to occur. I define the second condition as a way of reimagining the world and our position as Māori within the world, drawing on a different epistemology and unleashing the creative spirit. This condition is what enables an alternative vision, it fuels the dreams of alternative possibilities. The third is concerned with ways in which different ideas, social categories, and tendencies intersect, the coming together of disparate ideas, the events, the historical moment. This condition creates opportunities, it provides the moments where tactics can be deployed. The fourth I have defined simply as movement or disturbance, the distracting counterhegemonic movements or tendencies, the competing movements that transverse sites of struggle, the unstable movements that occur when the status quo is disturbed. The fifth is the concept of structure, the underlying code of imperialism, of power relations. This condition is grounded in reproducing material realities and legitimating inequalities and marginality.

What I am suggesting by privileging these layers over others is that separately, together, and in combination with other ideas, these five dimensions help map the conceptual terrain of struggle. The categorical terms being used are not of the same type and have not been motivated by a particular "model." Rather, they reflect the multiple positions, spaces, discourses, languages, histories, textures, and world-views that are being contested, struggled over, resisted, and reformulated by Māori.

In writing a "cartography" of the struggles facing Third World women, Chandra Mohanty (1991) has said that "the world (is) transversed with intersecting lines." Along such intersecting lines are ideas, categories, or tensions that often connect with each other in different ways. They are not necessarily oppositions or dualisms. They create and are created by conditions that are inherently unstable, arbitrary and uncontrollable. She also argued that one of the key features of struggle is the "simultaneity" of oppressions that are fundamental to the experience of social and political marginality. Intersections can be conceptualized as lines that intersect or meet other lines and also as spaces that are created at the points where intersecting lines meet. Spaces created by intersecting ideas, tendencies, or issues are sites of struggle that offer possibilities for people to resist.

Making space within such sites has become a characteristic of many Māori struggles in education, health, research, and social justice. What is slightly different between this notion and the idea of struggles in the margins is that, when attached to a political idea such as *rangatiratanga*, often translated as sovereignty or self-determination, then all space in New Zealand can be regarded as Māori space. This takes the struggle out of specifically "Māori contexts" and into the spaces once regarded as the domain of the "settler" or Pakeha community, such as large institutions like universities, where Māori really are a small minority. Rather than see ourselves as existing in the margins as minorities, resistance initiatives have assumed that Aotearoa New Zealand is "our place," all of it, and that there is little difference, except in the mind, between, for example, a Te Kohanga Reo, where Māori are the majority but the state is there, and a university, where the Māori are the minority and the state is there.

Whereas we can conceive of space geographically and politically, it is important to claim those spaces that are still taken for granted as being possessed by the West. Such spaces are concerned with intellectual, theoretical, and imaginative spaces. One of these is a space called Kaupapa Māori. This concept has emerged from lessons learned through Te Kohanga Reo and Kura Kaupapa Māori and has been developed as a theory in action by Māori people. Graham Smith (1995) has argued for Kaupapa Māori as an intervention into theoretical spaces, particularly within the sphere of education. Kaupapa Māori research refers to

Māori struggles to claim research as a space within which Māori can also operate. Given the history of the Western research gaze of indigenous peoples, it may seem unusual that Māori should take hold of the idea of research and attempt to apply it to our own questions. There are imperatives that have forced that on us, such as the constant need to prove our own history and to prove the worth of our language and values.

Māori and other indigenous peoples, however, also have their own questions and curiosities; they have imaginations and ways of knowing that they seek to expand and apply. Searching for solutions is very much part of a struggle to survive, it is represented within our own traditions, for example, through creation stories, values, and practices. The concept of "searching" is embedded in our world-views. Researching in this sense, then, is not something owned by the West, or by an institution or discipline. Research begins as a social, intellectual, and imaginative activity. It has become disciplined and institutionalized with certain approaches empowered over others and accorded a legitimacy but it begins with human curiosity and a desire to solve problems. It is, at its core, an activity of hope.

One of the criticisms made of educators who have been concerned about the emancipatory potential of schooling is that they have often ignored or diminished the role in social agency of such qualities as hope, optimism, and the need to strive for utopian goals. As summarized by McLaren (1995):

> Some radical educators have, in fact, argued that the notion of hope as the basis of a language of possibility is really nothing more than a "trick of counter hegemony," and that hope is employed for ideological effect rather than for sound theoretical reasons. In other words hope as a vision of possibility contains no immanent political project and as such has to be sacrificed on the altar of empirical reality. [p. 121]

I have stated previously the sense of noisy optimism that has been a characteristic of Māori politics. Here, I argue for the importance in Māori struggles of the imagination and of the capacity shown by Māori to constantly imagine and reimagine, to create and recreate our world. The capacity of colonized peoples to continue to imagine and to create our own worlds was the focus of quite systematic imperial and colonial practices that are encapsulated in the concept of dehumanization. The dehumanizing tendencies within imperial and colonial practices are deeply encoded. They constantly deny that colonized people actually have ideas of our own, can create new ideas, and have a rich knowledge base from which to draw.

I would not claim that, on its own, imagination is a critical tool or contains within it a political project that is connected inherently to emancipation. What I would argue is that if they are to work, to be effective, political projects must also touch on, appeal to, make space for, and release forces that are creative and imaginative. This point is made in Smith's (1995) identification of the significant elements within Kaupapa Māori. He argues that the *kaupapa* has to "grab people" emotionally; it has to excite them and "turn them on" to new possibilities.

The danger in such forces is that they do not necessarily lead to emancipatory outcomes. They are inherently uncontrollable, which is possibly why this aspect is excluded from decolonization type programs and other attempts at planned resistance. However, there is a point in the politics of decolonization where leaps of imagination can connect the disparate, fragmented pieces of a puzzle, ones that have different shadings, different shapes, and different images within them, and say that "these pieces belong together." The imagination allows us to strive for goals that transcend material, empirical realities. For colonized peoples, this is important because the cycle of colonialism is just that: a cycle with no end point, no emancipation. The material locates us within a world of dehumanizing tendencies, one that is constantly reflected back on us. To imagine a different world is to imagine us as different people in the world. To imagine is to believe in different possibilities, ones that we can create.

Decolonization must offer a language of possibility, a way out of colonialism. The writing of Māori, of other indigenous peoples and of anti/postcolonial writers would suggest, quite clearly, that that language of possibility exists within our own alternative, oppositional ways of knowing. Even though these may not be seen to connect with current socioeconomic realities, the fact that we adhere to, that we can imagine a connection suggests a resistance to being classified according to the definitions of a dominant group. Furthermore, the language of possibility, a language that can be controlled by those who have possession of it, allows us to make plans, to make strategic choices, to theorize solutions. Imagining a different world, or reimagining the world, is a way into theorizing why the world as it currently is is unjust and posing alternatives to such a world from within our own world-views.

Implications for Researchers: Choosing the Margins

The metaphor of the margin has been a very powerful metaphor in the social sciences and humanities for understanding social inequality, oppression, disadvantage, and power. It is used alongside other similar concepts such borders, boundaries, bridges, center-periphery, and insider/outsider to demarcate people in spatial terms as well as in socioeconomic, political, and cultural ones. Anthropology uses the term "liminal" to capture some of the elements that are lived by people in the margins. Gloria Ladson-Billings (2000) uses the term in this way, "Thus the work of the liminal perspective is to reveal the ways that dominant perspectives distort the realities of the other in an effort to maintain power relations that continue to disadvantage those who are locked out of the mainstream" (p. 259).

Feminists and minority scholars (such as African American writers) have worked the metaphor of the margin, the hyphen, or the border into social theories of oppression and marginalization and of resistance and possibility (Fine, 1992; hooks, 1984). Gloria Anzaldúa (1987), for example, writes of the border where she grew up literally at the border between the United States and Mexico and figuratively at the border and intersection between languages, between home and school, between having and not having, and as a site for positive identity formation. African American writer bell hooks (1984) wrote of the radical possibility of "choosing the margins" as a site of belonging as much as a site of struggle and resistance.

The critical issue hooks and other writers such as Stuart Hall have identified is that meaningful, rich, diverse, interesting lives are lived in the margins; these are not empty spaces occupied by people whose lives don't matter or people who spend their lives on the margins trying to escape. Many groups who end up there choose the margins, in the sense of creating cultures and identities out of the margins (for example, the deaf community, gay and lesbian communities, minority ethnic groups, and indigenous groups).

There are also researchers, scholars, and academics who actively choose the margins, who choose to study people marginalized by society, who themselves have come from the margins, or who see their intellectual purpose as being scholars who will work for, with, and alongside communities who occupy the margins of society. If one is interested in society, then it is often in the margins that aspects of a society are revealed as microcosms of the larger picture or as examples of a society's underbelly. In a research sense, having a commitment to social justice, to changing the conditions and relations that exists in the margins is understood as being "socially interested" or as having a "standpoint."

For researchers who come from the communities concerned, it may also be understood as "insider" research. Kaupapa Māori research can be understood in this way as an approach to research that is socially interested, that takes a position, for example, that Māori language, knowledge, and culture are valid and legitimate, and has a standpoint from which research is developed, conducted, analyzed, interpreted, and assessed. Some of these approaches are also referred to as critical research, as social justice research and as community action research. There are also specific methodologies that have been developed out of the work these approaches have initiated. Participatory action research, Kaupapa Māori research, oral histories, critical race theory, and testimonio are just some examples of methodologies that have been created as research tools that work with marginalized communities, that facilitate the expression of marginalized voices, and that attempt to represent the experience of marginalization in genuine and authentic ways.

Focusing on researching with marginalized groups foregrounds many of the issues that are faced by researchers working in the face of inequality and social injustice. As leading researchers in the social justice area have already established, it is crucial that researchers working in this critical research tradition pay particular attention to matters that impact on the integrity of research and the researcher, are continuously developing their understandings of ethics and community sensibilities, and are critically examining their research practices (Cram, 2001; Denzin & Lincoln, 2000; Fine, 1992; Rigney, 1999).

A third dimension to doing research in the margins is that the researchers who choose to study with and for marginalized communities are often in the margins themselves in their own institutions, disciplines, and research communities. It may be that the researchers come from a minority social group or perhaps their interest in and perceived support for marginalized communities unsettles the status quo or questions both implicitly and explicitly dominant approaches to research. Regardless, there is ample literature from feminist and minority group scholars that shows that doing work with marginalized groups or about their concerns can have a significant negative impact on careers and therefore on the perceived expertise and intellectual authority of the researchers concerned.

Māori researchers and academics have also written of the impact of community needs and institutional demands on their work lives and approaches to work and life as a Māori person (A. Durie, 1995; Irwin, 1988). Although communities may want to work with a Māori researcher, they may be quite unaware of the risks that many academic researchers face when researching in the margins. Thus, communities have expectations that researchers should not be building their careers by studying "them," but researchers feel pressure from the academy to turn research into peer-reviewed publications. Increasingly, research is viewed as an activity that must be measured and assessed for quality as part of a researcher's performance, and an individual's performance is linked directly to a department's and institution's ranking. A researcher working for social justice is likely to be involved in hours of work that does not lead to a "quality" academic publication—they may contribute to major social change but their research ranking will not reflect their contribution to society.

There are also implications and risks for researchers who work within the insider frame. From one perspective, the known methodological risks are about the potential for bias, lack of distance, and lack of objectivity. From another research perspective, they are about the potential to see the trees but not the forest, to underplay the need for rigor and integrity as a researcher, and to mistake the research role with an advocacy role. There are other risks, however, in terms of the relationships and accountabilities to be carried by an insider researcher.

Unlike their colleagues, these extra responsibilities can be heavy, not just because of what people might say directly but because of what researchers imagine the community might be saying. It can be difficult, because of the magnitude and amount of urgent tasks that seem to require action and support. Researchers make strategic decisions to deal with the urgent, while sacrificing the research and ultimately their careers. Mentoring by other indigenous scholars who have made their way through the system can provide some support, although these senior scholars are few and far between and are not always the best exemplars themselves of how to balance a life and maintain research while working with communities to make a positive difference.

Many of the social issues and challenges that confront marginalized communities will also be part of the biography and social network of an insider indigenous researcher. Visiting relatives who are sick, looking after grandchildren or someone's teenage child, writing submissions, being the breadwinner for more than one household, being in constant mourning, having to rush home to deal with emergencies, and being at the constant call of a community are often very normal parts of life for an indigenous researcher who is also trying to make his or her way into a career. Although every researcher may claim to have similar responsibilities and at some point to have taken on similar burdens, there is a qualitative difference between the conditions of people living in marginalized communities and those in middle-class suburbia.

Marginalized Populations, Research, and Ethics

For researchers working with "human subjects or participants," the terms "marginalized and vulnerable peoples" appear in the literature in relation to research ethics. Marginalized populations are often described as groups who have little access to power (for example, women, ethnic minority groups, gay and lesbian communities, children and youth). Vulnerable populations are also marginalized from power but are considered particularly vulnerable because they have even less individual agency to provide informed consent. Vulnerable groups include prisoners, armed forces personnel, people who are mentally ill, children, some groups with disabilities, and groups who can be and are more likely to be vulnerable to coercion. The significant event from which Western sensibilities about research abuses with marginalized and vulnerable populations was heightened was the Holocaust and the research undertaken by Nazi doctors on Jewish, Roma (Gypsies), and other groups imprisoned in the death camps. The Nuremberg Code of Ethics emerged from this momentous legacy. According to David Weisstub (1998):

> The Nuremberg Legacy represents almost a mythic chapter in the history of understanding of research ethics. . . . Nuremberg is a distant collective memory. For most of us Nuremberg emerged as a code and a symbol both in its principles representing the foundations of civilized medical practice and research and in its symbolization of the triumph of the democratic ideal over fascism. [p. 217]

Code was formed from the ashes of the Holocaust through the Nuremberg Tribunal and was an attempt to ensure that the types of research carried out by Nazi scientists would never happen again. The code recognizes that there are likely to be groups of people who are especially vulnerable when it comes to research and that these groups would also most likely exist in the margins of society. It is also the first acknowledgment that there are some basic moral principles by which researchers must abide.

From an indigenous perspective, the Nuremberg Code came too late, as the history of research as exploitation was already embedded in European imperialism leading into the twentieth century. And for other groups of people such as women, African American males, and many indigenous communities, the existence of the Nuremberg Code has not prevented research abuses from occurring. A series of scandals have highlighted the ways in which marginalized and vulnerable groups continue to be exposed to unethical research. According to Tolich (2001), the Cervical Cancer Inquiry, which looked into New Zealand's "darkest hour" in research, came about primarily because of the efforts of two feminist investigators who persisted in their inquiries despite the blocks and barriers put before them by institutional and professional systems. It was only after the Cervical Cancer Inquiry that academic institutions in New Zealand were required by legislation (Statute 161 of the Education Act 1989) to institute policies and practices for conducting ethical research with human subjects.

The Nuremberg Code was later followed by the World Medical Association Declaration of Helsinki in 1964 and, in the United States, by the Belmont Report in 1979. These three documents are referred to as landmarks in establishing a history of ethical research conduct (Sugarman, Mastrioni, Kahn, & Jeffrey, 1998). There is a difference, however, between professional ethics codes of practice that are essentially self-monitoring and voluntary, legislated, or officially regulated codes of practice. The Nuremberg Code has rarely been used in legal cases (Weisstub, 1998). The Helsinki Declaration is a professional voluntary code for medical practitioners who belong to the World Medical Association. The Belmont Report was an official report of the U.S. Department of Heath, Education and Welfare. What is known in the United States as The Common Rule is a set of federal policies adopted by the major U.S. agencies that conduct or fund research with human subjects.

In New Zealand, there are several legal instruments that cover aspects of ethical research with human subjects, including the Education Act 1989, the Human Rights Act 1999, the Health and Disability Services Human Rights Code, and the Health Information Privacy Code. The Treaty of Waitangi is also incorporated into research and ethics policies, and consultation with Māori communities is part of some institutions requirements when the research involves Māori participants. New Zealand also has a National Ethics Advisory Committee, a National Bioethics Committee, and other specialized committees that deal with single issues such as reproductive birth technologies.

Why is this background important when discussing issues that relate to indigenous peoples? There is one significant reason and three other contextual purposes. The significant reason is to establish the case history, in a sense, for why Māori as peoples need to be recognized as a marginalized group. The literature uses the word "populations" rather than "peoples," and there is a distinction in international law between these two terms. As a marginalized population, Māori are basically just another group or set of individuals and communities. As peoples, Māori have claims to self-determination. There is a risk that in fragmenting small groups of Māori into categories of marginalization and vulnerability we lose sight of the overall picture of Māori as an indigenous and marginalized people in New Zealand. The risk becomes especially important in discussions about the role of the Treaty of Waitangi in protecting Māori rights to develop as Māori and to be treated as equal citizens.

The contextual issues and history are important because research is an international activity conducted across the globe by researchers from different nations, institutions, disciplines, and approaches. The norms of research conduct are developed in this environment. Furthermore, legal precedents established in other Western jurisdictions such as the United States, Britain, Canada, and Australia have weight in the New Zealand context, especially if the issue is related to indigenous communities. Finally, science and technology are making rapid advances into areas that challenge existing notions of ethics on a broad scale, and Māori attempts to articulate and have recognized a different knowledge and ethical system are in a race against time. In this context, being better informed is an important protection.

On-Going Marginalization of Māori

Recent public discourses on the place of Māori and the Treaty of Waitangi position non-Māori as victims of discrimination because of the perceived extra special rights that Māori have to be consulted, to have our language and culture recognized, and to have Treaty of Waitangi protections built into legislation and policy frameworks. It would be quite fair to say that Māori have struggled a long time to make such inroads as part of making the Treaty of Waitangi "real" as the foundational instrument of the nation. Māori have also seen this process as being necessary to fulfill their visions of self-determination and to fulfill and benefit from the rights of citizenship.

It is this last point about citizenship that brings us back to the question of marginalization. In almost every social index, Māori are disproportionately represented as disadvantaged, even when statistical analyses control for class factors such as income levels. Furthermore, the long-term systemic nature of disadvantage has constituted patterns of participation by Māori people in society that are different from mainstream Pakeha norms and consequently tend to challenge taken-for-granted policies and practices of institutions. One obvious example is the impact of underachievement at secondary school, on adult second-chance learning, and on the average age of Māori in postgraduate education.

Māori participation rates in tertiary education is one of the highest in the Organisation for Economic Co-operation and Development, but the level at which Māori are participating is at a low second-chance level and is a direct consequence of the failure of schooling to deliver achievement to Māori. Many Māori students enter tertiary education through bridging programs, they tend to be older, they are more likely to be women, they tend to be part-time students in comparison to non-Māori, and it takes them much longer to complete a degree qualification. Furthermore, they have a disproportionately higher take-up rate for loans and because they are less likely on completion to move into higher-paying positions, they take longer to repay their loans. In sum, the pattern of participation in society reinforces disadvantage.

Whether one drives through New Zealand literally or as a figurative journey to understand social in/equality, Māori communities are on the margins of the economy and society. In the late 1980s, New Zealand began a significant neoliberal program of structural adjustment, of deregulation and reregulation of the economy and major reforms of education, health, and the welfare system (Kearns & Joseph, 1997; Kelsey, 1997; Moran, 1999).

The neoliberal agenda and the continuous process of reform has had a profound effect on New Zealand society; after two decades, it has produced a generation of young people for whom the neoliberal ideologies are normal and taken for granted. In education, neoliberalism is marked by a discourse of education as a marketplace with parents and students as consumers and clients, teachers and schools as self-managing providers of services, and curriculum knowledge as a commodity that can be traded in or traded up for social goodies such as well-being and social status.

The reform process redesigned the way schools were administered, redesigned the role of the principal government agency that was responsible for education, created a new agency to review and assess school performance, created a new curriculum framework, created a new qualifications framework and a new agency to accredit qualifications and institutions, created a user pays system for postsecondary education, and created a competitive environment through its funding arrangements. Private providers of postsecondary education and training were, until recently, able to compete with public institutions for public funding and aspire to attain degree-granting status.

In the neoliberal concept of the individual, Māori people in the 1980s presented a potential risk to the legitimacy of the new vision because Māori aspirations were deeply located in history, in cultural differences, and in the values of collectivity; even the Māori concept of family or whanau seemed threatening. When the neoliberal agenda was implemented, however, Māori communities were already embarked on their own educational revolution. The forward momentum of Māori development at that time has played a significant role in challenging the reform agenda to accommodate or at least attempt to make space for Māori aspirations. Jane Kelsey has argued that at times Māori were the only group in New Zealand society actually contesting the reforms in any serious way.

The development of Te Kohanga Reo sparked and continues to inspire the development of a range of Māori initiatives in education that have developed as alternative models within and outside the current system from early childhood to postsecondary tertiary education. The alternative models include Kura Kaupapa Māori, Māori language immersion schools that developed outside the state and were included as a separate category of education in the Education Amendment Act 1989, and Wananga or tribal degree-granting institutions that were also included as a category of the Education Amendment Act of 1989.

These alternatives were Māori-initiated institutions based on different conceptions of what education was about. They were community efforts that challenged the taken-for-granted hegemony of schooling and, as argued by Graham Smith (2000), revolutionized Māori thinking by demonstrating that Māori people could free their minds from the colonizer, and exercise agency in a purposeful, tactical, and constructive way. These educational alternatives did not begin with active state support, and even after they were included in legislation there was no supportive infrastructure to assist them. In the case of the Wananga, the three institutions took a claim to the Waitangi Tribunal related to capital expenditure. The tribunal ruled in their favor, and two of the Wananga have now settled their claim with the crown and have resources to develop their capital infrastructure.

I want to emphasize that the Māori development momentum was already in progress when the neoliberal reform process began. This meant that Māori had a platform for challenging those aspects of the reform process that seemed to threaten Māori development and a platform for engaging with the process in order to influence change.

This is not to say that the reform process welcomed Māori participation. On the contrary, Māori had to make serious demands to be included or to be heard. At times, overseas experts were brought in to dismiss Māori concerns or show how those concerns would be addressed by the new structures.

Nor can we say that Māori were particularly well organized or mobilized. In fact, the early reforms that privatized the state industries, such as forestry, created massive Māori unemployment and a high degree of community stress. The significance of the revolutionized thinking created by the development of Te Kohanga Reo was that in the absence of organized resistance, there was enough criticism to provide a counterhegemonic possibility and to have it voiced at every opportunity available. The point is that if Māori had been in disarray without any alternative models, the reform process would have run a different and likely a more devastating course. As it was, the reform process has had a disproportionately negative impact on Māori communities, widening disparities between Māori and non-Māori in educational achievement, health, and economic status.

What has become even clearer in the twenty-first century is the way in which policies aimed at Māori continue to resonate and recycle colonizing narratives. The discourse might change subtly, with terms shifting from Māori to *whanau*, *hapu*, *iwi*, to urban Māori and *iwi* Māori, and the unit of problem definition might change from tribes to *whanau*, from Māori women to Māori parents, from Māori providers to Māori consultants, but the underlying racialized tensions remain constant. The subtext is that Māori are responsible for their own predicament as a colonized people and that citizenship for Māori is a "privilege" for which we must be eternally grateful. Marginalization is a consequence of colonization, and the price for social inclusion is still expected to be the abandonment of being "Māori."

The impact of this sustained narrative on Māori is both a growing fragmentation within communities alongside a parallel urgency to redevelop and recenter ourselves around common baseline symbols and aspirations, for example, as in Mason Durie's three conceptualizations of "living as Māori, being a citizen of the world and Māori well-being and good health" (Durie, 2004, p. 66). The tension between fragmentation and coming together is an almost impossible situation and, in many cases, at our most vulnerable points, fractures occur, families fragment, core relationships between parents and children break down, and Māori people become alienated from themselves and from their extended families and communities.

It is neither accidental nor genetic that Māori mental health issues have risen dramatically in the last two decades so that they rank as one of the most important health issues for Māori. Marginalization as a process, as well as a state of affairs, impacts at multiple levels and sites.

Māori people are marginalized from mainstream New Zealand society. Some are able to choose the margins by embracing their Māori identities and participating in Māori society and culture. Some are alienated from Māori society. This occurs through a range of mechanisms or social, economic, and political processes. It may simply be that geographic distance from their home is a barrier to participation or that the loss of Māori language and culture is seen as a barrier. Some, by virtue of being institutionalized or enveloped into a system of care and protection, are removed from their social and cultural supports. Other groups (for example, those who have come together around a special interest) may find themselves excluded or alienated from existing Māori power structures but still function as Māori. Then there are probably those who are alienated from Māori and mainstream society (for example, people who have committed crimes against their own communities may never be welcomed back home; they have, in effect, been excluded from their own society).

Researchers in the Margins

As stated earlier, researchers who choose to do research in the margins are at risk of becoming marginalized themselves in their careers and workplaces. One strategy for overcoming this predicament is to embrace the work and commit to building a career from that place. As writers such as bell hooks and Gloria Anzaldúa have argued, the margins are also sites of possibilities that are exciting and "on the edge." Cultures are created and reshaped, people who are often seen by the mainstream as dangerous, unruly, disrespectful of the status quo, and distrustful of established institutions are also innovative; they are able to design their own solutions, they challenge research and society to find the right solutions.

Those who work in the margins need research strategies that enable them to survive, to do good research, to be active in building community capacities, to maintain their integrity, manage community expectations of them, and mediate their different relationships. Kaupapa Māori research developed out of this challenge. As Graham Smith, Leonie Pihama, and others who write in this tradition have emphasized, Kaupapa Māori research encourages Māori researchers to take being Māori as a given, to think critically and address structural relations of power, to build on cultural values and systems, and to contribute research back to communities that are transformative.

There are strategies that researchers can use that will enable them to build strong research relationships with different communities. There are also skills and principles that Māori researchers have learned through experience work well with Māori if practiced in sensitive and nuanced ways. These might be as simple as focusing on building good relationships and "showing one's face" as the first step in a relationship. But they are also about building networks of people who have stronger links into communities and building community capacities so that people can do the research themselves.

One of the anxieties that researchers may have is that when communities have the power to determine their own research they might not choose a Māori researcher even if they have all the right skills. That is a risk and a challenge. Many communities would want to choose the best researcher available or the researcher from their own community or area. Often their choice is brokered by a funding agency, more precisely a government-funding agency that may not know of Māori researchers or may not prefer a Māori researcher.

Experienced community organizations are also learning what they need from researchers, both Māori and non-Māori. In other indigenous contexts, some tribal nations in North America have protocols for researchers and their tribal structures have specialist research directors who manage all research on their nation. What is possibly very different in Aotearoa New Zealand is the growing capacity of Māori researchers across many different fields and disciplines. In the New Zealand context, Māori scholars can assemble quite large and multidisciplinary research collaborations, there are a growing number of independent Māori researchers working with communities, and there are funding agencies eager to support Māori research capacity development.

In what he calls a "sociology of absences," legal sociologist Boaventura de Sousa Santos (2004) calls for an ecology of knowledge/s that enables alternative ways of knowing and scientific knowledge to coexist and argues that there can be no global social justice without global cognitive justice. At the heart of this engagement in social justice and indigenous research are questions about knowledge, education, participation, and development. There are enduring questions about power relations, agency and structure, ethics and methodologies. Research is simply one site at which these issues intersect. Research is important because it is the process for knowledge production; it is the way we constantly expand knowledge. Research for social justice expands and improves the conditions for justice; it is an intellectual, cognitive, and moral project, often fraught, never complete but worthwhile.

References

Anzaldúa, G. (1987). *Borderlands/La Frontera: The new mestiza*. San Francisco: Aunt Lute.

Cram, F. (2001). Rangahau Māori: Tona tika, tona pono—The validity and integrity of Māori research. In M. Tolich (Ed.), *Research ethics in Aotearoa New Zealand* (pp. 35–52). Auckland: Pearson Education.

de Sousa Santos, B. (2004). World social forum: Toward a counter-hegemonic globalisation. In J. Sen, A. Anand, A. Escobar, & P. Waterman (Eds.), *The world social forum challenges empire* (pp. 235–245). New Delhi, India: Viveka.

Denzin, N. K., & Lincoln, Y. S. (2000). The discipline and practice of qualitative research. In N. Denzin. & Y. S. Lincoln (Eds.), *Handbook of qualitative research* (2nd ed., pp. 1–28). Thousand Oaks, CA: Sage.

Durie, A. (1995). Keeping an open mind: A challenge for Māori academics in a time of political change. Keynote address, Matawhanui Hui, Massey University, Palmerston North, New Zealand.

Durie, M. (2004). *Whaiora Māori health development*. Auckland: Oxford University Press.

Fine, M. (1992). *Disruptive voices*. Ann Arbor: University of Michigan Press.

hooks, b. (1984). *Feminist theory: From margin to center*. Boston: South End Press.

Irwin, K. (1988). Māori, feminist, academic. *Sites, 17*, 30–38.

Kearns, R. A., & Joseph, A. (1997). Restructuring health and rural communities in New Zealand. *Progress in Human Geography, 21*, 18–32.

Kelsey, J. (1997). *The New Zealand experiment*. Auckland: Auckland University Press.

Ladson-Billings, G. (2000). Racialised discourse and ethnic epistemologies. In N. K. Denzin & Y. S. Linclon (Eds.), *Handbook of qualitative research* (2nd ed., pp. 257–278). Thousand Oaks, CA: Sage.

Maniapoto, R. (1864). Retrieved from http://www.treatyofwaitangi.govt.nz/casestudies/waikatotainui.php

McLaren, P. (1995). *Critical pedagogy and predatory culture*. London: Routledge.

Mohanty, C. (1991). Cartographies of struggles: Third World women and the politics of feminism. In C. Mohanty, A. Russo, & L. Torres (Eds.), *Third World women and the politics of feminism* (pp.1–47). Bloomington: Indiana University Press.

Moran, W. (1999). Democracy and geography in the reregulation of New Zealand. In D. B. Knight & A. E. Joseph (Eds.), *Restructuring societies: Insights from the social sciences* (pp. 33-58). Ottawa, Canada: Carleton University Press.

Pihama, L. (2005). Asserting indigenous theories of change. In J. Baker (Ed.), *Sovereignty matters: Locations of contestation and possibility in indigenous struggles for self-determination* (pp. 191–210). Lincoln: University of Nebraska Press.

Rigney, D. (1999). Internationalization of an indigenous anticolonial cultural critique of research methodologies. A guide to indigenist research methodology and its principles. *Wicazo SA Review, Fall*, 109–121.

Smith, G. H. (1995). The cultural politics of making space. Seminar presentation, Winter Seminar Series, Education Department, University of Auckland, New Zealand.

Smith, G. H. (2000). Māori education: Revolution and transformative action. *Canadian Journal of Native Education*, 6, 57–72.

Smith, G. H. (2004). Mai i te maramatanga kit e putanga mai o te tahuritanga: From conscientization to transformation. *Journal of Educational Perspectives* (College of Education, University of Hawaii at Manoa), *37*, 1, 46–52.

Sugarman, J., Mastrioni, A. C., Kahn, C. & Jeffrey, P. (1998). *Ethics of research with human subjects. Selected policies and resources*. Baltimore, MD: University Publishing Group.

Tolich, M. (2001). Beyond an unfortunate experiment: Ethics for small town New Zealand. In M. Tolich (Ed.), *Research ethics in Aotearoa New Zealand* (pp. 2–13). Auckland: Pearson Education.

Weisstub, D. (Ed.). (1998). *Research on human subjects: Ethics, law and social policy*. New York: Pergamon.

Chapter 20

Thinking *Through* Theory

Contemplating Indigenous Situated Research and Policy

Margaret Kovach

Cree scholar Neal McLeod introduces *wîsahkêcâhk* in his 2007 book *Cree Narrative Memory. wîsahkêcâhk* is known in Plains Cree culture as the transformer. *wîsahkêcâhk* stories tell of the transformer deftly moving through the terrain of Cree narrative expressing itself, then re-imagining itself, in the consciousness of the Cree as the culture re-affirms itself generation upon generation. *wîsahkêcâhk* invites the imaginings of those who participate in Cree society and the understandings that the transformer inspires. "With regard to *wîsahkêcâhk*, there are many voices and many perspectives" (McLeod, 2007, p. 99). In these stories, as McLeod states, the nature of the transformer is only limited by the imagination of those who sit spellbound in the midst of its mystery. The transformer stirs us to think, and then think again. In the immediacy of a routinely fashioned life *wîsahkêcâhk* waits to visit, arriving with the intentionality of the paradoxically aloof provocateur and, in doing so, stops us short. Whether prompting a jarring halt in daily 'business as usual' or a less startling lull, when the transformer visits we notice. *wîsahkêcâhk* medicine does not so much direct as offer pause to listen to what we know, consider what we do not know, and think about what it is, exactly,

Originally published in *Qualitative Inquiry Outside the Academy,* edited by Norman K. Denzin and Michael D. Giardina, pp. 92–106. Republished in *Qualitative Inquiry—Past, Present, and Future: A Critical Reader,* edited by Norman K. Denzin and Michael D. Giardina, pp. 372–386. Left Coast Press, Inc.

that we are doing. If I were a Cree storyteller, and if this were a research story told by a fire, it would be in broaching theory talk that I would halt the flow of words, sit silent for a moment, knowing that at any moment *wîsahkêcâhk* will be entering the circle.

Absorbed in completing this writing task, I am not paying attention to my immediate situatedness, which is a desk cluttered with journal articles, books, orange Post-it notes, yellow highlighter pens, and an assortment of coffee cups from this most recent writing venture. Moving my mouse, I nudge Neil McLeod's *Cree Narrative Memory* against Kerry E. Howell's *The Philosophy of Methodology* perilously positioned amid the muddle on my desk. The nudge causes a chain reaction, the books slide, my coffee mug topples, and hot java smudges a red-inked underlined note on my essay outline—"theory moves through research."

Theory in qualitative research is a certainty, but like the intangible *wîsahkêcâhk* that moves with a maverick's covertness, theory in research can perplex. This is unfortunate, as the nature of theory implies suppositions that when left unquestioned flourish—particularly when the consenting majority favors a normative theory. Stringer (2014) states that theory is not necessarily right or wrong, "but that it focuses on particular aspects of the situation and interests them in particular ways" (p. 38). Whether theory impels a felt experience of liberation or oppression, whether it is contested or accepted, theory as both form and substance subsists through research that informs policy.

Indigenous peoples endure so-called 'capacity building' policy that is largely born of outsider imaginings built upon specious theoretical suppositions of what is and isn't good for Indigenous people. If the Indigenous voice is not being heard in the research theory that shapes Indigenous policy development, whose voice, then, is being relied upon? How trustworthy is this voice in offering an accounting of Indigenous people's lives? To omit the Indigenous voice in the theory-research-policy relationship is to be complicit in reproduction of dubious policy development. Theory unexamined, valorized through research and manifested in policy, poses, indeed has posed, great risk for Indigenous people. However, such a conjecture assumes that research, as a theory-laden exercise, does impact policy.

Klemperer, Theisens, and Kaiser (2001) offer this perspective on the linkage between research and policy:

> In our experience, the relationship between policy making and policy research resembles "dancing in the dark", where the dancers do not completely see each other, the movements are complex, and the environment influences the flow of the dance. (p. 197)

Klemperer et al. (2001) go on to illustrate specific ways in which research factors into the policy process. Citing Carol H. Weiss's work, the authors articulate different ways that research influences policy development. This typology includes: a) "Problem-solving research"; b) "Political uses of research"; and c) "Research used for enlightening purposes" (p. 200). Problem-solving research is specific research focused on a particular issue as a means to help develop and clarify policy on that issue. Political use of research involves the use of research to support political opinions already established. Finally, research for enlightening purposes helps give greater insight to a policy concern and "may help in the process of shaping ideas or conceptualizations of the problem" (p. 200).

Policy within Indigenous education (primary, secondary, and tertiary) is a good example of the theory, research, and policy dynamic in action. Policy discourse in Indigenous education in Canada is more often than not geared toward closing the Aboriginal "achievement gap." Certainly, this has merit given that a report on *Bridging the Aboriginal Education Gap in Saskatchewan* by economist Eric Howe "shows that a North American Indian male who drops out of school has lifetime earnings of only $362,023. If he just completes high school his earnings more than double" (Howe, 2011, p. 8). For a non-Aboriginal male in Saskatchewan who drops out of high school his lifetime earnings are $693,273 (Howe, 2011). The *Campaign 2000 "2011 Report Card on Child and Family Poverty in Canada"* (Family Service Toronto, 2011) reports that the child poverty rate for 1996–2006 for children under 18 living in low income two parent families was 52% for Aboriginal families, while for all children it was 18%. Education is, as Blair Stonechild puts forth in his appropriately titled book, *The New Buffalo: The Struggle for Aboriginal Post-secondary Education in Canada*, critical to addressing such inequities. The difficulty is that the Indigenous student achievement gap discourse tends to be motivated by an economic imperative loaded with deficit theorizing.

An aware Canadian only has to consider the recent Conservative federal government's proposed bill on First Nations education, *Working Together for First Nations Students*. The research found in the policy guide for this initiative, *Developing a First Nations Education Action: Discussion Guide* (Aboriginal Affairs and Northern Development Canada, 2012), cites achievement gap research using "lag behind" (p. 1) language to describe First Nations student abilities. The proposed response is that tighter funding, limited jurisdiction, and increased controls by the federal government are what is going to make the difference in graduation rates of First Nations students. Assembly of First Nations Chief Shawn Atleo stated in a recent interview that the new bill "is on the verge of potentially imposing an 'assimilationist' educational system on aboriginal children that repeats the mistakes of residential school" (Kennedy, 2013, para. 1). Aboriginal columnist Doug Cuthand from the *Saskatoon Star Phoenix* made this comment: "It's an old fashioned, top-down colonial approach that was supposed to have been put to bed 40 years ago with the adoption of the First Nations policy of Indian control of Indian Education" (Cuthand, 2013, A1). Strength-based theorizing that considers the possibility of anti-racist, culturally responsive schooling, based upon the strength of Indigenous cultural values, as a way to encourage student engagement is not what is being privileged in this approach. The power of culture, as articulated by the kokums and mosoms, is not being heard.

Within an Indigenous context, policy, and the research that informs policy, has often been from the outside looking in. In focusing on research, much has been extractive and has worked to mummify Indigenous culture. This has left a lingering distaste of research by Indigenous peoples (Tuhiwai Smith, 2013; Denzin & Lincoln, 2005). The production and reproduction of research laden with assumptions about Indigenous people has arisen from non-Indigenous situated, one-eyed seeing theorizing. Such theorizing has been the bane of the Indigenous community. Given the impact of theory manifested in research and policy, it is imperative, right at the start, that researchers are clear on what assumptions are being put out there in the form of theory. Unpacking how theory functions in research is useful in showcasing its pervasiveness.

Unpacking Theory

Traveling into the abstract language of research theory, I am reminded of a document I came across a number of years ago when I was an undergraduate post-secondary student. The report, entitled *What Was Said? The Taking Control Project*, was an inquiry into post-secondary education. In the 1986 report Cree educator Sid Fiddler posed a question pertinent then and relevant now to my research instructor self. I now appreciate this as a *wîsahkêcâhk* question. He asked: "How can you relate what is being taught to what the hell is happening on the reserve?" (cited in Stalwick, 1986, p. 7). He prefaced this question by pointing out that the abstract nature of education can hinder the inclusion of community knowledge. Knowing the risks, it remains necessary to venture into the fray of 'the abstract' so as to examine how theory is implicated in research.

I would like to differentiate between what is understood as a conceptual framework or paradigm in qualitative research and methodology. A framework or paradigm for qualitative inquiry can be described as an "an interrelated set of assumptions, concepts, values, and practices that comprise a way of viewing reality" (Schwandt, 2007, p. 122). A framework, or paradigm, includes broad, abstract assumptions and actions related to research. Examples of qualitative frameworks include positivism, transformative, constructivism, and, increasingly, the recognition of an Indigenous/Indigenist paradigm. Methodology can be described as relating to a specific research project and is the process by which a researcher goes about responding to the research question (Howard, 2013; Stringer, 2014). Examples of methodology include participatory action, feminism, grounded theory, and Indigenous methodology. The qualitative framework or paradigm and methodology are connected, but for the purposes of this discussion, theory will be situated within a discourse on methodology. This makes explicit an additional assumption of this commentary—methodology involves both theory and methods.

In this section, three definitional terms will be relied upon to describe and differentiate research theory. The use of definitional terms within the production and reproduction of theory can arguably work to oversimplify intrinsic complexities that surround the articulation of theory in research. However, I am including definitional terms in this chapter because I find them useful in unpacking what is meant by theory in research methodology and how theory is located within methodology, including the design, methods, and analysis in research. Finally, I find these definitions useful in making visible how research is permeated with theory and how, when unleashed from the 'laboratory,' this research influences the policy and practice that flow from it.

The following definitions are presented in a linear fashion, but the appearance of theory in research is not a linear process. While admitting to the possibility of oversimplifying the complexity of theory, I do fully respect that research theory travels through *wîsahkêcâhk* territory, where switchbacks, detours, and any number of alternative routes may be part of the terrain. In fact, I find the language of flux and movement associated with an Indigenous paradigm to be a more precise descriptor of the nature of theory in research.

The definitional terms used to describe ways that theory makes appearance in most qualitative methodologies include: a) *personal theory* (situatedness); b) *framework theory*; and c) *substantive (or substantiated) theory*. The terminology used in this section is borrowed from qualitative research (Howell, 2013; Schwandt, 2007). It is noted that there is a range of methodologies within qualitative inquiry and that these definitional terms can be found among approaches of an interpretive tradition. *Substantive theory*, in particular, is a term found in grounded theory (Charmaz, 2006). It ought to be noted that perspectives on the role of theory and subjectivities in qualitative methodology can differ. In referencing the work of Anfara and Mertz (2006), Mansor Abu Talib (2010) puts forward that researchers approach theory in qualitative research in various ways. This ranges from those who acknowledge the role of theory (Guba & Lincoln, 1994) to those who argue that theory "does not typically have a solid relationship with qualitative research (Merriam, 1997; Schwandt, 2007)" (Tavallaei & Abu Talib, 2010, p. 571).

Personal theory is the pre-existing beliefs and assumptions that a researcher brings to a research project. Howell (2013), who utilizes the term "personal theorizing" (p. 27), describes this as understandings that an individual holds arising from his or her individual experience. I am beginning with personal theory because it is most closely associated with one's own embodied, situated knowledges that exist before and beyond any particular research project. In qualitative research the subjectivity of personal situatedness is recognized as valid knowledge (Finlay, 2002; Richardson & St. Pierre, 2005). The process of participant reflection and centrality of life narrative in research appears in one of the earliest qualitative research projects, a study of the Polish peasant in Europe and America (1918–1920), by sociologists Thomas and Znaniecki. This study had its origins at the Chicago school of sociology in the early 1900s (Abbott & Egloff, 2008) and is cited as one of the first qualitative studies insisting upon the inclusion of subjectivity in a socially situated life. "The idea of 'the self' in *The Polish Peasant* is relational, situational and sequential, with writing a life, seriality and temporality seen as essential for gauging the processes of social becoming" (Stanley, 2010, p. 147).

As qualitative methodologies have progressed from their early ethnographic roots (early 1900s) to more positivist leanings (1960s) to more critically transformative strategies found in current approaches, there has been an invitation to reveal the situatedness and positionality of both participant and researcher in research (Denzin & Lincoln, 2005). As Richardson and St. Pierre (2005) suggest, critical self-reflection "evokes new questions about the self and subject; remind[s] us that our work is grounded, contextual, and rhizomatic; and demystif[ies] the research/writing process" (p. 965). They say that honoring one's own situatedness through self-situating "can evoke deeper parts of the self, heal wounds, enhance the sense of self—or even alter one's sense of identity" (p. 965). Finlay (2002) suggests that critical reflexivity is inseparable from contemporary qualitative inquiry and "is now the defining feature of qualitative research (Banister et al., 1994)" (p. 211). Personal theory is the life knowledge (including beliefs) that we bring to the research.

A *framework theory* is a focus on, and alignment with, a set of beliefs and assumptions associated with qualitative research methodologies. It is closely associated with what Guba and Lincoln (1994) reference as a paradigm or set of "basic beliefs" (p. 107). In his book, *Action Research*, Ernest T. Stringer uses the term "theory of the *method*" (2014, p. 39). The consideration of a framework theory generally occurs at the front-end of a specific research project and is, commonly, a theoretical orientation formalized in existing literature. The term *formal theory* in this context is synonymous with established theory found in research discourse. Examples include feminist, post-modernist, relativist, critical theory. The framework theory in this context is that which has often been defined in previous theoretical, customarily academic, writings. Those in the academy who have had the privilege to represent themselves have historically defined and established such theories. A framework theory emerges from a particular cultural context and from a particular voice.

Critical theory is an example of a framework theory. It is a particular theoretical perspective that assists in focusing research in a particular way. Bohman (2013) offers this perspective on critical theory, "A critical theory provides the descriptive and normative bases for social inquiry aimed at decreasing domination and increasing freedom in all their forms" (para. 1). Thus, research that integrates a critical theory perspective will have as a focus power and privilege. Often critical theory is associated with decolonizing research.

The choice of framework theory is quite significant because it is foundational in guiding research method choice and analysis. The framework theory is more often than not linked with personal theory in qualitative methodologies because researchers, being human, tend to gravitate toward theoretical framing that is congruent with (i.e., not repellent to) their own personal belief system. While the use of established theories in qualitative methodologies is the norm, there exists space for the establishment of emergent framework theories, of which Indigenous theory is an example.

Substantive theory has arisen from the methodological enterprise and language of grounded theory methodology. Substantive theory differentiates from personal theory and framework theory in that substantive theory emerges from the data of a specific research project. In articulating what is meant by substantive theory, grounded theorist Kathy Charmaz (2006) offers this description:

> Most grounded theories are substantive theories because they address delimited problems in specific substantive areas such as a study of how newly disabled young people reconstruct their identities. (p. 8)

Howell (2013) defines substantive theory as "derived from data analysis" and includes "rich conceptualizations of specific situations" (p. 27). Substantive theory, then, is closely associated with data and occurs in the research phase when one is working with the data to make meaning. One's own personal theory and subjectivities are implicated in the building of substantive theory within a singular research project. This is based upon the argument that research subjectivities can never be divorced from one's research choices and interpretations. Furthermore, the framework theory that is applied within a research design will impact the substantive theory arising from the data.

Theoretical choices in research shape-shift and evolve according to experience and knowledge (Howell, 2013). As Charmaz's (2010) states: "The theory [grounded or substantive] *depends* on the researcher's view: it does not and cannot stand outside of it" (p. 130). In a well-considered research design, there is evidence of a relationship between personal theory, framework theory, and situated theory.

Revealing how an aspect of a phenomenon functions in relationship to the larger phenomenon is instrumental in discerning its significance. Knowing the function of firewood in building a fire helps clarify its import, and so tending to the firewood is rudimentary. In much the same way, knowing the different forms that theory takes in research is basic to appreciating its role. Theory as form then becomes less of an enigma and a more transparent process. In considering personal theory, framework theory, and substantive theory as form (or a 'place-saver') the task then is to consider the 'type' or substance of theory being proposed. The next section references Indigenous theory to more specifically consider theory as that which focuses on a situation in a specific way Stringer (2014) and that which understands a situation from a particular perspective. Indigenous theory is a particular theoretical orientation with specific attributes and characteristics. A main argument throughout has been the importance of Indigenous situated voice in the theory-research-policy dynamic. Indigenous theory has much to offer here.

Indigenous Theory

Within Indigenous methodologies, an Indigenous theory can be useful in demystifying and concretely grounding methodology in Indigenous situated knowledge. The rationale for briefly addressing Indigenous theory is to illustrate that: a) an Indigenous theoretical perspective in research is possible and b) Indigenous theory is a viable theoretical approach well positioned to situate Indigenous experience. Personal theory (or situatedness) is valued within Indigenous philosophy and, thus, Indigenous theory. Consequently, the assumptions arising from this theoretical perspective (Indigenous theory) are grounded within Indigeneity itself, thereby offering an Indigenous insider-out approach to research.

The term *Indigenous paradigm* is common to Indigenous research and is used to articulate an Indigenous belief system. As with other qualitative paradigms (e.g., transformative, constructivist) an Indigenous research paradigm can be described as a set of assumptions, values, and practices that comprise an approach or perspective. Indigenist or Indigenous methodologies are founded upon this paradigm (Kovach, 2010; Wilson, 2008). Because of their paradigmatic orientation, Indigenous methodologies are well positioned to integrate theory steeped in Indigenous philosophy.

Indigenous philosophy and, subsequently, Indigenous theory are of an ancient, but ever evolving, set of beliefs and practices arising from tribal cultures. Writings on the nature and characteristics of Indigenous philosophy have seen growth within academic publication, including writing by such authors as Vine Deloria, Jr., Willie Ermine, Leroy Little Bear, and Marie Battiste. Much of this writing, documenting Indigenous community-based knowledges, shows a shared set of beliefs among Indigenous peoples globally. Such beliefs include the acknowledgment of process, wholeness, and the collective. In his article, *Jagged Worldviews Colliding*, Blackfoot scholar Leroy Little Bear (2000) writes:

> Arising out of the Aboriginal philosophy of constant motion or flux is the value of wholeness or totality. The value of wholeness speaks to the totality of creation, the group as opposed to the individual, the forest opposed to the individual trees. It focuses on the totality of the constant flux rather than the individual trees. (p. 79)

Of the totality, flux, and collectivity, Mohawk scholar Brant Castellano (2000) delineates the esteem assigned to spiritual, experiential, and holistic knowledges and the significance of oral transmission within Indigenous beliefs and practices. Within the metaphysics of Indigeneity, the symbiosis of individual and collective endure.

Perkins (2007) identifies several components of Indigenous theory while reminding that definitional categories and components are themselves antagonist toward the holistic nature of Indigenous theory. These components include: the "concept of harmony or balance"; "importance of place and history"; "experience, practice, and process"; the holistic and collective nature of Indigeneity; and "the cyclical and genealogical nature of time" (p. 64). Māori scholar Graham Hingangaroa Smith further conveys specific characteristics of Indigenous theory. According to Smith (cited in Kovach, 2010) Indigenous theory is culturally contextualized, born of community, articulated by a theorist knowledgeable of Indigenous worldview; change orientated; transferable, but not universal; flexible; theoretically engaged, not isolationist; critical; and accessible.

Threaded throughout an Indigenous theoretical perspective is the value of personal knowledge and the practice of communicating what has been learned. Vine Deloria, Jr. (as cited in Deloria, Jr., & Wildcat, 2001) had this to say about why Indigenous people relate personal experience: "We share our failure and successes so that we know who we are and so that we have confidence when we do things" (p. 46). Through this connection there is empathy and support, along with concrete practical guidance. Knowledge is personally situated but collectively sourced. Deloria, Jr., went on to say that tribal knowledges help us "to see our place and our responsibility within the movement of history as it is experienced by community" (p. 46). Collective notions of place, responsibility, and history anchor personal understandings and actions.

Personal situatedness allows for acknowledgement of kinship and community in personal realizations. The practice and protocol of self-situating with the purpose of acknowledging those who have held us up is increasingly found within research and scholarship by Indigenous authors (Cardinal, 2001; Coram, 2011; Debassige, 2010; Iwama, 2009). Within community, the protocol of introduction is a sign of respect and functions as a way for others to situate who we are within kinship and community systems.

The value of personal theory or situatedness within Indigenous theory asks, or rather requires, that Indigenous experience be included. In and of itself, this is a remedial, restitutional, and radical proposition. In Indigenous theory the totality of theory, in all its forms, is valued. Indeed a criterion of an Indigenous framework theory is to place oneself within one's own life and social context. Further, it is the articulation of personal theory and framework theory steeped in Indigeneity that ultimately leads to situated theory with an Indigenous sensibility.

The *wîsahkêcâhk* Hypothesis

In connecting back to policy, the absence of Indigenous situated theorizing has led to a ground swell of both research and policy promoting a deficit theorizing approach to Indigenous people. Such research and policy initiatives have pierced the Indigenous community with a 'gap' focused, victim-blaming sting. In the third edition of *The SAGE Dictionary of Qualitative Inquiry*, Schwandt (2007) speaks to the uses of theory. Here he quotes R. Alford's arguments that research responds to both theoretical and empirical questions. The theoretical questions posed include "Why did something happen? What explains this? Why did these events occur? What do they mean?" (p. 293). If we were to consider, for example, the experience of Indigenous student engagement in Canadian educational institutions, how would an Indigenous theory respond to these theoretical questions: How may this be different from the existing normative perspective? Would this shift thinking? In shifting thinking, would actions change? Would knowing the myriad ways that theory functions in research help to demystify how deficit theorizing of Indigenous peoples perseveres?

Research and policy impacting Indigenous communities have never been apolitical, nor have they been atheoretical. Whether visible or not, both are inevitably imbued with suppositions and conjectures. This essay offers some big picture connections. It begins with the premise that there is a connection between theory, research, and policy. In reflecting upon unexamined theory in an Indigenous context, we see that more often than not outsider theorizing in research and policy has diminished rather than upheld Indigenous peoples. Unpacking the different forms that theory takes in research—as in personal, framework, and substantive theory—offers insight into its persuasiveness. Moving toward an Indigenous theory, as a particular approach, provides a way forward toward a more fully Indigenous situated theorizing.

Within Indigenous country, for too long theorizing of Indigenous people, culture, and experience has occurred from an outsider situated vantage point. As research involving Indigenous peoples continues to be highly fundable, the production line, drive-through approach often trumps a more meditative one. All too frequently, it seems as if it is the same old song until there is a shift in energy—a book topples, coffee spills. Alertness expands and responsive intensifies. *wîsahkêcâhk*—the transformer—has entered the room. *wîsahkêcâhk* has the potential to trouble even the most theoretically complacent researcher, and in doing so, changes things. The shrewd transformer interrupts the habitual and makes space for us to pause, reflect, think, and think again. And in the often stagnant, deficit theorizing of Indigenous peoples in research and policy discourse, both thinking again and changing things couldn't hurt.

References

Aboriginal Affairs and Northern Development Canada. (2012). *Developing a First Nation Education Act: Discussion Guide.* Ottawa: Canada.

Abott, A & Egloff, R. (2008). The polish peasant in Oberlin and Chicago: The intellectual trajectory of W. I. Thomas. *American Sociologist 39* (4), 217–258.

Abu Talib, M. (2010). A general perspective on role of theory in qualitative research. *The Journal of International Social Research, 3*(11), 570–577.

Anfara, V., & Mertz, N. T. (2006). *Theoretical frameworks in qualitative research*. Thousand Oaks, CA: Sage.

Bannister, P. Burman, E., Parker, I., & Tindall, C. (1994). *Qualitative methods in psychology: A research guide*. Buckingham, UK: Open University Press.

Bohman, J., (2013). Critical theory. In E. N. Zalta (Ed.), *The Stanford encyclopedia of philosophy* (Spring 2013 ed.). Retrieved from plato.stanford.edu/archives/spr2013/entries/critical-theory

Brant Castellano, M. (2000). Updating Aboriginal traditions of knowledge. In G. J. Sefa Dei, B. L. Hall, & D. G. Rosenberg (Eds.), *Indigenous knowledges in global contexts: multiple readings of our world* (pp. 21–36). Toronto: University of Toronto Press.

Cardinal, L. (2001). What is an Indigenous perspective? *Canadian Journal of Native Education, 25*(2), 180–182.

Charmaz, K. (2006). *Constructing grounded theory: A practical guide through qualitative analysis*. Thousand Oaks, CA: Sage.

Coram, S. (2011). Rethinking Indigenous research approval. *Qualitative Research Journal, 11* (2), pp. 38–47.

Cuthand, D. (2013, October 25). Aboriginal Education Act a regression to 1950s. *The Saskatoon Star Pheonix*, A13.

Debassige, B. (2010). Re-conceptualizing Anshinaabe mino-bimaadiziwin (the good life) as research methodology: A spirit centred way in Anishinaabe research. *Canadian Journal of Native Education, 33*(1), 11–28.

Deloria, Jr., V., & Wildcat, D. R. (2001). *Power and place: Indian education in America*. Golden, CO: American Indian Graduate Centre and Fulcrum Resources.

Denzin, N., & Lincoln, Y. (2005). Introduction: The discipline and practice of qualitative research. In N. Denzin & Y. Lincoln (Eds.), *The SAGE handbook of qualitative research* (3rd ed., pp. 1–32). Thousand Oaks, CA: Sage.

Family Service Toronto (2012). *2011 report card on child and family poverty in Canada: Revisiting family security in insecure times*. www.campaign2000.ca/reportCards/national/2011EnglishRreportCard.pdf (accessed February 4, 2014).

Finlay, L. (2002). Negotiating the swamp: The opportunity and challenge of reflexivity in research practice. *Qualitative Research, 2*(2), 209–230.

Guba, E. G., & Lincoln, Y. S. (1994). Competing paradigms in qualitative research. In N. Denzin & Y. Lincoln (Eds.), *Handbook of qualitative research* (pp. 105–117). Thousand Oaks, CA: Sage.

Howe, E. (2011). *Bridging the Aboriginal education gap in Saskatchewan*. Retrieved from www.gdins.org/node/230

Howell, K. E. (2013). *An introduction to the philosophy of methodology*. London: Sage.

Iwama, M., Marshall, M., Marshall, A., & Bartlett, C. (2009). Two-eyed seeing and the language of healing in community based research. *Canadian Journal of Native Education, 32*(2), 3–23.

Kennedy, M. (2013, October 10). Stephen Harper's First Nation Education Act might continue assimilation, Shawn Atleo says [Postmedia News]. Retrieved from www.canada.com/life/Stephen+Harper+First+Nation+Education+might+continue+assimilation+Shawn+Atleo+says/9007822/story.html

Klemperer, A., Theisens, H., & Kaiser, F. (2001). Dancing in the dark: The relationship between policy research and policy making in Dutch higher education. *Comparative Education Review—Special Issue on the Relationship Between Theorists/Researchers and Policy Makers/Practioners, 45*(2), 197–219.

Kovach, M. (2010). *Indigenous methodologies: Characteristics, conversations, and contexts.* Toronto: University of Toronto Press.

Little Bear, L. (2000). Jagged worldviews colliding. In M. Battiste (Ed.), *Reclaiming Indigenous voices and vision* (pp. 77–85). Vancouver: UBC Press.

McLeod, N. (2007). *Cree narrative memory—From treaties to contemporary times.* Saskatoon, Canada: Purich.

Merriam, S. B. (1997). *Qualitative research and case study in education.* San Francisco: Jossey-Bass.

Perkins, U. (2007). Pono and the *Koru*: Toward Indigneous theory in Pacific island literature. *Hulili: Multidisciplinary Research on Hawaiian Well-being, 4*(1), 59–65.

Richardson, L., & St. Pierre, E. (2005). Writing: A method of inquiry. In N. Denzin & Y. S. Lincoln (Eds), *The SAGE handbook of qualitative research* (3rd ed., pp. 959–978). Thousand Oaks, CA: Sage.

Schwandt, T. A. (2007). *The Sage dictionary of qualitative inquiry.* (3rd ed.) Thousand Oaks, CA: Sage.

Stalwick, H. (1986). *Study guide no. 1—What was said. Taking Control Project.* Regina, Canada: University of Regina.

Stanley, L. (2010). To the letter: Thomas and Znaniecki's *The Polish Peasant* and writing a life, sociologically. *Life Writing*, 7(3), 149–151.

Stonechild, B. (2006). *The new buffalo: The struggle for Aboriginal post-secondary education in Canada.* Winnipeg, Canada: University of Manitoba Press.

Stringer, E. T. (2014). *Action research.* (4th ed.). Thousand Oaks, CA: Sage.

Tavallaei, M., & Abu Talib, M. (2010). A general perspective on role of theory in qualitative research. *The Journal of International Social Research, 3*(11), 570–577.

Tuhiwai Smith, L. (2013). *Decolonizing methodologies: Research and Indigenous Peoples* (2nd ed.). London: Zed Books.

Wilson, S. (2008). *Research is ceremony: Indigenous research methods.* Winnipeg, Canada: Fernwood.

Chapter 21

Indigenous Researchers and Epistemic Violence

César A. Cisneros Puebla

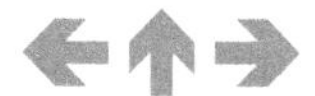

Our knowledge about the social world has been tremendously useless when dealing with the urgency of social justice, social change, and democracy. We have created diverse kinds of sociologies and humanities to analyze and interpret our subjectivity and the miseries that provoke the ambition of power and inequality. As human beings, our 21st century is bringing us a portrait of those negative dimensions of ourselves that never have changed: it looks like our world nowadays is just a globalized way to eternalize poverty, injustice, and inequality. In what ways have the social sciences and humanities contributed to keeping the status quo? In this chapter I will explore what role the current division of scientific labor has played in the construction of the order of our daily activities as researchers. My emphasis will be on Indigenous knowledges and the ways to move to other conceptual coordinates our concerns and questions.

We have learned to do sociology of knowledge and technology (Gouldner, 1976; Latour, 1987), sociology of social movements (Offe, 1985; Touraine, 1985), and sociology of daily life of other

Originally published in *Qualitative Inquiry Outside the Academy*, edited by Norman K. Denzin and Michael D. Giardina, pp. 164–178. Republished in *Qualitative Inquiry—Past, Present, and Future: A Critical Reader*, edited by Norman K. Denzin and Michael D. Giardina, pp. 387–401.

people (Schwartz & Jacobs 1979). But a sociology of our own practices as researchers, as scientists, as persons of flesh and blood, is still pending. We don't really know too much about ourselves as researchers, and/or as human beings, and how we came to be what we are. But today such a sociology of ourselves is more necessary than ever. Have we become what we are thanks to some educational and scientific institutions? Are we doing what we do having the presumptions and suppositions that we have without doubts? In some ways, the personal pathways of becoming a researcher, scientist, activist, or practitioner of any discipline are mysterious and hidden. Becoming a researcher or scientist and acting in consequence of that is equally a matter of speculation and suspicion in specific scenarios. Sometimes, for opportunistic reasons, as the president of the International Social Science Council says (ISSC, 2010, p. vi), social scientists "did not understand how their own creation worked." With no doubt, our "scientific" concepts are everywhere, and common citizens use them to understand their situation. Also, our social programs, ones based on our "scientific methods," have been around the world for decades, having some real consequences in specific areas. But is our creation what we dreamed?

To do a sociology of ourselves (and our work) is not just necessary, but urgent, from the perspective of creating useful knowledge to change the current situation. Our contribution to global social change is highly valued. We cannot let down the trust that society has in us: knowledge about ourselves and the consequences of our work and actions is the best guarantee for the future of our endeavor. As scientists and/or public intellectuals (Gergen, 2009) we must always know what side we are on. Our personal pathways into social sciences are carved in very specific social, historical, and geopolitical contexts. Obviously, becoming a social scientist in Germany is not comparable to becoming one in Peru. What is more, producing theory and doing social science research along the Rhine River differs from doing so in the Amazon River basin. As social scientists, we live together on a symbolic dimension of words and practices, but we inhabit different worlds. There are not meaningful comparisons between such human realities.

Knowing more about ourselves is not just describing our feelings and desires in a sort of autobiography or autoethnography. This is not what I am writing about. I am talking about putting our critical thought on the historic dimensions of what we are in the context of modernity. As a Latin American scholar, I must say that "my" modernity has a colonial past of its own dating back to the 16th century. Collecting and sharing stories of researchers around the world as to how and why they do what they do would allow us to enhance our awareness about the limits of our methods and approaches, the historical circumstances of our epistemologies, and the geopolitics of our knowledge. Knowing more about ourselves in historical, geopolitical, and epistemological views is our major current challenge. But knowing more about ourselves is also a matter of ethics and responsibilities. Gaining awareness of the historical dimensions of our theories, concepts, approaches, and methods leads us to an insightful moment of recognizing how contested our certitudes and taken-for-granted beliefs are in the encounter with other cultures and knowledges—encounters where the otherness has been eliminated and such process can be shown in critical ways (Dussel, 1995).

Human civilization is shaped by the conjunction of thousands of different trajectories. Such trajectories must be seen from the perspectives of conflict, domination, and inequality. Each society has its own rhythm, pattern, obstacles, problems, solutions, wars, and social memories. As social scientists, we need to find our place in the struggle between dominators and dominated, right and left, past and future, core and peripheries, and superior and inferior perspectives. Certainly, we must recognize that we are dealing with knowledge production in societies that treat humans unequally. After centuries of domination of some countries, people, classes, and races over other countries, people, classes, and races, we are still asking ourselves how such international inequality has been possible and continues to be so. The question about how such a global social order was constructed is still unanswered, although we have several theories about it. Different theories and their associated political and social movements continue to act and look for a new society based on their suppositions and principles.

Nevertheless, the negation of Otherness has been the principal equilibrium. For centuries, our modernity has included much ignorance about Otherness because the only way of knowing was to eliminate, subordinate, and/or oppress our differences from the Other. Mignolo (1995) has shown how the narrative of modernity needs the notion of "primitives" to create the spatial colonial difference and define the identities of supposed superior and inferior human beings. The colonization of the Americas was based on such terrible assumptions, and the effects of such narratives have been substantial, leading to different ways of producing societies and creating knowledge. And, of course, the coloniality of power also had and still has influence in the ways science is organized and institutionalized in each society.

Core and Peripheries in the Knowledge Divide

Monaterios (2008) has shown that postcolonial primary theoretical sources operate from different historical and cognitive perspectives. The South Asian Subaltern Studies group and scholars such as Fanon, Glissant, Said, Bhabha, and Spivak have framed the origin of modernity in the 18th century. In contrast, based on such Indigenous and non-institutionalized thinkers as Mariátegui and Rivera Cusicanqui, among others, postcolonial Latin American thinkers such as Dussel, Quijano, and Mignolo (to mention but a few) tend to frame the experiences of modernity in the 16th century; the conceptual debates are rooted in our conceptual legacies.

Although it is important to recognize that Spivak (1995) has provided us a way of thinking to deconstruct the legacy of colonialism and show that the subaltern can speak, and Bhabha (1995) has enriched our perspectives with concepts as hybridity to analyze cultural dominance, the postcolonial turn has brought us to other perspectives to analyze our actions regarding cultural products, ethics, conquerors and conquered, knowledge, values, and traditions. Without a doubt, the three "As" (Africa, Asia, and America) are still opposed to the one "E" (Europe) in thinking about subaltern cultures and oppressed groups from a long historical perspective. Among the "As" each "A" is thought to belong to the First Nations, the aboriginal people and civilizations. But we need to think critically about whether to include the islands and the archipelagos in the histories of resistance and struggle against dominion. From Africa, Asia, and America the subaltern voices must be listened so that we can embrace the emerging possibility of new histories and geographies.

The distinction between core and peripheries was first established as a consequence of the colonial world. Such a world of languages, practices, and performances created diverse cognitive processes. According to Quijano (2000), the modern idea of race emerged with the colonization of America: it is a mental category of modernity. It was created as an instrument of basic social and racial classification as "a way of granting legitimacy to the relations of domination imposed by … conquest" (p. 534). Coloniality of power is a main category that leads us to think in critical ways about how the imposition of the idea of race is and has been an instrument of domination. In a worldwide vision, the narratives of the oppressed must be integrated to let us overcome the accomplice of silence that generates the permanence of the status quo. Believe it or not, the practices linked to the original "modern" idea of race are still everywhere and their subtle presence assures different practices of domination in diverse social, emotional, and cognitive human spheres.

From a Latin American postcolonial perspective and analyzing the global capitalism's dynamics, Quijano (2000) proposes that we include conflict, domination, and exploitation as the basic elements to be considered to study the changes on such social dimensions as work, race, sex, natural resources, authority, governance, and public authority. We can definitely produce very critical approaches to deconstruct the dominant ideas of not just race but also sex, work, nature, authority, and governance, revealing in the process how deeply colonized thoughts and feelings are located in our minds and souls. In such direction, coloniality of power is an important category when thinking about the social geography of capitalism.

The knowledge divide can be seen as a historical consequence of the global dynamics of capitalism, dividing the world into the core and the peripheries. This knowledge divide also classifies social science researchers into core and peripheries. It is possible to think about coloniality of scientific labor as the coloniality that determined the geographic distribution of each one of us in the integrated forms of labor control in global capitalism. Nowadays, the core and peripheries are economically, socially, and technologically obvious when comparing social structures and countries in worldwide perspectives: their differences are apparent from the very first moment. Regardless of their colonial pasts, Africa, Asia, and America—in the sense they are discussed here—share similar processes of creation and institutionalization of knowledge: Indigenous, native voices and beliefs were silenced during colonization. 'Core' is producing theory and methods, and 'peripheries' are consuming and reproducing them. We can think about the postcolonial, decolonizing, and Indigenous knowledge systems discussion (Smith, 1999) as a kind of rebellion against such a distribution. We live together on a planet, but we inhabit different worlds. Global coloniality (Escobar, 2004) is marginalizing and even suppressing the knowledge and culture of subaltern groups; it seems like this oppression will never end. Being social researchers with the marks and traces of ancestral knowledge on the soul allows us to build on the strong shoulders of giants to create new life perspectives. But in the knowledge divide context, the only valid premises and concepts are those based in the dominant, colonial and Western societies. Still today, people from the center are not able to see the peripheries as formed by active actors seeking their own presence and with their own language in the worldwide knowledge production process. Such is natural given the long duration of colonializing ways of seeing, but the opposite is coming very fast: people from the center are changing their minds and souls to see what is coming from the colonized world. And not just listening to the oppressed colonialized voices of "other" researchers as a fake way of being "cool."

Globalized Knowledge and Domination

Coloniality of power is useful to understand how science is organized and institutionalized in each society, but can also be used to understand the current division of scientific labor. If social research methods created by Europeans and North Americans have become a sort of general knowledge (Ryen & Gobo, 2011, p. 411), it is convenient to remind ourselves that there is no context-free knowledge and no power-free interest. In social sciences and humanities, it is a mistake to think in terms of universal knowledge beyond any cultural differences. Nevertheless, questioning the assumed existence of globalized methodology or globalized knowledge leads us to criticize the illusion of homogeneous practices and uniform thinking everywhere around the world. Globalized knowledge means—particularly in social science research—domination of Anglo-American legacies, concepts, and methodologies over the peripheral world with their potentially innovative own conceptual legacies and Indigenous epistemologies.

Using a Mexican example, I would like to illustrate the effects of such ideas on the division of scientific labor in the context of globalized knowledge. In a brief essay, Maerk (2009) discusses what he calls "cover-science" as practiced in social sciences and humanities in Latin America. In his view, scholars in Latin America just copy foreign theories, concepts, and methods. He recalls what the Mexican-Spaniard philosopher Jose Gaos coined as "imperialism of categories," referring to categories that originated from other cultures, especially Europe, and are used to characterize processes of social, economic, and political orders in Latin America with no changes or adaptations. Maerk's analysis is not just based on his epistemological perspective but also in fieldwork he conducted in Mexico when doing empirical research. In his words (p. 186):

> Latin American and other scholars from the "global South" commit the error of "universalizing" the local knowledge of supposedly "great authors": Max Weber analyses and describes the bureaucrat of the "old continent"; Joseph Schumpeter focuses on the innovative European, but mainly British capitalist; Jürgen Habermas directs his attention to the industrialized First World society, in particular to the German society; and Pierre Bordieu studies mainly the French socio-cultural and socio-political condition. Instead of recognizing the singular character of each of these theories, there is a strong tendency in Latin America to believe that any of the resident capitalists is a capitalist in the sense of Schumpeter or Weber, or that the relation between the public and the private in Mexico or Brazil is similar to the one we find in Germany, as assessed by Habermas.

Undoubtedly, there is pendant discussion about globalized knowledge in the sense of validity, reliability, transparency, applicability, replicability, and originality when dealing with concepts and theories in social science and humanities. However, a particular and unique quality of Latin American researchers is the epistemological perspectives we embrace. Such epistemology is full of historical perspectives and political action on the issues researchers are dealing with. From the stance of sociology of science, this uniqueness is due to the differences in the social contexts in which knowledge is produced in each country. But is that quality just singular to Latin America? Are there not similar epistemological perspectives in Asia and Africa? In any case, why are the "great authors" necessary to understand such local, regional, or national circumstances and/or processes when their concepts are not linked to such local, regional, or national circumstances and/or processes?

Hence, the geographical closeness of Mexico and the United States offers an interesting case. Abend (2006) provides an interesting example from Mexican social science that could inspire similar explorations in other countries to create an international debate about practices and uniqueness of doing science and creating knowledge. The more noticeable difference Abend discovered in his analysis by comparing contributions in journals published in the period of 1995–2001 is related to the way Mexican scientists are testing theory or thinking about the dialogue between theory and data. Abend's sample of articles was drawn from the most cited and most prestigious journals in each country: in the United States, the *American Journal of Sociology* and the *American Sociological Review*; in Mexico, *Estudios Sociológicos* and *Revista Mexicana de Sociología*. Based on the social conditioning of scientific knowledge, Abend reminds us that Mexican and American sociologies are epistemologically, semantically, and perceptually incommensurable because of the unique understandings of what theory is, the role of subjectivity, and ethical neutrality. With respect to the differences between Mexican and American approaches to doing sociological research, Abend notes "an empirical sociology of epistemologies would constitute a step forward in the agenda of the sociology of knowledge, as it would further our understanding of the social conditioning of scientific knowledge" (2006, p. 32). Abend's analysis reinforces Maerk's annotation of Mexican sociologists just "copying" theories and concepts.

Let me ask once again but in different words: Is a "Mexican" way of doing sociology particular to just that country or is it also the favorite way of working in other developing countries? Referring to foreign authors' concepts without referring to data collected by native researchers seems to be a general practice to validate inquiry in the academia. "Doing theory" in such a way is just reproducing ideas and arguments in the recreational fiction of "universal" applicability of some sociological concepts, regardless of their historical and cultural situations. Could we reflect and produce some critical stances about what it means to be "doing theory" in different countries and diverse cultural worlds? "Doing theory" in the sense of making quotes of such "great authors" is, here in this chapter and from this desk, and I would assume from other desks and parts of the world, totally unacceptable.

Let me insist: globalized knowledge means, in the field of qualitative research in particular, domination of Anglo-American legacies, concepts, and methodologies over the peripheral world with their own potentially innovative conceptual legacies and Indigenous epistemologies. I must note that it is not the responsibility of any acclaimed and classical "great author" or the contemporary and still alive "great authors" being copied as in the described way of "cover-science" to change this practice. In another context, compare qualitative research and music, to follow the idea on doing "cover-science" as playing "covers": there is a potential dilemma for those musicians who decide to keep their traditional instruments and explore the richness of their own culture versus only playing ¨covers¨ of great American or European hits. As with the globalized musical world, the scientific world must be aware of its unity and diversity. It is important to recognize the different narratives we are able to listen to.

As I have elsewhere pointed out (see Cisneros Puebla, 2008), the narratives that are told about the history and development of qualitative research are deeply grounded in the experience of North America, and it is only very recently that the diversity of qualitative research history and experiences has come to light. A rich discussion is emerging regarding our position as global qualitative researchers based on various reflections from different perspectives about the dominance of Anglo-American legacies (Alasuutari, 2004; Cisneros Puebla et al., 2006; Mruck, Cisneros

Puebla, & Faux, 2005). Hsiung (2012, p. 5), for example, following Alasuutari (2004), has suggested that the "globalization of qualitative research … is emerging as a subfield where qualitative researchers in the periphery have begun challenging the domination of the Anglo-American core."

Thinking specifically about qualitative research, I believe we need a shift in the current division of scientific labor that sees scholarship in the core producing theory and methods, while those in the peripheries consume and reproduce it. More attention needs to be paid to the indigenization of qualitative research in the peripheral countries. Kathy Charmaz (2012), for instance, is currently leading a query around the ways grounded theory methodologies have been adopted by non-English-speaking researchers, and Gobo (2011) is questioning whether Indigenous methodologies and participatory action research are effective ways to escape methodological colonialism.

Geopolitically speaking, it would be valuable to explore what contributions in the peripheries could be taken in a globalized world of qualitative research to be integrated and practiced in the core. Once again, the music example could be a wonderful analogy to our practices as researchers: is the current division of scientific labor control eternal and non-changeable? It would be interesting to testify about the peripheries producing theory and methods and the core consuming and reproducing it. If qualitative scholars in the core could shift their roles from producers to consumers, the divide would change drastically, and our discussion would be freely moving away from colonial dimensions.

Indigenization and Epistemic Violence

We can assume that indigenization of knowledge consists of creatively adapting concepts, methods, and approaches to a culture different to that where such concepts, methods, and approaches were created. Communication between cultures is a very complex issue, but regarding knowledge production, we can follow the route that recognizes a second-generation indigenization phenomenon that refers to how Indigenous people are being educated in local universities in the peripheries; in previous generations, that took place in the centers. Huntington (1996) asserts that around the globe, education and democracy are leading to indigenization. Discussing cultural backlash, he quotes Roland Dore:

> The first "modernizer" or "post-independence" generation has often received its training in foreign (Western) universities in a Western cosmopolitan language. Partly because they first go abroad as impressionable teenagers, their absorption of Western values and lifestyles may well be profound. (p. 38)

This second-generation indigenization phenomenon occurred mainly (Maerk 2009, p. 188) in "societies under colonial rule until the twentieth century, e.g., in the Anglophone and Francophone Caribbean, in Africa, in the Middle East, and in parts of Asia." Maerk mentions the case of the Guyanese historian, Walter Rodney, comparing the Trinidadian Eric Williams, the French Martinican Aimé Césaire, and the African American W. E. B. Du Bois to highlight that second-generation members are mainly inclined to produce local knowledge rooted in their own cultural context and benefit and to be masters of what had been done for their predecessors.

But we need to identify that this is just one side of the phenomenon! Given the asymmetrical hierarchy Indigenous persons maintain with the non-Indigenous, the complex world of unfair subordination is reproduced and the dominion the colonizer performs to the colonized, or the power the conqueror executes to the conquered, appears as eternal "naturalized" social relationships difficult to be destroyed.

Developing autochthonous research methods is decisive to overcome the epistemic—and I would add racial—violence. Walker (2013, p. 302) has recognized such violence when Indigenous peoples in colonized countries "are told that scholarly research must focus primarily on 'linear intellectual analysis.'" But it is also crucial to enrich our practices as researchers by getting into new ways of experiencing relationships and human interactions. Ancestral knowledge around the world is still waiting to be listened to in the horizon to change our presence on the planet. As in the case of the music, just to follow the analogy once again, any ethno-musicologist would be able to testify how some rhythms, sounds, instruments, scales, and tunes have been provided to the "globalized musical sphere" because they have been produced in the very marginal societal areas or in the deep subaltern social structure. Yet why have colonized qualitative researchers not been listened to by their colleagues when producing their own approaches or Indigenous methods? Is it just a consequence of the quality of their products? Or is it a result of the lack of integrity, validity, reliability, transparency, applicability, and/or replicability accorded to the dominant Western epistemology? Such questions must to be answered by all people involved in the field: experts, students, novices, senior researchers, funding agencies, practitioners, "great authors" and "small authors," from the core and from the peripheries, from the North and South and from the West and East.

The personal pathways of becoming researcher, scientist, activist, or practitioner of any discipline will no longer be mysterious and hidden if we develop efforts to create a movement to emphasize the multiple and complex connection between the self and the social. Such a complex connection should be analyzed even if hurts. Recently, Garot (2013) has questioned himself in his role as white male ethnographer in the context of how he is acting the colonialized self of some clandestine actors by using some of Fanon's ideas. And his example will hopefully call attention to how it will be possible to do research after the postcolonial turn if we are able to bring the discussion to final consequences. What are such lasting consequences?

- Understand that the current division of scientific labor can't be eternal
- Deconstruct the very basic concepts of our certitude, certainty, evidence, and truth
- Destroy the asymmetrical hierarchy of knowledge and practices
- Recognize that epistemic violence has silenced other ways of knowing
- Re-examine the role of Indigenous and native methods in knowledge production
- Transform the relationship between core and peripheries
- Integrate the Asian and Latin American postcolonial thoughts

- Produce a critical sociology of knowledge
- Create a network of critical and Indigenous methodology
- Create and perform the decolonized self in daily life

'Indigenize' has different meanings depending on what area of the world we are located in. Rivera Cusicanqui (2010) has a powerful and meaningful voice from Aymara culture and legacies. She argues for a political economy of knowledge instead of a geopolitics of knowledge—the prevailing thread in postcolonial literature—because such discussion is not leading to social justice or human rights. As a non-institutionalized Bolivian thinker, her interesting approach should be considered by others. However, for me, doing science as Indigenous is not just related to *indigeneity*: it is a kind of critical awareness about our own beliefs' and thoughts' limits in the realm of a decolonized geopolitics of knowledge and language. I am not as Indigenous as Rivera Cusicanqui, but I can't accept being mestizo because of the accumulated violence such words contain. In colonialism, as our Aymara non-institutionalized thinker has told us, the words do not express anything—the words hide. As a colonial word, 'mestizo' hides multiple processes.

In this last part I am talking about myself through dialogue with postcolonial thinkers. In the end, we need to define ourselves within the globalization of qualitative research to acknowledge we are persons of flesh and blood, with culture, history, and language. Other voices from Asia and Africa are necessary to go beyond any limitation—to cultivate our analysis of the hidden and deep epistemic violence nested in the current division of scientific labor worldwide.

Acknowledgments

A previous and preliminary version was presented as a paper at the 2013 International Congress of Qualitative Research, hosted by the University of Illinois, Urbana-Champaign in May 2013, and was published as "The Journey Ends: An Epilogue" in: D. Mertens, F. Cram, & B. Chilisa (Eds.), *Indigenous pathways into social research. Voices of a new generation* (pp. 395–402). Walnut Creek, CA: Left Coast Press, Inc.

References

Abend, G. (2006). Styles of sociological thought: Sociologies, epistemologies, and the Mexican and U.S. quests for truth. *Sociological Theory, 24*, 141.

Alasuutari, P. (2004). The globalization of qualitative research. In G. Gobo, C. Seale, J. F. Gubrium, & David Silverman (Eds.), *Qualitative research practice* (pp. 595–608). Thousand Oaks, CA: Sage.

Bhabha, H. (1995) Interview with cultural theorist Homi Bhabha by W. J. T. Mitchell. (1995). *Artforum, 33*(7), 80–84.

Charmaz, K. (2012). Grounded theory in global perspective. Paper presented as part of the panel Challenges for Qualitative Inquiry as a Global Endeavor I: Methodological Issues, at the Eighth International Congress on Qualitative Inquiry, University of Illinois, Urbana-Champaign, May 18, 2012.

Cisneros Puebla, C. (2008). On the roots of qualitative research. In J. Zelger, M. Raich, & P. Schober (Eds.), *GABEK III. Organisationen und ihre wissensnetze* (pp. 53–75). Innsbruck, Austria: Studien Verlag.

Cisneros Puebla, C. A., Figaredo, D. D., Faux, R., Kölbl, C., & Packer, M. (2006). About qualitative research epistemologies and peripheries. *Forum Qualitative Sozialforschung/ Forum: Qualitative Social Research*, 7, Art. 44. nbn-resolving.de/urn:nbn:de:0114-fqs060444 (accessed January 13, 2012).

Dussel, E. (1995). *The invention of the Americas: Eclipse of "the Other" and the myth of modernity*. New York: Continuum.

Escobar, A. (2004). Beyond the Third World: Imperial globality, global coloniality, and antiglobalization social movements. *Third World Quarterly, 25*, 207–230.

Garot, R. (2013). The psycho-affective echoes of colonialism in fieldwork relations [21 paragraphs]. *Forum Qualitative Sozialforschung/Forum: Qualitative Social Research, 15*(1), Art. 12. www.qualitative-research.net/index.php/fqs/article/view/2102/3624 (accessed December 3, 2013).

Gergen, K. (2009). *Relational being: Beyond self and community*, New York: Oxford University Press.

Gobo, G. (2011). Globalizing methodology? The encounter between local methodologies. *International Journal of Social Research Methodology, 14*, 417–437.

Gouldner, A. W. (1976). *The dialectic of ideology and technology: The origins, grammar, and future of ideology*. London: Macmillan Press.

Hsiung, P-C. (2012). The globalization of qualitative research: Challenging Anglo-American domination and local hegemonic discourse. *Forum Qualitative Sozialforschung (Forum: Qualitative Social Research), 13*, Art. 21. nbn-resolving.de/urn:nbn:de:0114-fqs1201216 (accessed February 23, 2012).

Huntington, S. P. (1996). The West: Unique, not universal. *Foreign Affairs, 6*, 28–46.

ISSC Report. (2010). *World social science report. Knowledge divide*. Paris: ISSC, UNESCO.

Latour, B. (1987). *Science in action: How to follow scientists and engineers through society*. Cambridge, MA: Harvard University Press.

Maerk, J. (2009). Overcoming cover-science in Latin American social sciences and humanities—An intervention. In M-L. Frick & A. Oberprantacher (Eds.), *Power and justice in international relations: Interdisciplinary approaches to global challenges. Essays in honor of Hans Köchler* (pp. 185–192). Farnham, UK: Ashgate.

Mignolo, W. D. (1995). *The darker side of the renaissance: Literacy, territoriality and colonization*. Ann Arbor: University of Michigan Press.

Monaterios, E. (2008). Uncertain modernities: Amerindian epistemologies and the reorienting of culture. In S. Castro-Klaren (Ed.), *A companion to Latin American literature and culture* (pp. 553–570). Malden, MA: Wiley-Blackwell.

Mruck, K., Cisneros Puebla, C. A., & Faux, R. (2005). Editorial: About qualitative research centers and peripheries. *Forum Qualitative Sozialforschung (Forum: Qualitative Social Research), 6*, Art. 49. nbn-resolving.de/urn:nbn:de:0114-fqs0503491 (accessed February 23, 2012).

Offe, C. (1985). New social movements: Challenging the boundaries of institutional politics. *Social Research, 52*, 817–868.

Quijano, A. (2000). Coloniality of power, Eurocentrism and Latin America. *Nepantla, 3*, 533–580.

Rivera Cusicanqui, S. (2010). *Ch'ixinakax utxiwa : Una reflexión sobre prácticas y discursos descolonizadores*. Buenos Aires: Tinta Limón.

Ryen, A., & Gobo, G. (2011). Managing the decline of globalized methodology. *International Journal of Social Research Methodology, 14*, 411–415.

Schwartz, H., & Jacobs, J. (1979). *Qualitative sociology: A method to the madness*. New York: Free Press.

Smith, L. T. (1999). *Decolonising methodologies: Research and Indigenous peoples*. New York: Zed Books.

Spivak, G. C. (1995). Can the subaltern speak? In B. Ashcroft, G. Griffiths, and H. Tiffen (Eds.), *Post-colonial studies reader* (pp. 24–28). London: Routledge.

Touraine, A. (1985). An introduction to the study of new social movements. *Social Research, 52*, 749–487.

Walker, P. (2013). Research in relationship with humans, the spirit world, and the natural world. In D. Mertens, F. Cram, & B. Chilisa (Eds.), *Indigenous pathways into social research. Voices of a New Generation* (pp. 299–315). Walnut Creek, CA: Left Coast Press, Inc.

Chapter 22

Freeing Ourselves

An Indigenous Response to Neo-Colonial Dominance in Research, Classrooms, Schools, and Education Systems

Russell Bishop

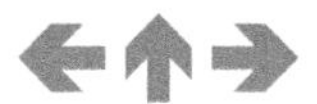

This then is the great humanistic and historical task of the oppressed: to liberate themselves and their oppressors as well. The oppressors, who oppress, exploit and rape by virtue of their power, cannot find in this power the strength to liberate either the oppressed or themselves. Only power that springs from the weakness of the oppressed will be sufficiently strong to free both.

—Freire (1972, p. 21)

Introduction

This chapter draws from the work that I have been doing over the past 25 years in the field of Māori and Indigenous education within the frame of kaupapa Māori theory. This journey over time has led me from researching the impact of colonization on my mother's Māori family to an appreciation of just what researching in Māori contexts involves. What I learned from that analysis was then extrapolated to re-theorize the marginalization of Māori students in

Originally published in *Qualitative Inquiry Outside the Academy,* edited by Norman K. Denzin and Michael D. Giardina, pp. 146–163. Republished in *Qualitative Inquiry—Past, Present, and Future: A Critical Reader,* edited by Norman K. Denzin and Michael D. Giardina, pp. 402–420. Left Coast Press, Inc.

mainstream secondary school classrooms. From this understanding, a means of supporting teachers and leaders to reposition themselves discursively and create caring and learning relationships within mainstream classrooms was developed. From these theoretical beginnings a large-scale classroom-based, school-reform project grew and eventually developed into a comprehensive approach towards theory- or principle-based education reform that is being implemented in 49 of the 320 secondary schools in New Zealand.

Fundamental to this theorizing and practice were the understandings promoted by Paulo Freire over 40 years ago, that the answers to the conditions that oppressed peoples found themselves in was not to be found in the language or epistemologies of the oppressors, but rather in that of the oppressed. This realization was confirmed when I understood that researching in Māori contexts needed to be conducted dialogically within the world view and understandings of the people with whom I was working. This realization also led me to understand how dialogue in its widest sense is crucial for developing a means whereby Māori students would be able to participate successfully in education.

Kaupapa Māori Responses

The major challenges facing education in New Zealand today are the ongoing and increasing social, economic, and political disparities within our nation, primarily between the descendants of the European colonizers (Pakeha) and the Indigenous Māori people. Māori have higher levels of unemployment (especially among youth), are more likely to be employed in low paying employment, have much higher levels of incarceration, mental and physical illness, and poverty than do the rest of the population, and are generally under-represented in the positive social and economic indicators of the society. These disparities are also reflected at all levels of the education system.[1]

Along with those of other indigenous peoples in the world who have suffered the impact of colonialism, these disparities reflect major and ongoing power imbalances that, along with socio-economic and political marginalization, have seen major culture and language loss among Māori people, particularly over the past century. This marginalization, culture and language loss, and the ethnic revitalization that has developed from within Māori culture itself in response is the major focus of this chapter. This chapter will demonstrate how theorizing and practice that have grown from within Māori epistemologies have been applied in a number of settings as counter-narratives to the dominant discourses in New Zealand.

Māori People Address the Problem of Educational Disparities

Frustrated with the lack of an effective system response to the problem of educational disparities and language and culture loss, in a Freirean sense, Māori people have undertaken their own response which grew out of the wider ethnic revitalization movement that developed among Māori people in New Zealand during their massive post World War II urbanization. This response initially saw the growth of a discourse of proactive theory and practice, broadly termed *kaupapa* (agenda, philosophy) Māori. Kaupapa Māori seeks to operationalize Māori people's aspirations to restructure power relationships at all levels in society to the point where partners can be autonomous and interact from this position rather than from one of subordination or dominance as has been the situation since the time of the signing of the Treaty of Waitangi in 1840 when the new nation of New Zealand was established. This theorizing drew together an emerging political consciousness among Māori people that promoted the revitalization of Māori cultural epistemologies as a philosophical and productive counter-narrative to the hegemony of neo-colonial discourses. In reference to kaupapa Māori in education, G. Smith (1997) explained this as occurring when "Māori communities armed with the new critical understandings of the shortcomings of the state and structural analyses began to assert transformative actions to deal with the twin crises of language demise and educational underachievement for themselves" (p. 171).

Elaborating on this point in 2003, Smith (2003) identified that the aim was to move from reactive grievance to proactive politics, from negative to positive motivations, from 'decolonization,' which locates the colonizer at the center of the debate, to 'consciousness raising' "which puts Māori at the centre" (p. 2). In short, to promote self-determination (*tino rangatiratanga*) by and for Māori people (Bishop, 1996; Durie, 1995, 1998; G. Smith, 1997; L Smith, 1999), which in Durie's (1995) terms "captures a sense of Māori ownership and active control over the future" (p. 16). However, this call for self-determination is clearly understood by Māori people as being relative, not absolute; that is, it is self-determination in *relation to others*. In Young's (2004) terms, such an approach identifies "a quest for an institutional context of non-domination" (p. 187). To ensure non-domination, "relations must be regulated both by institutions in which they all participate and by ongoing negotiations among them" (Young, 2004, p. 177). Therefore, educational institutional leaders and practitioners should structure and conduct their practices in such a way as to seek to mediate potential tensions by actively minimizing domination, co-ordinating actions, resolving conflicts, and negotiating relationships. In Young's terms, this is an education where power is shared between self-determining individuals within non-dominating relations of interdependence.

Early examples of kaupapa Māori theorizing in practice included the growth of Māori medium education institutions such as Te Kohanga Reo (Māori medium elementary schools), Kura Kaupapa Māori (Māori medium primary schools), Wharekura (Māori medium secondary schools), and Waananga Māori (Māori tertiary institutions). As G. Smith (2003) explains, Māori communities "were so concerned with the loss of Māori language, knowledge and culture that they took matters into their own hands and set up their own learning institutions at pre-school, elementary school, secondary school and tertiary levels" (pp. 6–7). Despite facing many problems, these new institutions continue to make inroads into the general culture of New Zealand to the extent that they are now immutable elements of the wider society.

Simultaneously, a number of other initiatives grew within the philosophical frame of kaupapa Māori. This chapter looks at three examples of how this author was involved in an indigenous people's initiative to *free ourselves* from neo-colonial oppression by creating counter-narratives to the dominant discourses around research, classroom practices, and school and system organization. The chapter also highlights how such an approach has redirected the actions of members of the 'oppressor' groups to discursively reposition themselves through an ongoing process of conscientization in relation to the representations of Māori as a minoritized group.

Kaupapa Māori Research Approaches

An early example of a Kaupapa Māori project was an investigation of what constituted effective approaches to researching in Māori settings undertaken by the author (Bishop, 1996, 2005). In this project, the centrality of the process of establishing extended family-like relationships, understood in Māori as *whanaungatanga*, were used metaphorically as a research strategy to ensure that issues of initiation, benefits, representation, legitimation, and accountability were not being dominated by the researcher's agenda, concerns, and interests within the research process.

In this sense, *whanaungatanga* means that groups (be they of research or classroom participants) are constituted as if they were a *whanau*, or extended family. Metge (1990) explains that to use the term *whanau*, whether literally or metaphorically, is to identify a series of rights and responsibilities, commitments and obligations, and supports that are fundamental to the collectivity. These are the *tikanga* (customs) of the *whanau*; warm interpersonal interactions, group solidarity, shared responsibility for one another, cheerful cooperation for group ends, corporate responsibility for group property, material or non-material (e.g., knowledge) items and issues. These attributes can be summed up in the words *aroha* (love in the broadest sense, including mutuality), *awhi* (helpfulness), *manaaki* (hospitality), and *tiaki* (guidance).

What is central to developing research (and classroom) relationships in this manner is that the *whanau* is a location for communication, for sharing outcomes, and for constructing shared common understandings and meanings. In other words, it is the context within which research (or classroom) activities can take place effectively. In such contexts, individuals have responsibilities to care for and to nurture other members of the group, while still adhering to the *kaupapa* (agenda, purpose) of the group. The group will operate to avoid singling out particular individuals for comment and attention and to avoid embarrassing individuals who are not yet succeeding within the group, and group products and achievement frequently take the form of group rather than individual performance.

This approach gave voice to a culturally positioned means of developing interviewing so as to collaboratively construct research stories (Collaborative Storying; see Connelly and Clandinin, 1990) in a culturally conscious and connected manner by focusing on the researcher's connectedness, engagement, and involvement with others in order to promote self-determination, agency, and the voice of those involved in the interaction (Bishop & Glynn, 1999; Bishop, 2005). Indeed, establishing and maintaining extended family (*whanau)* type relationships is a fundamental, often extensive and ongoing part of the research process that precedes and contextualizes all other activities. This re-ordering of what constitutes the research relationship is undertaken not on terms of or within understandings constructed by the researcher; instead *whanaungatanga* (establishing relationships within Māori discursive practices) uses Māori cultural practices and means of sense-making, such as *hui* (Māori formal meetings), found in Māori decision-making processes in Māori formal meetings on *marae* (Māori formal meeting settings), other extended family settings, and informal day-to-day practices (Bishop, 2005: Salmond, 1975), to set the pattern for research relationships.

Kaupapa Māori in Mainstream/Public School Classrooms

The above-described understanding was then extrapolated to classroom settings (Bishop & Glynn, 1999). This extrapolation suggested that a pedagogy that would be effective for Māori students in mainstream schools would be one that was understandable in Māori epistemological terms, would address the on-going power imbalances and racism that exist in neo-colonial New Zealand, and would create a context that would re-order the relationships between teachers and students in classrooms and mainstream/public schools. In other words, just as *whanau* relationships, *whanaungatanga* re-orders what constitutes the research relationship in classrooms; relationships could also be re-ordered using this organizing metaphor. Similarly, this re-ordering of the pedagogic relationship need not be within the cultural understandings or constructions of the teacher, but instead, processes of *whanaungatanga* that use Māori language, cultural understandings, decision-making processes, means of sense-making, and students' prior knowledge and language would create a pedagogic approach that would more effectively support Māori students' engagement and learning. Such a pedagogy would develop caring and learning relationships that would be culturally responsive (Gay, 2010) and culturally sustaining (Paris, 2012). In this pedagogic approach, power would be shared between self-determining individuals within non-dominating relations of interdependence (Young, 2004); the maintenance and promotion of Māori culture and language would be central; learning would be interactive, dialogic, and spiralling; and participants would be connected and committed to one another through the process of co-constructing shared common understandings and meanings. Drawing on Gay (2010), Villegas and Lucas (2002)—who identify the importance of a culturally responsive pedagogy—and Sidorkin (2002) and Cummins (1996)—who propose that relations ontologically precede all other concerns in education—I have termed such a pattern Culturally Responsive Pedagogy of Relations (see Bishop, 2008).

How such a pedagogy could be operationalized was then investigated by interviewing Māori students, their families, principals, and teachers in 2001 (Bishop & Berryman, 2006), in 2004–2005, and again in 2007 (Bishop et al., 2007). The interviews were undertaken within the Collaborative Storying approach described above that sought to address the self determination of Māori secondary school students by talking with them and other participants in their education about their understandings of what is involved in limiting and/or improving their educational achievement. These narratives of experience became the foundation of a research and development project called *Te Kotahitanga: Improving the Educational Achievement of Māori students in Mainstream Schools* (Bishop et al., 2003, 2007, 2011), which has been implemented in 49 secondary schools with some 32,000 students, 14,000 of whom were Māori, and 2,000 teachers.

The process of Collaborative Storying from a range of engaged and non-engaged Māori students (as defined by their schools) in five non-structurally modified mainstream secondary schools was very similar to *testimonio* in that it is the intention of the direct narrator (research participant) to use an interlocutor (the researcher) to bring his, her, or their situation to the attention of an audience "to which he or she would normally not have access because of their very condition of subalternity to which the *testimonio* bears witness" (Beverly, 2000, p. 556). In this research, the students were able to have their narratives about their experiences of schooling shared with teachers who otherwise might not have access to them. These vicarious experiences proved to be a very powerful means of facilitating teachers' critical reflections on the part they themselves might be playing in the low attendance, retention, and achievement of Māori students in their classrooms.

Such an approach is consistent with Ryan (1999), who suggests that a solution to the one-sidedness of representations that are promoted by the dominance of the powerful—in this case, pathologizing discourses—is to portray events as were done in the collaborative stories of the Māori students, in terms of "competing discourses rather than as simply the projection of inappropriate images" (p. 187). He suggests that this approach, rather than seeking the truth, or "real pictures," allows for previously marginalized discourses "to emerge and compete on equal terms with previously dominant discourses" (p. 187).

In these recounts of experience, in contrast to the majority of their teachers who tended to dwell upon the problems of what they saw as the children's deficiencies, Māori students clearly identified that the main influence on their educational achievement was the quality of the in-class relationships and interactions they had with their teachers. Most of their teachers were reproducing society-wide power imbalances by explaining Māori students' learning difficulties in deficit terms, the results being the perpetuation of their use of pathologizing practices, which in turn perpetuated the persistent pattern of educational disparities. Such discursive positioning created contexts for learning that Māori students described as being negative and harmful to their developing positive identities for themselves. In addition, relationships between Māori students and their teachers were characterized by teachers having low expectations of Māori students' ability to learn. As a result, Māori students behaved inappropriately and absented themselves from classroom interactions they found to be unacceptable, resulting in a general breakdown in the classroom being a place of concentrated learning for all. This breakdown in relationships creates a downward spiral of lowering teacher expectations, as seen in low levels of the cognitive challenge in lessons, a concentration on the use of traditional transmission pedagogies, less use of effective discursive interactions in classrooms by the teachers, and a consequent lack of engagement and attendance by Māori students in the lessons and learning.

In contrast, the Māori student interviewees explained how teachers could create an alternative context for learning in which Māori students' educational achievement could improve by teachers changing the ways they related to and interacted with Māori students in their classrooms. It was suggested that if teachers were supported to understand the impact of negative, deficit theorizing and subsequent practice on their relationships with students in their classrooms and learn to (re)theorize their actions in ways that were culturally responsive to their students, they would understand how they could be agentic, which in turn would refocus their attentions on the teaching-learning relationship. As a result, teachers would have higher expectations of their students, which would lead to greater engagement by students with learning. In effect, the context that Māori students saw as being supportive of their learning was one where teachers establish caring and learning classroom relationships that they described in terms of whanau-like relationships, *whanaungatanga*.[2]

Based on these observations, Bishop et al. (2003) developed an Effective Teaching Profile (ETP). Fundamental to the ETP is teachers' understanding of the need to reject deficit theorizing as a means of explaining Māori students' low educational achievement levels, and taking an agentic position in their theorizing about their practice. In order to help teachers change their practice the professional development program was developed. It provides teachers with professional learning opportunities where they can critically evaluate where they discursively position themselves when constructing their own images, principles, and practices in relation to Māori and other minoritized students in their classrooms. Teachers are provided with ongoing opportunities to consider the implications of their discursive positioning on their own agency and for

Māori students' learning. Teachers are then able to express their professional commitment and responsibility for bringing about change in Indigenous and other minoritized students' educational achievement by accepting professional responsibility for the learning of all of their students, not just those whom they can relate to readily.

As Mazarno, Waters, and McNulty (2005) identified, most educational innovations do not address the "existing framework of perceptions and beliefs, or paradigm, as part of the change process—an ontological approach" (p. 162), but rather assume "that innovation is assimilated into existing beliefs and perceptions" (p. 162). They go on to suggest that reforms that are more likely to succeed are those that are fundamentally ontological in nature, providing participants with an "experience of their paradigms as constructed realities, and an experience of consciousness other than the 'I' embedded in their paradigms" (p. 162). In other words, reforms need to provide teachers with experiences of how discourses can determine their subsequent relationships and interactions. This insight is something pointed out by several theories from a range of perspectives as widely divergent as Bruner (1996) and Foucault (1972). Hence the focus in Te Kotahitanga on rejecting deficit theorizing, for as Sleeter (2005) suggests with reference to American schooling:

> It is true that low expectations for students of color and students from poverty communities, buttressed by taken-for-granted acceptance of the deficit ideology, has been a rampant and persistent problem for a long time … therefore, empowering teachers without addressing the deficit ideology may well aggravate the problem. (p. 2)

In effect, if we think that other people have deficiencies, then our actions will tend to follow our thinking and the relationships we develop, and the interactions we have with these people will tend to be negative and unproductive (Valencia, 1997). That is, despite teachers being well-meaning and with the best intentions in the world, if teachers are led to believe that students with whom they are interacting are deficient, they will respond to them negatively. We were told time and again by interview participants in 2001 (Bishop & Berryman, 2006) and again in 2007 (Bishop et al., 2007) that negative, deficit thinking on the part of teachers was fundamental to the development of negative relations and interactions between the students and their teachers, resulting in frustration and anger for all concerned.

Therefore, far from positioning teachers as having deficiencies, or creating a false dichotomy between teachers being agents and teachers working with a model that 'regulates' them, the learning opportunities offered to teachers in the professional development program provides them with ongoing opportunities to undertake what Davies and Harre (1990) called *discursive repositioning*. This means that they are offered opportunities to draw explanations and subsequent practices from alternative discourses that offer them solutions instead of those that reinforce problems and barriers. Evidence of the effectiveness of this approach is to be found in surveys and interviews conducted with teachers in the project (Bishop et al., 2007, 2011; Meyer et al., 2010; Sleeter, 2011) that demonstrate teachers' appreciation of an approach that offers activities that enable them to experience cognitive dissonance of the sort described by Timperley, Wilson, Barrar, and Fung (2007) in that it is undertaken in a respectful manner that supports teachers as learners. In this way, the program draws from Māori epistemologies by using the metaphor of a 'koha' to explain the process of discursive (re)positioning within the project. A koha is literally a gift that is placed on a *marae* (cultural meeting place) by the visitors (in this case the external professional developers) for the hosts (the teachers) to respond as they see fit. It is up to the hosts to determine themselves if they will accept the gift or not. The visitors cannot impose the gift upon the hosts. However, once the gift has been picked up there is an expectation from the visitors that it will be looked after with respect and cared for in a manner that demonstrates reciprocal responsibility, thus emphasizing the connectedness between host and visitors once the ritualized process of gift giving and receiving has been undertaken.

These central understandings are then manifested in these teachers' classrooms when effective teachers demonstrate on a daily basis that: they care for the students as culturally located individuals; they have high expectations for students' learning; they are able to manage their classrooms and curriculum so as to promote learning; they are able to engage in a range of discursive learning interactions with students or facilitate students to engage with others in these ways; they know a range of strategies that can facilitate learning interactions; they collaboratively promote, monitor, and reflect upon students' learning outcomes so as to modify their instructional practices in ways that will lead to improvements in Māori student achievement; and they share this knowledge with the students (Bishop & Berryman, 2006).

The most recent analyses of the effect of the implementation of the ETP through the professional development program show that the schools who are the most effective implementers of the ETP see Māori student schooling experiences improve dramatically. In addition, participation, engagement, retention, and achievement all show positive gains compared to a comparison group of schools (Bishop et al., 2011; Meyer et al., 2010).

Example 3: Freeing Public Schools and the Education System

The third example is about developing a model for freeing public schools and the education system that supports them from neo-colonial dominance by scaling up; that is, by extending and sustaining effective, Indigenous-based education reform as opposed to education reform that is based on dominant group understandings. Scaling up such education reform has the potential to have a major impact on the disparities that exist in society, because deepening and expanding the benefits of effective education reform programs will change the status quo of historical, ongoing, and seemingly immutable disparities. Nevertheless, claiming that educational reform on its own can cure historical disparities is not the purpose of this chapter; rather, it is clear that educational reform can play a major part in a comprehensive approach to addressing social, economic, and political disparities.

Current approaches to scaling up educational reform have not worked for Indigenous and minoritized students. Most attempts are short term, poorly funded at the outset, and often abandoned before any real changes can be seen, soon to be replaced by some "bold new initiative." In contrast, the model identified in this chapter suggests that educational reforms need to have built into them, from the very outset, those dimensions that will see them sustained in the original sites and spread to others. These elements will allow educational reforms to be scaled up with the confidence that the reform will not only be able to be sustained in existing and new sites, but that, above all, will work to reduce disparities and realize the potential of those students currently not well served by education. Put simply, educational reforms that can be sustained and extended can have an impact on educational and social disparities through increasing the educational opportunities for students previously denied these options, on a scale currently not available in most Western countries.

GPILSEO: A Model for Cultural and Structural Reform

The GPILSEO reform model is based on Coburn's (2003) analysis of conditions necessary for taking a project to scale. This analysis was used by Bishop and O'Sullivan (2005) and Bishop, O'Sullivan, and Berryman (2010) as a useful starting heuristic for considering how to successfully implement and take an educational reform project to scale in a large number of classrooms and schools, and to sustain the achievement gains made in these classrooms and schools. The central understanding of this model is that a reform initiative must have a series of dimensions present from the very outset, at a variety of levels—classrooms, schools, and within the wider system—in order that educational reform can be successful.

In order to ensure achievement gains are made by target students and that these gains are sustainable, the following elements should be present in the reform initiative *from the very outset.* These elements need to include: a means of establishing a school-wide GOAL and vision for improving the targeted students' educational achievement; a means of developing a new PEDAGOGY to depth so that it becomes habitual; a means of developing new INSTITUTIONS and structures to support the in-class initiatives; a means of developing LEADERSHIP that is responsive, transformative, pro-active, and distributed; a means of SPREADING the reform to include all teachers, parents, community members, and external agencies; a means of EVALUATING the progress of the reform in the school by developing appropriate tools and measures of progress; and a means of creating opportunities for the school to take OWNERSHIP of the reform in such a way that the original objectives of the reform are protected and sustained.

For example, in classrooms for a reform initiative to bring about sustainable change, there must be, from the very outset: a *goal* on improving targeted students' (in this case, Māori) participation, engagement, and achievement in the classroom; a means of implementing a *relational pedagogy* to depth so that new ways of relating and interacting are organized and instituted; a means of developing new institutions, such as structured collaborative decision making sessions, so that new ways of relating and interacting are organized and instituted; a means of developing distributed leadership within the classroom where students can participate in the co-construction of curriculum content and learning processes; a means whereby the new classroom relationships and interactions are spread in order to include all students; a means of monitoring and evaluating the progress of all students so as to inform practice; and above all, a means whereby the teachers and their students know about and take ownership of the reform, its aims, objectives, and outcomes.

At a school level there needs to be: a focus on improving all targeted students' achievement across the school; a culturally responsive pedagogy of relations developed across all classrooms that informs relations and interactions at all levels in school and community; time and space created for the development of new institutions within the school, such as induction hui, observations and feedback sessions, structured collaborative decision-making meetings about future pedagogic interactions based on evidence of student progress, and shadow-coaching of specific goals in the classroom—and structures such as timetables and personnel organization need to support this reform; leadership that is responsive to the needs of the reform, pro-active in setting targets and goals, and distributed to allow power sharing; a means whereby all staff can join the reform and for parents and community to be included into the reform; a means whereby in-school facilitators, researchers, and teachers are able to use appropriate instruments to gather evidence/data to monitor the implementation of the reform so as to provide data for formative and summative purposes; and a means whereby the whole school, including the board of trustees, can take ownership of the reform. Ownership is seen when there has been a culture shift so that teacher learning is central to the school and systems, and structures and institutions are developed to support teacher learning—in this way, addressing both culturalist and structuralist concerns at the school level.

The need for system-wide reform: a national policy focus and resource allocation sufficient to raise the achievement of the target students and reduce disparities; a means whereby pre-service teacher education is aligned with in-service professional development so that each supports the other in implementing new relational pedagogies; a review of funding so that salaries for in-school professional developers can be built into schools' staffing allocations and schooling organizations to provide ongoing, interactive, and embedded reform; national level support and professional development for leaders to promote distributed leadership models; collaboration between policy funders, researchers, and practitioners; national level support for evaluation and monitoring that is ongoing and interactive, and that informs policy; national level support for integrated research and professional development that provide data for formative and summative purposes; national ownership of the problem; and the provision of sufficient funding and resources to see solutions in a defined period of time and in an ongoing, embedded manner.

This model therefore encompasses the need to address both culturalist and structuralist positions at the three levels of classroom, school, and system by creating a means of changing the classroom, the culture of the school, and the education system. Cultural change concerns are addressed through goal setting, the development of appropriate pedagogies to depth and the support this requires, and the taking of ownership of the whole reform at each level. Structural concerns are addressed by the development of new institutions; responsive and distributed leadership; the spread of the reform to include all involved; the development of data-management systems within the school to support the reform; and the taking of ownership by the teachers, school, and policy makers of both the cultural and structural changes necessary to reform education to address educational disparities. In this way education can play its part in removing the key contributing factors to poverty among Māori and other minoritized peoples in Aotearoa/New Zealand. Structural concerns are also addressed at a system-wide level when schools are supported at a national level to implement these structural changes.

So overall, this chapter records the development of a means where, just as Paolo Freire predicted it should, educational reform has grown out of the power of the oppressed. It commenced by our initially wresting control over what constitutes research into Māori peoples' lives from the dominant groups. It then meant that we could use this control to establish professional development for teachers that makes sense to Māori students and not just to the teachers (although that happens as well) and then design a model to expand this process to a large number of sites in New Zealand.

Notes

1 In comparison to majority culture students (in New Zealand these students are primarily of European descent): the overall academic achievement levels of Māori students is low; their rate of suspension from school is three times higher; they are over-represented in special education programs for behavioral issues; enrollment in pre-school programs is in lower proportions than other groups; they tend to be over-represented in low stream education classes; they are more likely than other students to be found in vocational curriculum streams; they leave school earlier with less formal qualifications and enroll in tertiary education in lower proportions. For example: 23% of Māori boys and 35% of Māori girls achieved university entrance, compared to 47% and 60% for their non-Māori counterparts in 2009; in 2010, Māori students were twice as likely to leave school at the age of 15 than Pakeha students; only 28% of Māori boys and 41% of Māori girls left school in 2009 with a level 3 qualification or above, compared to 49% and 65% of their non-Māori counterparts (Ministry of Education, 2010a); in 2009, the retention rate to age 17 was 45.8% for Māori , compared to 72.2% of non-Māori; Māori suspension rate is 3.6 times higher than that of Pakeha (Ministry of Education, 2009); and while 89.4% of Māori new entrants had attended pre-school programs in 2010, 98.1% of Pakeha/European new entrants had done so (Ministry of Education, 2010b).

2 See Bishop & Berryman (2006) for details of these analyses by Māori students.

References

Beverley, J. (2000). Testimonio, subalternity, and narrative authority. In N. K. Denzin & Y. S. Lincoln (Eds.), *Handbook of qualitative research* (2nd ed., pp. 555–565). Thousand Oaks, CA: Sage.

Bishop, R. (1996). *Collaborative research stories: Whakawhanaungatanga*. Palmerston North, New Zealand: Dunmore Press.

Bishop, R. (2005). Freeing ourselves from neo-colonial domination in research: A kaupapa Māori approach to creating knowledge. In N. K. Denzin & Y. S. Lincoln (Eds.), *The Sage handbook of qualitative research* (3rd ed., pp. 109–138). Thousand Oaks, CA: Sage.

Bishop R. (2008). Te Kotahitanga: Kaupapa Māori in mainstream classrooms. In N. K. Denzin, Y. S. Lincoln, & L. T. Smith (Eds.), *Handbook of critical and Indigenous methodologies* (pp. 439–458). Thousand Oaks, CA: Sage.

Bishop, R., & Glynn, T. (1999). *Culture counts: Changing power relations in education*. Palmerston North, New Zealand: Dunmore Press.

Bishop, R., & O'Sullivan, D. (2005). *Taking a reform project to scale: Considering the conditions that promote sustainability and spread of reform*. A monograph prepared with the support of Nga Pae o te Maramatanga, The National Institute for Research Excellence in Māori Development and Advancement. Unpublished manuscript.

Bishop, R., & Berryman, M. (2006). *Culture speaks: Cultural relationships and classroom learning*. Wellington, New Zealand: Huia.

Bishop, R., O'Sullivan, D., & Berryman, M. (2010). *Scaling up education reform: Addressing the politics of disparity*. Wellington, New Zealand: NZCER Press.

Bishop, R., Berryman, M., Tiakiwai, S., & Richardson, C. (2003). *Te Kotahitanga: The experiences of year 9 and 10 Māori students in mainstream classrooms*. Wellington, New Zealand: Ministry of Education.

Bishop, R., Berryman, M., Cavanagh, T., & Teddy, L. (2007). *Te Kotahitanga Phase 3 whanaungatanga: Establishing a culturally responsive pedagogy of relations in mainstream secondary school classrooms*. Wellington, New Zealand: Ministry of Education.

Bishop, R., Berryman, M., Wearmouth, J., Peter, M., & Clapham, S. (2011). *Te Kotahitanga: Maintaining, replicating and sustaining change*. Wellington, New Zealand: Ministry of Education.

Bruner, J. (1996). *The culture of education*. Cambridge, MA: Harvard University Press.

Coburn, C. (2003). Rethinking scale: Moving beyond numbers to deep and lasting change. *Educational Researcher, 32*(6), 3–12.

Connelly, F. M., & Clandinin, D. J. (1990). Stories of experience and narrative inquiry. *Educational Researcher, 19*(5), 2–14

Cummins, J. (1996). *Negotiating identities: Education for empowerment in a diverse society.* Los Angeles: California Association for Bilingual Education.

Davies, B., & Harre, R. (1990). Positioning: The discursive production of selves. *Journal of the Theory of Social Behaviour, 20*, 43–65.

Durie, M. (1995). *Principles for the development of Māori policy.* Paper presented at the Māori Policy Development Conference, Wellington, New Zealand.

Durie, M. (1998). *Te mana, te kawanatanga: The politics of Māori self-determination.* Auckland, New Zealand: Oxford University Press.

Foucault, M. (1972). *The archaeology of knowledge.* New York: Pantheon.

Freire, P. (1972). *Pedagogy of the oppressed.* New York: Continuum.

Gay, G. (2010). *Culturally responsive teaching: Theory, research and practice* (2nd ed.). New York: Teachers College Press.

Marzano, R. J., Waters, T., & McNulty, B. A. (2005). *School leadership that works: From research to results.* Alexandria, VA: Association for Supervision and Curriculum Development.

Metge, J. (1990). Te rito o te harakeke: Conceptions of the Whanaau. *Journal of the Polynesian Society, 99*(1), 55–91.

Meyer, L. H., Penetito, W., Hynds, A., Savage, C., Hindle, R., & Sleeter, C. (2010). *Evaluation of Te Kotahitanga: 2004–2008.* Wellington, New Zealand: Ministry of Education.

Ministry of Education. (2009). Statement of intent: 2009–2014. Retrieved from www.minedu.govt.nz/theministry/publicationsandresources/statementofintent/soi2009.aspx

Ministry of Education. (2010a). *Participation and attainment of Māori students in National Certification of Educational Achievement.* Wellington, New Zealand: Education Counts, Ministry of Education. Retrieved from www.educationcounts.govt.nz/statistics/schooling/ncea-attainment/ncea-achievement-data-roll-based/participation-and-attainment-of-Māori -students-in-national-certificate-of-educational-achievement

Ministry of Education. (2010b). *Education counts: Teaching staff.* Retrieved from www.educationcounts.govt.nz/statistics/schooling/teaching_staff

Organisation for Economic Co-operation and Development. (2007). *Education at a glance 2007: OECD indicators.* Paris: OECD.

Paris, D., (2012), Culturally sustaining pedagogy: A needed change in stance, terminology, and practice. *Educational Researcher, 41*(3), 93–97.

Ryan, J. (1999). *Race and ethnicity in multi-ethnic schools: A critical case study.* Clevedon, UK: Multilingual Matters.

Salmond, A. (1975). *Hui: A study of Māori ceremonial greetings.* Auckland, New Zealand: Reed & Methuen.

Sidorkin, A. M. (2002). *Learning relations: Impure education, deschooled schools, and dialogue with evil.* New York: Peter Lang.

Sleeter, C. (2005). *Un-standardizing curriculum: Multicultural teaching in the standards-based classroom.* New York: Teachers College Press.

Sleeter, C., (Ed.). (2011). *Professional development for culturally responsive and relationship-based pedagogy* (1st ed.). New York: Peter Lang.

Smith, G. H. (1997). *Kaupapa Māori as transformative praxis.* Unpublished doctoral dissertation, University of Auckland, Auckland, New Zealand.

Smith, G. H. (2003). *Indigenous struggle for the transformation of education and schooling.* Keynote address to the Alaskan Federation of Natives (AFN) Convention. Anchorage, Alaska.

Smith, L. T. (1999). *Decolonizing methodologies: Research and indigenous peoples.* London: Zed Books.

Timperley, H., Wilson, A., Barrar, H., & Fung, I. (2007). *Teacher professional learning and development: Best evidence synthesis iteration (BES).* Wellington, New Zealand: Ministry of Education.

Valencia, R. R. (1997). *The evolution of deficit thinking: Educational thought and practice.* London: Falmer Press.

Villegas, A. M., & Lucas, T. (2002). *Educating culturally responsive teachers: A coherent approach.* New York: State University of New York Press.

Young, I. M. (2004). Two concepts of self determination. In S. May, T. Mahood, & J, Squires (Eds.), *Ethnicity, nationalism and minority rights* (pp. 176–198). Cambridge, UK: Cambridge University Press.

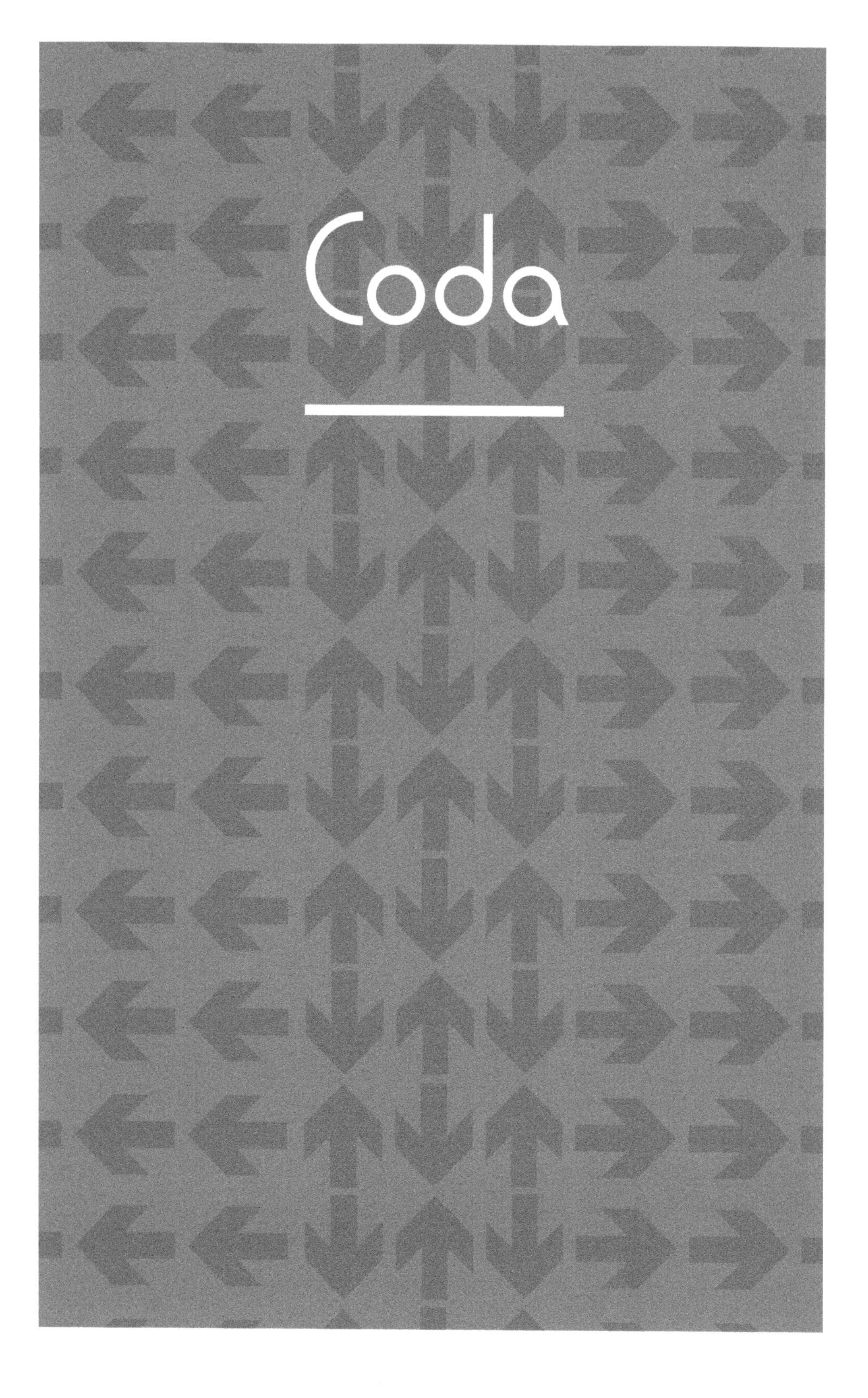
Coda

Chapter 23

Are You Serious?

Playing, Performing, and Producing an Academic Self

Laura L. Ellingson

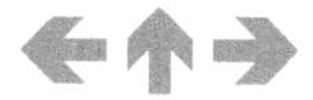

The world of play favors exuberance, license, abandon. Shenanigans are allowed, strategies can be tried, selves can be revised.

—Ackerman (1999, p. 6)

Ackerman's description of play bears little resemblance to any description of academic life that I have ever encountered; indeed, it is nearly antithetical to the staid and serious, antique patina of the ivory tower. Even gentler, more contemporary notions of universities as collaborative spaces for teaching scholars and engaged learners seldom go so far as to incorporate exuberance and license.

I don't know about you, but I can't remember the last shenanigan I participated in, and I seldom act with abandon as a professor, researcher, and knowledge constructor.

What a shame.

I propose that the dominant metaphor of qualitative research as work—fieldwork, working with data, producing a body of

Originally published in *Global Dimensions of Qualitative Inquiry*, edited by Norman K. Denzin and Michael D. Giardina, pp. 195–209. Laura L. Ellingson. © 2013 Left Coast Press, Inc., Walnut Creek, CA. Republished in *Qualitative Inquiry—Past, Present, and Future: A Critical Reader*, edited by Norman K. Denzin and Michael D. Giardina, pp. 423–437. Left Coast Press, Inc.

work, working toward a conclusion, "I put a lot of work into developing that typology," her work uses critical theory—may be productively reframed through conscious efforts to incorporate playful attitudes and playful techniques into qualitative research. The metaphor of work is limited by its connotations of capitalism, status, stress, and fatigue, all of which are deemphasized by the notion of play. In this chapter, I demonstrate how playing with participants, data, and representation creates opportunities for humane, profound, and pragmatic research processes.

A few caveats.

I am not arguing here that faculty need time off from work in the face of ever-growing demands at institutions decimated by draconian budget cuts and pressured to produce students/customers with specific job skills—although that case needs to be made. Nor am I suggesting play as an important pedagogy for teaching, although others have written about that topic and more remains to be said (Farné, 2005). Finally, I do not mean to imply that qualitative researchers or our products are monolithic; rich variations in our use of theory, epistemology, ontology, and methods constitute a distinct strength of our field. Instead, I suggest that our reasonable desire for academic legitimacy has led our community to deemphasize a crucial sense of playfulness within—rather than as a break from—our research processes.

Taking Work Seriously

How did researchers become so serious? It is due at least in part to self-selection bias. Adherence to rules and hard work overcame the lure of play a long time ago for those of us who were attracted to the idea of graduate school in the social sciences, education, or allied health fields. We fulfilled requirements, filled out forms, followed procedures, jumped through hoops. We worked hard to earn the right to call ourselves researchers, and among the hard workers who strive to justify daily their place in the academy are feminists who want to be taken seriously as both cultural critics and knowledge producers. Explained one feminist scholar:

> Feminisms work. And then work more. Feminist work is occupied with women's rights: in homes and in offices, with bodies, with technology, with health, and with politics. The feminisms

> of the past three hundred years have all been inextricably entangled with these matters of gravity and importance. As such, there has been no playtime in feminism. (Chess, 2009, para. 3)

The lack of playtime has become largely taken for granted as normal in academia. Even those who embrace artistic, narrative, performative, and autoethnographic forms of representation regularly speak of work, struggle, trauma, loss, and frustration in carving out spaces for alternative logics (e.g., Denzin & Lincoln, 2011; Gergen & Gergen, 2012). Qualitative and interpretive researchers want the same thing other researchers want—jobs, tenure, and the space to pursue our passions in teaching and research. To gain access to the academy, we have framed qualitative research—including and especially what Richardson (2000) called "creative analytic practices" that embrace aesthetic and evocative ways of knowing—and ourselves as qualitative researchers as *serious*, that is, as worthy of inclusion in the academy. Because academic training still teaches us to think in terms of dichotomies—right/wrong, good/bad, mind/body, science/art, work/play—we turned away from the devalued side of the serious/frivolous dualism and celebrated our seriousness. But our over-emphasis on seriousness comes at a cost, one that many scholars recognize intuitively. I suspect that Lugones's longing for a playful self as a feminist researcher is easily recognizable to readers, feminist or not:

> I am also scared of ending up a *serious* human being, someone with no multi-dimensionality, with no fun in life, someone who is just someone who has had the fun constructed out of her. I am seriously scared of getting stuck in a "world" that constructs me that way. A world that I have no escape from and in which I cannot be playful. (Lugones, 1987, p. 15; emphasis added)

Seriousness may be important, but when taken to extremes that exclude playfulness, it becomes a barrier to constructing and sustaining productive and meaningful academic careers.

As with all dichotomies, the play/work boundary ultimately proves elusive: "As a binary, [work/play] often breaks down, blurring and marking a continually shifting set of distinctions" (Brooks & Bowker, 2002, p. 114). These blurred boundaries are apparent in qualitative research in which creative sparks and sudden critical insights form as much of our processes as rule-bound actions. Brooks and Bowker (2002) advise instead that we recognize "elements of play at work." paying attention to both opportunities and constraints imposed within work environments.

Thus far, I have asserted that qualitative researchers should be playful in our work, without posing work and play as mutually exclusive opposites. But I have not answered the question: What is play? Simply, "play is free movement within a more rigid structure" (Salen & Zimmerman, 2004, p. 304). Play is voluntary, not coerced, and is consciously engaged; that is, we know we are playing, and we choose to do it (Hinthorne & Schneider, 2012). Yet play also can incorporate a serious element. I have urged qualitative researchers to think of our forays into new methods of analysis and alternative forms of representation as more an adventure than a hassle and to engage in learning and experimentation as a form of serious play rather than as a series of trials and errors (Ellingson, 2009, p. 81). We can construct our methodological work as play(ful) and our play as (somewhat) serious. Serious play includes free movement plus the element of critical reflection. "Rather than simply engaging in an enjoyable, intrinsically motivated activity, serious play invokes conscious reflection on the activity itself in a way that directly connects the play space to real-life issues and concerns" (Hinthorne & Schneider, 2012, p. 2808). We can play seriously with our participants, data, and representations. As we move freely in creative spaces, we pause for reflection, particularly on the ways in which not only our minds and words but also our embodied selves enter into our play (Ellingson, 2012).

Playing at Work, Working at Play

In the remainder of this chapter, I discuss several ways in which qualitative researchers may embrace consciously a variety of playful elements in research processes, including passion and pleasure, deep attention, creativity, performance, and multiplicity.

Passion and Pleasure

Somewhere along the line, many of us forgot that we get to choose (some of) the games we play as scholars. We are a passionate lot: Ask most researchers a question about their current projects, and they will eagerly spout a wealth of facts, ideas, and possibilities embedded in their ongoing research. Passion guides our choices and drives us to continue with the often-frustrating processes of research (Reinharz, 1992). I have argued elsewhere that a sense of playfulness can turn study design into an experience of *wondering*, an enjoyable process of considering not only what would be expedient, theoretically sound, and methodologically rigorous, but also what would be satisfying, rewarding, and fun (Ellingson, 2009). I am not promoting mere self-indulgence; rather, I argue that making choices that satisfy the researcher's mind/body/soul self will yield more insightful findings. We are more motivated to continue the drudgery of typing field notes and transcriptions, asking yet another question, staring off into space for hours as our brains wrestle with thousands of details, building coherent themes, writing evocative narratives, and constructing compelling performances instead of settling for the simplest answers to our research questions. Lofland (1970, p. 35) called the premature stopping at surface answers "analytic interruptus," a failure to continue until we have delved below the surface to access the deeper meanings in our findings. We continue to play with pleasure long after we lack the energy to work.

I describe wondering as a playful process of asking questions about researchers' project goals, intended audiences, abilities and interests, data collection and ongoing analyses, topics of investigation, and choice of genres for representation. In this context, I also urge paying attention to one's own preferences and desires (Ellingson, 2009, pp. 75–77). Our passions—what we care about, what excites us—are important to pay attention to when harnessing the power of play. The following questions are meant to inspire a playful approach to the choices we make at the beginning stages and throughout the lengthy course of a qualitative research project:

- What is my favorite thing about my data? What makes me smile when I think of it? What makes me cry? What makes me angry?
- What would be fun to write?
- What process issues or ideas come up in my journaling that intrigue me?

- What strong emotions do I have about my participants, their stories, and our relationships?
- Whose research do I admire? Why?
- What about my study embarrasses me or makes me feel self-conscious? Why?
- What am I most proud of in my data?
- If one of my mentors asked me about my project, what would I want to tell her/him? (Ellingson, 2009, p. 76)

Wondering, that is, conscious consideration of ideas and free writing on possibilities, can be a playful approach to design and ongoing choices in the iterative processes of qualitative research. By consciously acknowledging our passions and preferences, we can harness the energies that come with affirming our passions as researchers. What we did naturally as children and perhaps do now in other contexts of our lives—as fans of musicians, theater, or sports; as family photographers, creative cooks, or involved parents (and aunts, uncles, grandparents, and chosen family); as engaged citizens at the local, national, and global levels—is to tie our passions to that in which we invest our time and energy. Passion and pleasure go hand in hand with play.

P(l)aying Attention

Ackerman (1999) defines deep play as the experience of a full immersion in which one becomes lost within the playful world created in the moment and, for a time, escapes the boundaries of the outside world. *All aspects of qualitative research benefit from such periods of playful immersion.* Being in the ethnographic field, keenly attentive to the grand narratives of culture, the norms of language, etiquette, and social roles, while simultaneously noting the minutest details of eye contact and gestures, can constitute a form of deeply meaningful play. As I observe and participate, I continually try to exceed my normal capacity for attention, to take note—literally with a pen and figuratively with my eyes, ears, mind, and gut—of the mundane details that swirl around me. Going for a personal best, I try to etch the phrases and inflections of a particular conversation into my brain for later recall. This form of play can become a test of my skills against the limits of perception and attention. Such moments stand out against the backdrop of average days of fieldwork (long after the rapt discovery of the honeymoon phase is over), during which, if I am honest, I often feel so bored that tears threaten and elaborate excuses about why I must leave the setting immediately take root in my mind, making attention to my participants a painful struggle. Turning observation and note-taking into play makes the experience not only more enjoyable but also far more productive than framing the process as work.

Deep play also enhances data analysis. Analyzing field notes, interview transcripts, and other qualitative materials can be tedious. But it also occasionally achieves a sense of such effortless flow that I am at play with my findings, happily stacking bits of language and description into this pile and that one, reconfiguring them to see how they best fit, like brightly colored building blocks arranged into a fresh architecture of patterns that illuminates complex phenomena. Deep play in data analysis is akin to what Eisenberg (1990) called jamming, a type of flow or transcendence, wherein the individual is joyfully subsumed into a group experience. For Eisenberg, jamming involves highly coordinated action with others, absent the normally expected shared interpersonal and organizational history and infrastructure. In data analysis, jamming can be thought of a surrender of the researcher-self to the process of organizing huge amounts of material into meaningful patterns or coherent narratives. In seeking order from chaos, I can at times be so fully immersed in playing with the data or materials that I attain a sense not of mastery over the materials but of the materials mastering me, making me part of the order that is being constructed. As with fieldwork, extensive periods of drudgery and boredom are necessary groundwork for these rare periods of playful sense-making, but these joyful interludes are what inspire me to continue my research.

Reflexivity benefits from playfulness as well. What is reflexivity but a continual playing with one's own sense of self in relation to one's participants and their space(s)? We are taught in methods courses to reflect on how our gender, race, religion, education, class, sexuality, and abilities contrast with and overlap with participants' social categories. Such reflections can become rote after a while if we are not attentive, yielding little but obligatory statements about researchers' standpoints. Yet deep play with categories—and with the very notion of dividing people based on certain characteristics and not others (see Bowker & Star, 2000)—tosses those categories, personalities, and spaces up into the mental air and down onto the page, over and over again, playing with possibilities. Such deep consideration is facilitated by embracing the patience of play, the willingness to try over and over again until the sculpture of blocks resembles the ethereal form just beyond your mind's grasp. When you come upon the insight, you recognize it as the one, the answer you have been waiting for, the final piece of the puzzle.

Playing Outside the Box

Along with passion and deep attention, research play sparks creativity and innovation. Play involves risk, a willingness to proceed into the unknown. When we try something different, we improvise. Improvising is critical to play, and this leads us to ask new questions, make connections among disparate topics of study, apply theories to new areas, and bridge interdisciplinary boundaries. I urge qualitative researchers to think of the theories, topics, and methods that they learned in graduate school as starting points, rather than career constraints. Tremendous creative energies emerge when we embrace learning new methodological skills not for the sake of mere novelty but as an opening to possibilities, an openness that we cannot sustain if we are too serious and not interested in play and adventure.

Ackerman (1999, p. 7) says: "Make-believe is at the heart of play, and also at the heart of much of what passes as work." If we take the term "make-believe" literally, we may make or construct a belief or a set of rules or a whole other world, and then we act as if we believe it/them to be true. As children, most of us played make-believe and constructed fantasy worlds of knights and dragons or cops and robbers. I remember play inspired by the *Little House on the Prairie* books in my friends' backyard (I had dibs on being the young Laura Ingalls Wilder, due to my name), being a family of birds in a nest my brothers and I made out of blankets and couch pillows in our living room, and recreating the worlds of our favorite TV shows with neighborhood kids (such as *CHiPs*, which featured handsome California Highway Patrol officers, and the campy 1970s version of *Battlestar Galactica*, where brave women and men named for Greek mythological characters charged about outer space blowing up anyone who threatened their community of intergalactic refugees).

Thinking back on the ways in which we seized on an idea, proposed basic rules of behavior, and then improvised an enjoyable coordinated performance of another world with friends, I draw inspiration for research. Our "make-believe" muscles may need to be toned after years of little use, but with practice, we can harness our ability to imagine other ways of being and doing. Such skills can aid our research in many ways. Imagination is necessary when constructing a performance or creative presentation of findings that is designed to educate, persuade, and support community groups, children, or other audiences. Imagination also comes into play when we contemplate our findings and generate novel solutions to ongoing problems or design culturally appropriate campaign messages for reaching underserved communities, or develop new models and extend theories. We have to ask ourselves and our collaborators, "What if we tried it this way?" and then be willing to make-believe our way through many ideas until we find one that best serves the goals of our research.

Playing the Fool

The trickster is a playful character who reveals us to ourselves by showing social norms in exaggerated, multiple, dichotomy-resistant ways: "Trickster is the mythic embodiment of ambiguity and ambivalence, doubleness and duplicity, contradiction and paradox" (Hyde, 1998, p. 7). The trickster offers double-vision:

> When I travel from one "world" to another, I have this image, this memory of myself as playful in this other "world." I can then be in a particular "world" and have a double image of myself as, for example, playful and as not playful. … I can have both images of myself and to the extent that I can materialize or animate both images at the same time I become an ambiguous being. This is very much a part of trickery and foolery. It is worth remembering that the trickster and the fool are significant characters

> in many non-dominant or outsider cultures. One then sees any particular "world" with these double edges and sees absurdity in them and so inhabits oneself differently. (Lugones, 1987, p. 13)

Frentz (2009) draws on Haraway's (1991) extension of the trickster as a "split self" or shape shifting character who generates embodied and located knowledge that decries detached objectivity and embraces specificity. Such "situated knowledges" may embrace a way of knowing and of communicating that knowledge to others within a third space of play. Here, the trickster character reveals the taken-for-granted constraints of the institutional context (e.g., health care, education) by playfully violating accepted rules of interaction, giving us the opportunity to see beyond the rigid either/or of the system (e.g., either physician or patient, teacher or student) to both/and, a doubling of vision that reveals what is usually hidden (e.g., physicians also have vulnerable bodies and patients may recognize significant symptoms in their bodies; teachers also are learners and students have knowledge to offer others).

My way of playing the fool—academically speaking—has been to participate in performances of The Ethnogs, FemNogs, Rip Tupp, and assorted others who have joined in a performance (e.g., a fan who gets rousted by security, curtain girl) (Ethnogs et al., 2011). Our performance of aging rock stars, women's liberationists/groupies, and band security detail illustrates what we call *automythography*:

> Automythography is the excavation of cultural myths (including beliefs, practices, and stereotypes) through the critical reading of narrative accounts, invented or experienced, of a particular period or about a set of events. We believe that scholars can learn about the myths that drive a certain group or era by creating and telling stories about that group or era. (Ethnogs et al., 2011, p. 673)

Our collaborative invention of a shared past casts a critical eye on rock music culture by ironically embodying exaggerated stereotypes of rock stars, groupies, and roadie/security guy.

While the knowledge generated by our performances is noteworthy, the sheer joy of performing our theme song,

"Ethnography Is a Way of Life"—complete with dancing, screaming fans—is the most meaningful aspect of our work for me. The joy I experienced was not only pleasurable but also instructive; my memories of the performances help me reflect on how I conduct ethnography. In particular, I question the quality of attention that I am able to give my participants and my ability to remain mindful and present with them while my busy mind whirls with theories, insights, and to-do lists. My ironic embodiment of the feminized role of a groupie—even with our backstory as radical women's liberationists—engenders a critique of my feminist standpoint and calls attention to my embodied presence as a woman whose White privilege intersects with her status as an above-the-knee amputee.

As we play the fool in academia, taken-for-granted aspects of academic culture, collegial friendships, rock music fandom, and ethnographic methods are revealed and opened up for questioning. Memories of our tremendous fun repeatedly enacting this performance within academic conference spaces (National Communication Association and International Congress of Qualitative Inquiry) are now made poignant by the sudden loss of our bandleader, Nick Trujillo, who passed away in October 2012. The loss of our friend remains too fresh, but I imagine that in time I will reflect and recognize more lessons on life, relationships, academia, and myself that Nick gifted me through his presence in my life.

What Do You Know? Epistemic Play

As a confirmed methodology geek, perhaps my favorite form of play involves moving fluidly along the methodological continuum, refusing a fixed state as an interpretive social scientist, feminist researcher, narrative ethnographer, grounded theory practitioner, or health care reform pragmatist. I openly embrace a multiplicity of paradigms, refusing to frame art and science as mutually exclusive or as at odds. Instead, I embrace a range of complementary methodologies, each of which is more suitable for some goals and questions than for others. We usually base our defense and promotion of a particular methodology by critiquing its perceived opposite, but we can instead embrace multiplicity without attacking other ways of knowing. Recalling the definition of play offered earlier, it focused on (relatively) free movement as critical to the experience of play. To move with significant freedom among methodological and epistemological possibilities, one must move beyond the art/science dichotomy.

Elsewhere, I have written at length about a continuum approach to mapping the field of qualitative methodology that constructs a nuanced range of possibilities in place of what traditionally have been constructed as the art/science dichotomy, linguistically reified by further oppositions such as hard/soft, quantitative/qualitative, positivist/interpretive, and statistics/stories (Ellingson, 2009). I proposed a qualitative continuum comprised of a vast and varied middle ground, with art and science representing only the extreme ends of the methodological and representational options.

Building on Ellis's (2004) representation of the two ends of the qualitative continuum (i.e., art and science) and the analytic mapping of the continuum developed in Ellis and Ellingson (2000), I envisioned the continuum as having three main areas, with infinite possibilities for blending and moving among them. The goals, questions, methods, writing styles, vocabularies, role(s) of researchers, and criteria for evaluation vary across the continuum as one moves from a realist/positivist social science stance on the far right, through a social constructionist middle ground, to an artistic/interpretive paradigm toward the left (Ellingson, 2009, 2011).

Each of these general approaches offers opportunities and constraints, and none are mutually exclusive. No firm boundaries delineate any regions of the continuum. Furthermore, terms of demarcation and description used throughout the continuum (e.g., interpretive, postpositivist) have proven inconsistent, suspect, and contestable; terminology in qualitative methods remains dramatically variable across disciplines, paradigms, and methodological communities, with new terms arising continually (Gubrium & Holstein, 1997; Lindlof & Taylor, 2010). At any point on the qualitative continuum, a set of assumptions about epistemology (i.e., about what knowledge is and what it means to create it) influences choices surrounding the collection of empirical materials and analysis methods, which, in turn, tend to foster (but do not require) particular forms of representation.

Engaging multigenre and multimedia analyses and representations within a qualitative research project is playful because no one standard of truth is enabled to emerge; the multiplicity of beauty, rigor, pragmatics, and theoretical insights offers up a range of truths (Denzin & Lincoln, 2011). Skipping along and across methodological and paradigmatic boundaries and threading among the many standards of truths may foster transformation of the very methodological rules by which we play. "Transformative play … occurs when the free movement of play alters the rigid structure in which it takes shape. The play doesn't just occupy and oppose the interstices of the system but actually transforms the space as a whole" (Salen & Zimmerman, 2004, p. 305).

Seemingly chaotic or contradictory maneuvers may thus generate insights into the limitations of the structures and enable us to break them down and re-create them to be better, more flexible, more spacious options, or simply further alternatives for qualitative researchers to play. Crystallization, a postmodern form of methodological triangulation, explicitly requires one or more forms of art and of science in order to multiply a research project's possible truths while denying the possibility of a single, conclusive truth (Ellingson, 2009). The transformative possibilities of serious play through crystallization and other multimethod, multigenre, multimedia, and multiparadigmatic frameworks give me hope for a qualitative community that comes together across software and stories, $p<.05$ and poetry, performance and pragmatics.

Conclusion

"Whoever wants to understand much must play much," claimed Gottfried Benn, an early 20th-century German physician (www.searchquotes.com), whose insightful statement on the linkages between play and understanding also aptly describes playful approaches to qualitative research and knowledge construction. The aspects of play described here—passion and pleasure, deep attention, creativity, performance, and multiplicity—offer hopeful possibilities for qualitative research processes that harness the power of exuberance and promote greater freedom of movement within existing and future structures.

References

Ackerman, D. (2000). *Deep play.* New York: Vintage.

Bowker, G. C. & Star, S. L. (2000). *Sorting things out: Classification and its consequences.* Cambridge, MA: MIT Press.

Brooks, L. J. & Bowker, G. (2002). Playing at work: Understanding the future of work practices at the institute for the future. *Information, Communication, and Society, 5*, 109–136.

Chess, S. (2009). How to play a feminist. *Thirdspace: A Journal of Feminist Theory and Culture, 9.* http://www.thirdspace.ca/journal/article/view/273/315 (accessed December 12, 2012).

Denzin, N. K. & Lincoln, Y. S. (2011). Introduction: The discipline and practice of qualitative research. In N. K. Denzin & Y. S. Lincoln (Eds.), *Handbook of qualitative research* (4th ed., pp. 1–19). Thousand Oaks, CA: Sage.

Eisenberg, E. M. (1990). Jamming: Transcendence through organizing. *Communication Research, 17*, 139–164.

Ellingson, L. L. (2009). *Engaging crystallization in qualitative research: An introduction.* Thousand Oaks, CA: Sage.

Ellingson, L. L. (2011). Analysis and representation across the continuum. In N. K. Denzin & Y. S. Lincoln (Eds.), *The SAGE handbook of qualitative research* (4th ed., pp. 595–610). Thousand Oaks, CA: Sage.

Ellingson, L. L. (2012). Interviewing as embodied communication. In J. Gubrium, J. Holstein, A. Marvasti, & K. M. Marvasti (Eds.), *Handbook of interview research* (2nd ed., pp. 525–539). Thousand Oaks, CA: Sage.

Ellis, C. (2004). *The ethnographic I: A methodological novel about autoethnography.* Walnut Creek, CA: AltaMira.

Ellis, C. & Ellingson, L. L. (2000). Qualitative methods. In E. F. Borgatta & R. J. V. Montgomery (Eds.), *Encyclopedia of sociology* (2nd ed., Vol. 4, pp. 2287–2296). New York: Macmillan Library Reference.

Ethnogs, The, The FemNogs, and Rip Tupp [Trujillo, N., Krizek, R., Sotirin, P., Ellingson, L. L., Mills, M., Drew, S., & Poulos, C.]. (2011). Constructing mythic identity and culture: A performance and critique of The Ethnogs. *Qualitative Inquiry, 17*, 664–674.

Farné, R. (2005). Pedagogy of play. *Topoi, 24*, 169–181.

Frentz, T. S. (2009). Split selves and situated knowledge: The trickster goes titanium. *Qualitative Inquiry, 15*, 820–842.

Gergen, M. M. & Gergen, K. (2012). *Playing with purpose: Adventures in performative social science.* Walnut Creek, CA: Left Coast Press, Inc.

Gubrium, J. & Holstein, J. (1997). *The new language of qualitative method.* New York: Oxford University Press.

Haraway, D. (1991). Situated knowledges: The science question in feminism and the privilege of partial perspective. In D. Haraway (Ed.), *Simians, cyborgs, and women: The reinvention of nature* (pp. 183–201). London: Routledge, Chapman and Hall.

Hinthorne, L. L. & Schneider, K. (2012). Playing with purpose: Using serious play to enhance participatory development communication in research. *International Journal of Communication, 6*, 2801–2824.

Hyde, L. (1998). *Trickster makes this world: Mischief, myth, and art.* New York: Farrar, Straus and Giroux.

Lindlof, T. R. & Taylor, B.C. (2010). *Qualitative communication research methods* (3rd ed.). Thousand Oaks, CA: Sage.

Lofland, J. (1970). Interactionist imagery and analytic interruptus. In T. Shibutani (Ed.), *Human nature and collective behavior: Papers in honor of Herbert Blumer* (pp. 35–45). New Brunswick, NJ: Transaction Books.

Lugones, M. (1987). Playfulness, world-traveling, and loving perception. *Hypatia, 2*, 3–19.

Richardson, L. (2000). Writing: A method of inquiry. In N. K. Denzin & Y. S. Lincoln (Eds.), *Handbook of qualitative research* (2nd ed., pp. 923–943). Thousand Oaks, CA: Sage.

Reinharz, S. (1992). *Feminist methods in social research.* New York: Oxford University Press.

Salen, K. & Zimmerman, E. (2004). *Rules of play.* Cambridge, MA: MIT Press.

Epilogue

Chapter 24

A Conversation about the Past, Present, and Future of Qualitative Inquiry

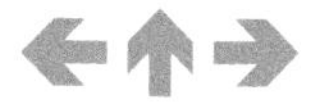

Michael D. Giardina
Norman K. Denzin
Svend Brinkmann
Marcelo Diversi
Maria del Consuelo Chapela Mendoza
Christopher Poulos
Elizabeth Adams St. Pierre

Proem

The qualitative inquiry community is vast and diverse, a collection of viewpoints that complicate and contest, provoke, and push the boundaries of the field. To close this volume, we have brought together scholars who have been at the forefront of their (inter)disciplines to engage in a critical discussion over the past, present, and future of qualitative inquiry. Their responses speak, whether directly or indirectly, to the four thematic sections organizing this volume, and suggest various points of agreement and

Qualitative Inquiry—Past, Present, and Future: A Critical Reader, edited by Norman K. Denzin and Michael D. Giardina, pp. 441–464.

disagreement about where we as a loosely connected global community might move in the future.

Each contributor was given a list of four questions via email and asked to offer brief responses based on his or her unique position to qualitative inquiry. The editors of the volume then created the narrative that follows based on these responses.

Past-Present-Future

Sifting through all of the responses, the thing that strikes us first is the diversity of responses, the disagreement—or, rather, the vastly different perspectives taken on this 'thing' we call qualitative inquiry.

MICHAEL: Let's start by looking back from where we've come. Generally speaking, what do you think are the most important developments in qualitative inquiry in the last ten years?

This may seem like a simple question, but given the broad spectrum of fields within which the invited contributors work, it is anything but.

MARCELO: At the macro-level, I think the International Congress of Qualitative Inquiry (ICQI) has been one of the most important developments of the last decade. From the very first gathering, it has become a community where qualitative inquiry moves from the margins to the center of ways of knowing. Most folks from humanities, social sciences, education, arts, and health fields finally had a gathering place where the pursuit of qualitative inquiry does not need to be explained, justified, defended, or validated in order to exist and thrive. I am well aware of gathering places for qualitative researchers that came before ICQI, and I was grateful for those spaces as a graduate student and junior faculty in the 1990s. But such places were largely discipline-bound and significantly smaller in number, scope, and reach. The ICQI has grown into a community, much larger than disciplinary and national boundaries, that sees qualitative inquiry as a way of being engaged in ideals of inclusiveness, equality, justice, human rights, and scholarship of liberation.

Just as importantly, in my view, is that critical and interpretive paradigms could finally challenge and coexist with the logical-positivist paradigm dominating qualitative inquiry since its formal beginnings in anthropology, ethnology, sociology, and other "human studies" (Dilthey, 1883/1989). Critical and interpretive paradigms continue to be pushed to the margins, perhaps even more so since the 9/11 attacks and the nefarious suspension of human and civil rights, in the guise of patriotism and security, that followed. Critique of American society, power, inequalities, and domestic and international policies tends to come from critical and interpretive paradigms in qualitative inquiry. We all know that power doesn't like resistance, so critical and interpretive paradigms in qualitative inquiry have increasingly become a target of retaliation and persecution. Voices of dissention are defamed, slandered, fired, un-hired, vilified, smeared. The bodies pile up: University of Colorado Boulder's Ward Churchill, DePaul University Chicago's Norman Finkelstein, and now Steven Salaita and his case against the University of Illinois, to mention some of the targets of the most egregious persecution against critical scholarship of the last decade. To be sure, ICQI is but one site of communion and resistance against the contemporary face of colonization. But it is a central one for those engaged in critical and interpretive qualitative inquiry. It has become a site for solidarity and hope that qualitative inquiry can help us imagine and co-construct a world with more justice and dignity for more people, even as neoliberal forces continue to erode academic freedom and critical inquiry. At a practical level, ICQI has also served to keep geographically and disciplinarily isolated qualitative researchers connected through the year-round work of Special Interest Groups (SIGs), guest-edited special issues in the congress journal, and the collaborations that get re-made and renewed at every gathering. Directly and indirectly, qualitative inquiry publications, workshops, and classes all over the world have benefited from ten years of ICQI. Even though contested in many cases, tenure and promotion to gate-keeping institutional positions have been granted in large part because of the bridges, connections, and legitimation ten years of ICQI have brought about.

I think this connection across disciplines and geopolitical boundaries is an essential development in the last ten years. This connection is essential in order to continue advancing qualitative inquiry as a way of being and knowing. And this connection is essential in order to resist, challenge, and provide alternatives to the new forms of narrative and thought control by the establishment—namely, the systemic and coordinated defunding of public higher education, the greater dependence on wealthy donors and corporatization this defunding has created, the financial burden on the current generation of college students for the profit of banks, the dismantling of humanities and arts, the subjugation of social sciences not singly focused on evidence-according-to-positivism, the perverse smear campaigns against intellectuals who speak truth to power, and the push toward a White-washed education that attempts to turn students into power-blind consumers instead of enlightened life-long learners and citizens. I imagine anyone reading this volume will be aware that many scholars have blazed similar trails before us. Many continue to do it now, including everyone involved in this volume. But only with a greater connection and collective work can we make critical qualitative inquiry a stronger voice for social justice and decolonization.

MARIA: Rather than identify a particular theoretical or methodological imperative, I prefer to start by locating the place, as conceived by critical geography (Harvey, 1996; Cresswell, 2013), from where I join this debate. This place is an intersection where positivism, biomedicine, neoliberal market, Latin American academy and its socio-historical context, health institutions, human individual and collective suffering, impotence, the human body, the critical geographic space, history, society, and Critical Qualitative Inquiry meet. In this place power struggles are paradigmatic of what 'uneven' means (Navarro, 1984; Laurell, 2010). The search for inequity seems to be a purpose, for example, through the use of epidemiology and fear-raising propaganda to control all aspects of everyday life and to produce consumers since before birth (Bauman, 2007; Le Breton, 2011); the development of technology accessible to the rich who expend resources to prevent, cure, and even elate for agony, seeking an unattainable goal of preventing disease and death, also offered, but not delivered, to the poor (Laurell, 2013); or the generation of all-life dependence to medical institution knowledge and paraphernalia. Positivism and biomedical approaches to disease disguise market and political interests over their production and invention (Blech, 2005; Gérvas and Pérez-Fernández, 2013; Gotzche, 2013). To maintain the state of things, in this place it is convenient to neglect and despise epistemological and methodological reflection under the premise that only objective, measurable evidence is respectable, truthful, and accountable (Habermas, 1987). Reflection, innovation, the search for new words, listening to people already expropriated of their voices by the levels of 'patients' or 'population' are what Bourdieu (1990) called 'heretical' and dangerous for field endurance.

In this place, epistemological and methodological innovation arrives, if at all, late, while researchers' working conditions diminish academics' possibility to produce, use, and communicate innovative methodologies. Also, overall neo-liberal hegemony has already infiltrated the academic space, making it more administrative, subject to scrutiny, less devoted to social justice or the production of knowledge, and more attached to political and market projects (De Sousa-Santos, 2004; Derridá, 2002; Giroux, 2009). Critical Health Qualitative Inquiry (CHQI) in this place is, relatively recently, imported; opportunities to conform solid and quality CHQI, teaching, innovation, and communication, are scarce. This does not help to raise CHQI's voice against the medical bunker (Chapela, 2013).

This place used to be proud of the 1918 Cordoba University Reforms (Tünnermann, 1996)—reforms that attained public, autonomous, free and committed-with-the-poor higher education and research. Nowadays, public and private universities use public resources to support private interests, increasingly loosing autonomy and identity. As a result of crippling free-market labor and administrative procedures, academic freedom is in siege (as Marcelo discussed with respect to, among others, Steven Salaita). Unless radical changes occur in overall social structures, it seems that for the next decade this place will be more tightly tethered to the market, positivism, biomedicine, neoliberal politics, and administration. However, critical projects can enhance and expand resistance and change possibilities.

Due to the place from where I am speaking, then, I do not dare to define THE MOST important CHQI developments in the last ten years; however, I find the following important developments:

Spread and positioning of the idea of Health Qualitative Inquiry (HQI) has occurred in the last decade. With very powerful exceptions, such as the work of social medicine researchers, some nurses, members of the International Association of Qualitative Inquiry or the Global or Iberoamerican

International Congresses of HQI, and others, during the last ten years attempts to produce QI research in health corresponded to the acceptance of the social determinants of health (SDH) by the World Health Organization and the need to produce information about these social determinants. HQI became mainly a discursive fashion often considered as an easy way to become *avant-garde*, thus neglecting the study and training of/in QI and its commitment to understanding. Medical researchers likewise produced their own interpretation of QI within their positivistic thinking; thus, in the medical literature appeared 'QI' papers structured as conventional medical papers, making commonplace the use of words such as 'phenomenological,' 'representation,' '*bricolage*,' evacuated from their meaning; making efforts to comply with samples; focusing on instruments (a favorite: focal groups); and interpreting with percentages with the aid of QI software—reporting, for example, results of twenty 'deep interviews' of two hours each; or other. Alongside that intentionality in research emerged an eagerness to learn quality HQI. For a place that neglects epistemological and methodological reflection, the idea of the need of reflection became refreshing and searched, changing for some teachers and researchers their epistemological positions and opening the possibility of methodological research.

Although very marginal in the place from where I am speaking, the idea of HQI in understanding social problems has begun to transcend traditional disciplines, to varying degrees of success. Some of the benefits of this change in direction are the need to question the traditional knowledge jail that prescribes that good researchers should follow one author or school of thought, the questioning of the condemnation of eclecticism present since the decade of 1960, and an opening for researchers to question their own work. Such a turn has impacted as well the development of alternatives to define health problems, the conception of health itself, and the search for better methodologies to understand health.

ELIZABETH: An important development that is unfortunate, I think, is how easily the positivism of the scientifically-based research (SBR), evidence-based research (EBR) movement reinforced the latent positivism that interpretive qualitative methodology—what I call 1980s qualitative methodology (for example, Denzin, 1989; Erickson, 1986; Lincoln & Guba, 1985)—could never quite rid itself of. For example, too many qualitative studies that claim to be "interpretive" or "constructionist" or "critical" still use concepts and practices like *bias, subjectivity* (as in "subjectivity statements"), *triangulation*, *systematicity, findings, coding data*, and so on. But after SBR, too much qualitative research, which was invented as resistance to positivist social science, became at least quasi-positivist. In education, the National Research Council's report, *Scientific Research in Education,* contributed to the resurgence of positivism, the scientizing of education, and, I believe, the rise of mixed methods research, which, as students outside my department at the University of Georgia and elsewhere always tell me, is a way to "sneak a few interviews into a quantitative study." I admit that I find much mixed methods research ontologically and epistemologically confused.

Of course, Institutional Review Boards that tried to turn qualitative studies into the quantitative studies they understood contributed to the positivization of qualitative methodology. But the publishing industry also contributed by cranking out book after book and article after article that explained exactly how to do qualitative research, thus turning it into methods-driven research. And, of course, university qualitative research courses do that, too—they use those textbooks.

In most of the qualitative studies I read, it's clear that researchers haven't studied much social theory;

typically, they just find "themes and patterns" in their data, after coding it, rather than doing a theoretical analysis. This isn't surprising because it's easier to teach and do methods-driven research than to teach and learn theory.

So I would sum up by saying that the mostly interpretive 1980s qualitative methodology that I studied as a doctoral student in the early 1990s, which had radical potential, has, in general, been reduced to quasi-positivist or positivist methods-driven research. There are exceptions, of course, but the on-the-ground, run-of-the-mill qualitative methodology that I encounter everywhere is positivist and almost atheoretical.

SVEND: I want to tack in a slightly different direction: for me it has been noteworthy to see how qualitative inquiry, around the world, is increasingly put to use for purposes that most people associated with the International Congress of Qualitative Inquiry would not agree with. I am thinking of focus group research, for example, used in marketing, where it furthers a consumerist capitalist ethos. Also, political parties use qualitative research in the current "market democracy" to chart the preferences and attitudes of citizen-consumers. Qualitative inquiry has, in this sense, become mainstream, with all the costs and benefits that follow.

Furthermore, it seems to me that qualitative inquiry is moving in three quite opposed directions at the same time. It is moving towards standardization with increased focus on coding and categorization, supported by the CAQDAS machinery. This trend can be called qualitative positivism, because it is supposed that the use of "the correct method" somehow guarantees scientific truth. A second trend is that, at the same time, it is also moving towards fragmentation with lots of new experimental practices that borrow from literature and the arts. A third trend is the politicalization of qualitative inquiry, involving activism and a social justice agenda.

The classical triad of the true, the beautiful, and the good seems to be involved, but the question is if qualitative inquiry can be all three things.

CHRIS: Focusing for a moment on a very specific methodological orientation, I would say that the emergence of autoethnography as a major methodology—no longer sidelined or marginalized by doubts about its power, efficacy, and legitimacy as a mode of qualitative inquiry—has had a powerful impact upon all other modes of qualitative inquiry. The voice of the researcher is no longer a muted voice. The standpoint of the researcher is now central to qualitative inquiry.

Relatedly, the myth of objectivity has been shattered. The researcher is no longer a bystander. (Never was, but...now we have made this explicit!) Experimentation with textual forms, poetry, performative writing—all the various "messy texts" and artistic renderings of the inquiry process and its "products"—has really taken center stage. Moreover, I do agree with what has been said about the continuing emergence of critical qualitative inquiry as a corrective to enactments of power. The ongoing development of approaches in which the phenomenon leads to the choice of method, rather than the researcher predetermining and grafting a preferred method onto the situation at hand, is also, as has been said, a development worth noting.

MICHAEL: Given these past developments and trends of which you speak, what do you think will be the major themes to emerge in the next ten years? Do you think we will continue to see a splintering of approaches? A more deeply political (and politicized) qualitative inquiry?

ELIZABETH: I'm not sure about "themes." During the next ten years, I think that what we call "qualitative methodology" will splinter, which it's been doing—there's nothing stable about it—and that's good. I think we'll continue to see interpretive research that resists positivism. I'm especially taken with the second edition of a wonderful book on interpretive research edited by Yanow and Schwartz-Shea (2013) in which they're trying to get political science to make the interpretive turn—the turn other disciplines claim to have made in the 1980s; talk about being paradigms behind! Clearly, interpretive inquiry is radical for fields that are solidly positivist.

But I think quasi-positivist and positivist qualitative research will proliferate because it's easy to do and useful for those who want uncomplicated answers. I also think we'll continue to see critical work organized around identity politics and social justice issues. And I think post qualitative research, which I'm especially interested in, will attract some researchers. Of course, I would say that post qualitative research is not qualitative research at all because it does not use the humanist subject or the logic of representation, so we'll have to see what gets done there.

The National Research Council's (2014) report, *Proposed Revisions to the Common Rule for the Protection of Human Subjects in the Behavioral and Social Sciences,* proposes recommendations that will, if adopted in the revision of the Common Rule, exempt most qualitative research from IRB review. This is a huge change that could really open up qualitative methodology again. But what I find scary is that so many of the qualitative researchers I talk with about the recommendations resist them. They've grown accustomed to the practices of formalization enforced by IRBs and think they're correct and good. They think it makes sense, for example, for someone doing an autoethnography to sign her own consent form. Positivism's normalizing, disciplinary power cannot be overestimated.

One thing I've learned during the last ten years is that it's very difficult for us to escape our training. If we learned, early on, positivist, methods-driven research that privileges, for example, practices of formalization and systematicity, we're going to think that's good research. If we studied poststructural theory and/or DeleuzoGuattarian transcendental empiricism early on, we're going to think that's good work. I think Brian Fay was right when he said that *we have been theorized,* made by theory, and so it's difficult to make these "turns." We really do have to re-think almost everything to "turn." Who wants to work so hard? In that regard, I learned during the SBR years that the romance of "talking across differences" is just that. A positivist and a Deleuzian are not thinking/living in the same world. It is highly unlikely they'll be able to "dialog" until they reach "consensus."

MARCELO: I'm going to answer Questions Two and Three at the same time here, so I'll just pass on my turn in the next round: the major themes of the next ten years and the major challenges/opportunities are, for me, directly linked: Survival. Higher education as social justice. Renewed paradigm wars. Movement-building. Perhaps these are not "themes" in a strict sense. But these are the main issues I see on the horizon for qualitative inquiry. From where I stand, and as far out as I can see from here, I think that the ever-increasing corporatization of higher education in many parts of the world will continue to promote the notion of validity and pose a threat to the legitimacy of qualitative inquiry. I think this is particularly true in the United States, given the systemic and intentional defunding of public higher education in the last decade or so. As our universities continue to get starved of public funds, and I believe the trend will pick up speed in the next decade, critical qualitative inquiry will be forced to construct more persuasive narratives of justification and legitimation as a mode of knowledge production.

I believe we will need to tailor these narratives according to the many different audiences and stakeholders involved in higher education, but with special care and attention to undergraduate students. If we manage to make critical and interpretive qualitative inquiry resonate with the very large body of undergraduate students this country has, the establishment may lose some of its power in constricting and White-coating knowledge. The conservative strategy to demonize scholarship that questions systems of power that justifies the oppression and inequalities of our days may find resistance in the very classrooms the establishment aims to control. I don't have an omnipresent standpoint, but my fifteen years of bringing critical and interpretive qualitative inquiry into my own classrooms lend verisimilitude to the notion that students are interested in learning about the power structure shaping and informing their own lives. And I know for a fact that I am not alone in this experience. Thanks to the new stages and venues for qualitative inquiry, the literature is filled with epiphanic moments of liberation and communion with Others in classes informed by critical inquiry.

Without the students, critical and interpretive qualitative inquiry will be hard-pressed to find substantive allies. Given that our electoral system has been rigged to favor big money and their interest groups, it is an illusion to think state legislators will reverse the privatization trend and recommit to putting "public" back in public higher education (where the largest slice of higher education happens) in the foreseeable future. We know we can't count on politicians in this money-is-free-speech historical moment. Who else can we count on to advance critical inquiry in the next decade? We know too well whose interests the mainstream media serve. They will continue to privilege narratives that justify profit over people, foment fear of the Other in order to keep us divided and blind to their plutocratic masters, and repeat easy us-versus-them soundbites to hide the nuances of power structures that benefit few at the expense of most. Social media can be a helpful medium, though the main platforms are securely in the hands of bottom-line corporations. We know we can't count on higher education professional administrators, whose salaries, contract fine-prints, and pay-off clauses resemble corporative incentives and not those of faculty and staff. Again, the evidence is clear for all to see. With shocking ease, the upper administration will sell out any faculty member who challenges the status quo as quickly as a donor can send an email. Once more, the recent un-hiring of Steven Salaita by the University of Illinois is telling of what is to come for those engaged in critical inquiry. If you are reading this and don't know the case, and care about the future of critical qualitative inquiry, I urge you to do some digging. It will give you a clear picture of what qualitative inquiry (and critical scholarship more generally) will be fighting against in the next decade.

MARIA: Similar to what Marcelo said, as a product of a state of siege constructed by hegemonic neoliberalism, in this place the battle will endure and can worsen. Therefore, present themes, such as transdisciplinarity inclusive research, development of a HCQI Latin-American identity, the enhancement of what has already started, decolonization, democratization, equity, social justice, suffering, mutual aid, and communality are likely to develop as means for resistance.

To let the problem, the question, the need for understanding define the method will probably become a central theme to approach health conventional thinking, to open ways to dialogue with critical positivist health researchers, and to the construction of research spaces in frontier, and to create frontiers, not mixtures or limits. This can yield in ways to persuade the health establishment and to erode the medical bunker; to show the effect of A-critical positivism to enhance disease; to reach the necessary voice for lobbying; to include people's voices in health decisions; to set the instruments in people's hands; to understand the healing power of CHQI (Chapela and Cerda, 2010); to help health personnel achieve more humanized working conditions; to include different knowledges, words, practices; to understand the human body, health, suffering, disease, care, living, and dying; to influence the media and public policies; to cherish, care and struggle for academic freedom and autonomous, free, public higher health education; and, indeed, to alleviate human suffering, even if all that happens just in a small way.

MICHAEL: I think we would find significant agreement with the political struggles mentioned above. So, moving in a different direction, what about specific methodological developments in qualitative inquiry?

SVEND: In my mind, there is an interesting trend towards integration of natural, human, and social sciences these years. Neuroscientists are collaborating with phenomenologists; anthropologists are working with biologists; brain, body, and culture are seen as entangled. Distinctions between *Verstehen* and *Erklären* that we thought were clear no longer hold. This is bound to make an impact on qualitative inquiry—and I am not thinking of the current discourse of "mixed methods," which is exactly just mixing *Verstehen* and *Erklären*, but rather inquiry that does not accept this distinction in the first place. Can what (some) natural scientists do be conceived of as qualitative inquiry? Should we invite biologists to our conferences? Some of them do conduct fieldwork, for example? What will we win and what will we lose by having this broader view of qualitative inquiry? I think that will be an exciting theme for us to discuss in the years to come.

CHRIS: I believe we are entering a period of even broader experimentation with textual form, while at the same time becoming more critical of power structures that mute voices and dampen participation. Democratic engagement and participatory, multi-vocal/multi-perspectival/inter-disciplinary/multi-disciplinary inquiry will carry the leading edge of our efforts. Critical qualitative inquiry will be at the forefront of our work. Autoethnography and performance ethnography will continue to develop and enrich our understanding of the human condition.

← ↑ →

MICHAEL: If the past (and present) is a messy landscape, what comes next? What are the greatest challenges and opportunities to/in qualitative inquiry in the present? Looking forward to the future?

SVEND: I believe a major challenge will be how to keep the field together, if it is true that it is moving in quite different directions at the same time. Will the term "qualitative inquiry" continue to be useful? Will it be emptied of content? Will it be a nice, positive term that can be used for less nice purposes? Should the field even be kept together—is that a goal in itself? Should we, like Elizabeth St. Pierre, acknowledge that we are moving to a situation of *post*-qualitative research? I am ambivalent, because I see that many disciplines (including my own: psychology), and also many nations, are only now arriving at some form of qualitative inquiry as a legitimate research practice. They are arriving at discussions and research practices that are useful locally, but these discussions were ended many years ago in other parts of the qualitative world. It is important that researchers do not feel inferior even if they have not read Derrida or Barad, but are doing their good-old-fashioned qualitative research projects, as long as these serve worthy purposes in local contexts.

ELIZABETH: My personal challenge is to encourage scholars to read and study theory(ies) so they have something to think with when they do research. I especially like Alecia Jackson and Liza Mazzei's lovely book, *Thinking with Theory in Qualitative Research*, that's moving in that direction. As a professor, I would really like for our students to study the history of empiricism and the philosophy of science *before* they study research methodology. And I would like for that work to begin at the master's level and not wait until it's almost too late at the doctoral level.

CHRIS: In my view, the "old guard" gatekeepers still want to tamp us down, but they cannot. Dead ideologies and dead epistemologies (for example, positivism) will try to maintain a grasp on power, but they will slip into the murky waters of irrelevance as phenomenologically driven qualitative inquiry continues to gain steam. Corporate colonization of the life world will continue to encroach on our universities. We will have to work very hard to hold the forces of corporatization at bay. Strong voices of resistance will need to be engaged.

MARIA: As Michael and Norman proposed for contesting neoliberalism, health inequity and medical-market will find their solutions in the streets (see Giardina & Denzin, 2013). The present situation of suffering is unbearable, fear to our lives and bodies is unsustainable, services are inaccessible or do not solve problems, medical markets and their alliances with scientific and medical institutions are day after day more visible. This situation, while terrible, can become an awareness opportunity to CHQI development for the next ten years. Awareness about the need for change for academics, for health services personnel, for people living in sustained suffering, even for institutions, is probably our main opportunity to meet HCQI challenges in the future. Other opportunities are an increasing interest in HQI: the strengthening of HCQI researchers and HCQI research groups with disposition to share and learn, the existence and recognition of some good, quality HQR, and the demand of research to meet the World Health Organization's social determinants of health goals.

As for the challenges, considering what I have said up to this point, the erosion of the positivist bio-medical bunker continues to be a main challenge. I will only briefly name some other challenges:

- Catch up with QI advances in other disciplines and world regions
- Develop a Latin American HQI identity and knowledge
- Prevent the spread of HQI that lacks quality
- Teach teachers, produce teaching materials
- Write, write, and write. To communicate, convince scholars to become *authors*
- Develop ways for accessible quality publishing
- Develop CHQI academic and solidarity groups and networks
- Think qualitative, look qualitative, live qualitative, trust qualitative
- Keep, cultivate, care, cherish, share, and find new places to plant, and protect, the CHQI seed
- Find methodological proposals that can fulfill the vacuum of positivistic-market-biomedical failure
- Produce a set of quality standards that can orient scholars in their search for quality and at the same time can be accepted and understood by the medical bunker
- Write with left and right hands. Use the right for conventional communication, and the left to learn, understand, share, and grow in freedom
- Put the instruments in people's hands

← ↑ →

MICHAEL: Since we are on the topic of 'the future,' what do you see as 'new' or 'emergent' methods of inquiry that are especially innovative or have the potential to impact the field in the years ahead?

MARIA: I will approach this question as a conclusion to my former arguments from the perspective of the place where I am situated. We all—academics, health personnel, people living our collective and individual lives—need to talk; we need to say what has been worrying us and we have not said before. We need to talk to produce autonomous information and understanding about suffering and health. We need to trace horizons of change and hope. We need to provoke narratives in their different expressions, in new ways, in old ways, collective, individual, performed, spoken, written, sung, painted, pictured, filmed, numbered, danced, or in any other way they can strengthen and make visible what we need to say; narratives written with right and left hands, two or many, as much as needed. Therefore, we need to advance in old and new ways to produce narratives where self and Other can construct frontiers, showing and encouraging 'leaning' (Pelias, 2011); narratives capable of telling about frontiers: the body, health, the hyphen community-institutions, self-Other, person-collectivity, society-history-space, life-death, suffering—transformative action. To search in the frontier requires labyrinthine methodologies, where the need for understanding constructs and reconstructs the method to observe, interpret, and communicate as many times as needed (Chapela, 2003). We, finally, require methodologies that can land and grow in the hands of people, and methodologies to make methodologies land and be at their hand so they can use them to help in their change decisions.

MARCELO: To build on what Maria just said, I think that decolonization has been emerging as a method of inquiry that has the potential to help qualitative inquiry fight the concerted attack on ways of knowing that defy, expose, and challenge the oligarchic establishment of our globalized times. Humanity and lived experience, the very objects and subjects of qualitative inquiry, are shaped by contemporary colonization by a resourceful minority over the much less resourceful majority. While the more traditional methods of colonization like violence and overt subjugation continue to be go-to tools, contemporary colonization relies heavily on narrative control through covert fear-mongering and shameless anti-intellectualism. Decolonization stands on the shoulders of Indigenous movements, critical theory, Third World feminism, cultural studies, and postcolonialism, and I don't want to give the impression that I think it is a better way of advancing qualitative inquiry. But to me, decolonizing inquiry seems to be a promising framework to examine our ever-increasing globalized humanity, to connect the dots between lived experience and power structures, biography and history, narratives that justify inequalities and narrative-makers, between injustice and our individual and collective responsibilities to stand up against it. Perhaps even more important, in my view, is the common ground/framework for imagining greater solidarity in the future that decolonizing inquiry seems to offer historically oppressed groups *and* social justice allies who come from more privileged backgrounds. At least to me, decolonizing inquiry has become a way of resisting oppression and imagining a more just future, of believing in the possibilities of liberatory education.

SVEND: At the same time, I also do no think that we should leave the traditional craft of inquiry behind; that is, work organized around practices of observation (fieldwork) and conversation (interviewing). These continue to be basic human skills that are knowledge-producing, and which are employed in qualitative inquiry. But, especially when communicating research, and with the ambition of reaching a larger audience, I believe that novels, plays, television documentaries, and so forth should be used to an increasing extent to make our work known.

CHRIS: To Svend's point, I believe that the quality of our writing and our voicing of our concerns, our knowledge, and our praxis will continue to increase. We must remain vigilant/watchful and deeply engaged in our efforts to overcome resistance to experimentation. We will need to engage our entire collective will to protect academic freedom, and to "show forth" the variety of methods of building evidence. As intellectuals, we are called to bring our work to the attention of the broader public. This is why I maintain hope for qualitative inquiry broadly, and autoethnography and ethnography more specifically. I believe it is accessible to audiences beyond academic publishing and presentation. We must work harder to reach the people! Our writing and our speaking should be put to good use to open up worlds of mutual understanding.

ELIZABETH: After the debacle of those years of SBR that, I'm afraid, have not unwound, I tried to open up some space for something different to happen with the concept *post qualitative inquiry*. I envisioned inquiry that might actually use the "post" approaches of the last century without trying to embed them in humanist, representationalist qualitative methodology—for example, some awkward combination of an interview study and a Foucaultian genealogy or a rhizoanalysis of interview data. I think *post qualitative* also gestures toward all the "new" work coming out of the flattened ontology of the ontological turn, which is quite Deleuzian—new empiricism, new materialism, the posthuman, the more-than-human, and so on.

But this inquiry demands an ontological turn, and we simply don't teach ontology, just like we don't teach empiricism or philosophy of science, so it's very

> difficult to do this work. I want to encourage people to study ontology and empiricism to see how we've thought them differently from Plato and the Stoics onward. If climate change in this age of the anthropocene isn't a wake-up call to think the nature of *being* differently, I don't know what is. There's a very real urgency in the ontological turn. We can't just continue to privilege human being.

By Way of a Conclusion

As our assembled colleagues make clear in the above dialogue, qualitative inquiry is being pulled in multiple directions at once: pushing the boundaries of both traditional social science and interpretive research; engaging in struggle against oppressive institutional and political machinations; balancing the need for deep theoretical engagement with a praxical approach to the research act; and striving to engage with (if not change) the landscape on which qualitative inquiry currently sits.

In this way, the epilogue to this volume leaves us with more questions than answers; it foretells coming struggles, opportunities, and points of contention. This is the heart of qualitative inquiry in the present (if not future) tense: a multitude of voices mobilized in the enactment of social change, in its myriad forms, for the betterment of all. Thus does the future hold immense promise, if we are there to pick up the call from those who have gone before us to go forth and change the world. *We have a job to do; let's get to it.*

References

Bauman, Z. (2007). *Consuming life.* Cambridge, MA: Polity Press.

Blech, J. (2005). *Los inventores de enfermedades. Cómo nos convierten en pacientes.* [Disease inventors. How they turn us into patients.] Barcelona, Spain: Destino.

Bourdieu, P. (1990). *Sociología y cultura.* [Sociology and cultura.] México: Grijalbo.

Chapela, M. C. (2003). *The construction of critical knowledge for the development of human health.* London: Institute of Education, University of London.

Chapela, M. C. (2013). Is it possible for critical social sciences to trespass the biomedical sciences bunker in a neoliberal era? *Cultural Studies ↔ Critical Methodologies, 16*(3) 504–509.

Chapela, M. C., & Cerda, A. (2010). Investigación cualitativa sanadora. [Healing Qualitative Inquiry.] In C. Martínez (Ed.), *Por los caminos de la investigación cualitativa. Exploraciones narrativas y reflexiones en el ámbito de la salud* (pp. 120–138). México: UAM-X.

Cresswell, T. (2013). *Geographic thought: A critical introduction.* Chichester, UK: Wiley-Blackwell.

CSDH. (2008). *Closing the gap in a generation: health equity through action on the social determinants of health. Final Report of the Commission on Social Determinants of Health.* Geneva: World Health Organization.

Denzin, N. K. (1989). *Interpretive interactionism.* Newbury Park, CA: Sage.

De Sousa-Santos, B. (2004). *La universidad en el siglo XXI. Para una reforma democrátic y emancipadora de la universidad.* [The university in the XXI Century. Towards a university democratic and emancipatory reform.] Madrid and Buenos Aires: Miño y Dávila, Laboratorio de Políticas Públicas.

Derrida, J. (2002). *La universidad sin condición.* [University without condition.] Madrid, Spain: Editorial Trotta.

Dilthey, W. (1991[1883]). *Introduction to the human sciences.* Princeton, NJ: Princeton University Press.

Erickson, F. (1986). Qualitative methods in research on teaching. In M. C. Wittrock (Ed.), *Handbook of research on teaching* (3rd ed.) (pp. 119–161). New York: Macmillan.

Gérvas, J., & Pérez-Fernández, M. (2013). *Sano y salvo.* [Safe and sane.] Barcelona, Spain: Los libros del Lince.

Giardina, M., & Denzin, N. (2013). Confronting neoliberalism: Toward a militant pedagogy of empowered citizenship. *Cultural Studies ↔ Critical Methodologies, 13*(6), 443–451.

Giroux, H. (2009). The rise of corporate university. *Cultural Studies ↔ Critical Methodologies, 9*(5), 669–695.

Gotzche, P. (2013). *Deadly medicines and organised crime: How big pharma has corrupted healthcare.* London: Radcliffe.

Habermas, J. (1987). *Knowledge and human interests.* Cambridge, UK: Polity Press.

Harvey, D. (1996). *Justice, nature, and the geography of difference.* Cambridge, MA: Blackwell.

Laurell, A. C. (2010). Revisando las políticas y discursos en salud en América Latina. [Reviewing health policies and discourses in Latin America.] *Medicina Social, 5* (1), 79–88.

Laurell, A. C. (2013). *Impacto del seguro popular en el sistema de salud mexicano.* [Impact of popular insurance within the Mexican health system.] Buenos Aires, Argentina: CLACSO-CROP.

Le Breton, D. (2011). *Adiós al cuerpo.* Ciudad de México: La Cifra Editorial. Original title 1999, *L'Adieu au corps.* Paris: Editions Métalié.

Lincoln, Y. S., & Guba, E. G. (1985). *Naturalistic inquiry.* Newbury Park, CA: Sage.

National Research Council. (2014). *Proposed revisions to the common rule for the protection of human subjects in the behavioral and social sciences.* Committee on Revisions to the Common Rule for the Protection of Human Subjects in Research in the Behavioral and Social Sciences. Board on Behavioral, Cognitive, and Sensory Sciences, Committee on National Statistics, Division of Behavioral and Social Sciences and Education. Washington, DC: The National Academies Press.

Navarro, V. (1984). *Lucha de clases, Estado y medicina.* [Class struggle, the state, and medicine.] México: Nueva Imagen.

Pelias, R. (2011). *Leaning: A poetics of personal relations.* Walnut Creek, CA: Left Coast Press, Inc.

Pérez-Álvarez, M. & González-Pardo, H. (2007). *La invención de trastornos mentales: ¿escuchando al fármaco o al paciente?* [Mental illness invention: listening to drugs or patients?] Madrid, España: Alianza Editorial.

St.Pierre, E. A. (2011). Post qualitative research: The critique and the coming after. In N. K. Denzin & Y. S. Lincoln (Eds.), *Sage handbook of qualitative inquiry* (4th ed., pp. 611–635). Thousand Oaks, CA: Sage.

Tünnermann, C. (1996). Breve historia del desarrollo de la Universidad en América Latina. [Brief history of the development of the university in Latin America.] In Conferencia Regional sobre Políticas y Estrategias para la transformación de la Educación Superior en América Latina y el Caribe. *La educación superior en el umbral del Siglo XXI* (pp. 11–38). Havana, Cuba: CRESALC.

Yanow, D., & Schwartz-Shea, P. (Eds.). (2013). *Interpretation and method: Empirical research methods and the interpretive turn* (2nd ed.). Armonk, NY: M.E. Sharpe.

Index

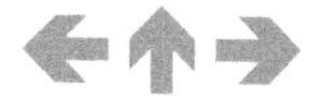

About the Editors and Authors

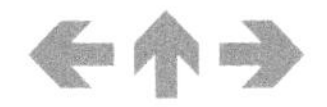

Editors

Norman K. Denzin (PhD, University of Iowa) is Distinguished Professor of Communications, College of Communications Scholar, and Research Professor of Communications, Sociology, and Humanities at the University of Illinois, Urbana-Champaign. One of the world's foremost authorities on qualitative research and cultural criticism, Denzin is the author or editor of more than two dozen books, including *The Qualitative Manifesto*; *Qualitative Inquiry Under Fire*; *Reading Race*; *Interpretive Ethnography*; *The Cinematic Society*; *The Voyeur's Gaze*; and *The Alcoholic Self.* He is past editor of *The Sociological Quarterly*, co-editor (with Yvonna S. Lincoln) of four editions of the landmark *Handbook of Qualitative Research*, co-editor (with Michael D. Giardina) of ten plenary volumes from the annual International Congress of Qualitative Inquiry, co-editor (with Lincoln) of the methods journal *Qualitative Inquiry*, founding editor of *Cultural Studies ↔ Critical Methodologies* and *International Review of Qualitative Research*, editor of three book series, and founding director of the International Congress of Qualitative Inquiry.

Michael D. Giardina (PhD, University of Illinois) is an Associate Professor of Sport, Media, and Politics and Associate Director of the Center for Sport, Health, and Equitable Development at Florida State University. He is the author of *Sport, Spectacle, and NASCAR Nation: Consumption and the Cultural Politics of Neoliberalism* (Palgrave, 2011, with Joshua Newman), which received the 2012 Outstanding Book Award from the North American Society for the Sociology of Sport (NASSS) and was named to the 2012 *CHOICE* Outstanding Academic Titles list, and *Sporting Pedagogies: Performing Culture & Identity in the Global Arena* (Peter Lang, 2005), which received the 2006 Outstanding Book Award from NASSS. He is also the editor or co-editor of more than a dozen books on qualitative inquiry, cultural studies, and interpretive research. He is Editor of the *Sociology of Sport Journal*, Special Issue Editor of *Cultural Studies ↔ Critical Methodologies*, and the Associate Director of the International Congress of Qualitative Inquiry.

Authors

Russell Bishop is Foundation Professor for Māori Education in the School of Education at the University of Waikato, Hamilton, New Zealand. He is also a qualified and experienced secondary school teacher. Prior to his present appointment he was a senior lecturer in Māori Education in the Education Department at the University of Otago and interim director for Otago University's Teacher Education program. His research experience in the area of collaborative storying as Kaupapa Māori has given rise to national and international publishing, including the books, *Collaborative Research Stories: Whakawhanaungatanga* (Dunmore Press, 1996); *Culture Counts: Changing Power Relationships in Classrooms* (Zed Books, 2003); *Pathologising Practices: The Impact of Deficit Thinking on Education* (Peter Lang, 2004), *Culture Speaks: Cultural Relationships and Classroom Learning* (Huia, 2007); and *Scaling Up Education Reform* (NZCER Press, 2012).

Svend Brinkmann is a Professor of Psychology at Aalborg University, Denmark, where he is Co-director of the Center for Qualitative Research. He is the author of many books, including *John Dewey—En introduktion* (*John Dewey: An Introduction*) (Copenhagen, Hans Reitzels Forlag, 2006) and *Psyken: Mellem synapser og samfund* (*Psyche: Between Synapses and Society*) (Aarhus University Press, 2009), and editor of such books as *InterViews: Learning the Craft of Qualitative Research Interviewing* (Sage, 2008; with Steiner Kvale).

Maria del Consuelo Chapela is a Professor at Universidad Autonoma Metropolitana in Mexico, where she conducts research on health promotion, medical education, multiculturalism, decolonization, and qualitative inquiry.

Clifford G. Christians is Research Professor Emeritus of Communications, Media Studies, and Journalism at the University of Illinois, Urbana-Champaign. One of the world's leading authorities on media and social ethics, Christians is the author or editor of numerous books, including *Good News: A Social Ethics and the Press* (Oxford University Press, 2003, with John Ferre and Mark Fackler), *Media Ethics: Cases and Moral Reasoning* (1st–10th editions) (Longman, 2011, with Mark Fackler, Kathy McKee, Peggy Kersehl, and Robert Woods), and *Communication Ethics and Universal Values* (Sage, 1997, with Michael Traber). He has also been a visiting scholar in philosophical ethics at Princeton University, in social ethics at the University of Chicago, and a PEW fellow in ethics at Oxford University. In 2004, he received the Paul J. Deutschmann Award for Excellence in Research from the Association for Education in Journalism and Mass Communication.

César A. Cisneros Puebla is a Professor in the Department of Sociology at Autonomous Metropolitan University-Iztapalapa, Mexico. He consults in the field of qualitative computing and research within South America and abroad, and has conducted research projects supported by the U.S. Centers for Disease Control and Prevention. He has been a visiting professor at the

International Institute for Qualitative Methodology, University of Alberta, Canada, and in the CAQDAS Networking Project at the University of Surrey, United Kingdom.

Cynthia B. Dillard is the Mary Frances Early Professor of Teacher Education at the University of Georgia. Her major research interests include critical multicultural education, spirituality in teaching and learning, epistemological concerns in research, and African/African America feminist studies. Most recently, her research has focused on Ghana, West Africa, where she established a preschool and was enstooled as Nana Mansa II, Queen Mother of Development, in the village of Mpeasem, Ghana, West Africa. She is the author of *On Spiritual Strivings: Transforming an African American Woman's Life* (SUNY Press, 2007) and *Learning to (Re)member the Things We've Learned to Forget: Endarkened Feminisms, Spirituality and the Sacred Nature of Research and Teaching* (Peter Lang, 2012).

Greg Dimitriadis is Professor and Associate Dean for Academic Affairs in the Graduate School of Education at University at Buffalo, the State University of New York. He is the author of *Performing Identity/Performing Culture: Hip Hop as Text, Pedagogy, and Lived Practice* (Peter Lang, 2001) and *Friendship, Cliques, and Gangs: Young Black Men Coming of Age in Urban America* (Teachers College Press, 2003), co-author of *Reading and Teaching the Postcolonial: From Baldwin to Basquiat and Beyond* (Teachers College Press, 2001) and *On Qualitative Inquiry* (Teachers College Press, 2004), and co-editor of *Promises to Keep: Cultural Studies, Democratic Education, and Public Life* (Routledge Falmer, 2003), *Learning to Labor in New Times* (Routledge Falmer, 2004), and *Race, Identity, and Representation in Education* (2nd edition) (Routledge Falmer, 2005).

Marcelo Diversi is Associate Professor of Human Development at Washington State University Vancouver. He is the author of *Betweener Talk: Decolonizing Knowledge Production, Pedagogy, and Praxis* (Left Coast Press, 2009; with Claudio Moreira), which received the 2010 Book of the Year Award, Division of

Ethnography, from the National Communication Association. He has also published more than a dozen articles on topics such as indigenous qualitative inquiry, youth culture, homelessness, and poverty.

Laura L. Ellingson is Professor and Director of Women's & Gender Studies at Santa Clara University. She is the author of *Engaging Crystallization in Qualitative Research: An Introduction* (Sage, 2009) and *Aunting: Cultural Practices that Sustain Family and Community Life* (Baylor University Press, 2010; with Patricia Sotirin), which received the Bonnie Ritter Outstanding Book Award, Feminist and Women's Studies Division, from the National Communication Association in 2012.

Charles R. Garoian is Director of the School of Visual Arts and Professor of Art Education at Penn State University. He is the author of *Spectacle Pedagogy: Art Politics, and Visual Culture* (SUNY Press, 2008; with Yvonne M. Gaudelius) and *Performing Pedagogy: Towards an Art of Politics* (SUNY Press, 1999). His scholarly articles can be found in *Leonardo*, *The Art Journal*, *The Journal of Aesthetic Education*, *Journal of Visual Arts Research*, *Journal of Social Theory in Art Education*, *Journal of Multicultural and Cross-Cultural Research in Art Education*, *Studies in Art Education*, *Teacher Education Quarterly*, and *School Arts Magazine*.

Henry A. Giroux holds the Global TV Network chair professorship at McMaster University in the English and Cultural Studies Department. His most recent books include: *America's Education Deficit and the War on Youth: Reform Beyond Electoral Politics* (Monthly Review Press, 2013), *Youth in Revolt: Reclaiming a Democratic Future* (Paradigm, 2013), *The Twilight of the Social: Resurgent Politics in an Age of Disposability* (Paradigm, 2012), *On Critical Pedagogy* (Continuum, 2011), and *Zombie Politics and Culture in the Age of Casino Capitalism* (Peter Lang, 2010).

H. L. (Bud) Goodall, Jr. was Professor and Director of Communication at the Hugh Downs School of Human Communication at Arizona State University, where he taught from 2004 until his death in 2012. Considered a pioneer in narrative ethnography in the field of communication, he was the author of many books and articles, from *Casing a Promised Land* (Southern Illinois University Press, 1989) to *Counter-Narrative* (Left Coast Press, 2010), but he was most proud of his ethnographic memoir *A Need to Know: The Clandestine History of a CIA Family* (Left Coast Press, 2006), wherein his personal quest for the truth about his father was realized. Diagnosed with stage 4 pancreatic cancer in the spring of 2011, he turned his attention to writing about living with cancer in a blog that remains available (along with other works) on his website: www.hlgoodall.com.

Jean Halley is Associate Professor of Sociology at the College of Staten Island of the City University of New York. She is the author of *Boundaries of Touch: Parenting and Adult-Child Intimacy* (University of Illinois Press, 2007), *The Parallel Lives of Women and Cows: Meat Markets* (2012), *Seeing White: An Introduction to White Privilege and Race* (Rowman & Littlefield, 2011; with Amy Eshleman and Ramya Vijaya), and editor of *The Affective Turn: Theorizing the Social* (Duke University Press, 2007, with Patricia Ticineto Clough).

George Kamberelis is Professor and Director of the School of Education at Colorado State University. He has conducted research on children's emerging and developing literacies, children's writing development, discourse and identity, language and cultural diversity, critical media literacy, and interpretive research methods. Among his many works, he is co-author (with Greg Dimitriadis) of *On Qualitative Inquiry: Approaches to Language and Literacy Research* (Teachers College Press, 2004) and *Focus Groups: From Structured Interviews to Collective Conversations* (Routledge, 2013; with Greg Dimitriadis).

Margaret Kovach is Associate Professor of Educational Foundations at the University of Saskatchewan, Canada. She is the author of *Indigenous Methodologies: Characteristics, Conversations, and Contexts* (University of Toronto Press, 2009). Her work has appeared in such journals as *Canadian Review of Social Policy*,

Canadian Journal of Native Education, and *First People Child & Family Review*.

Antjie Krog is a poet, writer, journalist, and Professor Extraordinary in the Faculty of Arts at the University of the Western Cape, South Africa. She has published twelve volumes of poetry in Afrikaans, two volumes in English, and two nonfiction books: *Country of My Skull* (Broadway Books, 2000), on the South African Truth and Reconciliation Commission, and *A Change of Tongue* (Zebra Press, 2013), about the transformation in South Africa after ten years. Her work has been translated into English, Dutch, Italian, French, Spanish, Swedish, Serbian, and Arabic. *Country of My Skull* is widely used at universities as part of the curriculum dealing with writing about the past. She was also asked to translate the autobiography of Nelson Mandela, *Long Walk to Freedom*, into Afrikaans. She has received numerous prestigious awards for nonfiction, translation, and poetry (in both Afrikaans and English), as well as the Award from the Hiroshima Foundation for Peace and Culture for the year 2000 and the Open Society Prize from the Central European University. Her most recent books include *There Was This Goat*, written with Nosisi Mpolweni and Kopano Ratele and published by KZN Press in March 2009, which investigates the Truth and Reconciliation Commission testimony of Notrose Nobomvu Konile, and *Begging to be Black* (Random House Struik, 2011), which mixes memoir and history, philosophy, and poetry.

Gloria Ladson-Billings is the Kellner Family Chair in Urban Education and Professor of Curriculum and Instruction and Educational Policy Studies at the University of Wisconsin-Madison, where she currently serves as Assistant Vice Chancellor for Academic Affairs. She is the author of numerous books, including *Dreamkeepers: Successful Teachers of African American Children* (Jossey-Bass, 1994); *Beyond the Big House: African American Educators on Teacher Education* (Teachers College Press, 2005); and *Crossing over to Canaan: The Journey of New Teachers in Diverse Classrooms* (Jossey-Bass, 2001). She is also the editor of such books as *Education Research in the Public Interest: Social*

Justice, Action, and Policy (Teachers College Press, 2006, with William F. Tate) and *City Kids, City Schools: More Reports from the Front Row* (New Press, 2007, with William Ayers, Gregory Michie, and Pedro Noguera). She has also served as president of the American Educational Research Association.

D. Soyini Madison is a Professor at Northwestern University in the Department of Performance Studies. She also holds appointments in the Department of African American Studies and the Department of Anthropology. She is the author of *Critical Ethnography: Methods, Ethics, and Performance*, co-editor of *The Sage Handbook of Performance Studies* (2006, with Judith Hamera) and editor of *The Woman That I Am: The Literature and Culture of Contemporary Women of Color* (PalgraveMacMillan, 1993). She lived and worked in Ghana, West Africa, as a senior Fulbright scholar conducting field research on the interconnections between traditional religion, political economy, and Indigenous performance tactics. She received a Rockefeller Foundation Fellowship for her most recent book, *Acts of Activism: Human Rights and Radical Performance* (Cambridge University Press, 2010), which is based on fieldwork in Ghana.

Annette Markham is Guest Professor in the Department of Informatics at Umeå University, Sweden, and Associate Professor in the Department of Aesthetics & Communication, Aarhus University, Denmark. She is the author of *Life Online: Researching Real Experiences in Virtual Space* (AltaMira Press, 1998) and editor of *Internet Inquiry: Conversations about Method* (Sage, 2009, with Nancy Baym).

Joseph A. Maxwell is Professor in the Graduate School of Education, College of Education and Human Development, at George Mason University. He is the author, most recently, of *Qualitative Research Design: An Interactive Approach* (2nd edition, Sage, 2005) and *A Realist Approach for Qualitative Research* (Sage, 2011). He has also published widely on qualitative research and evaluation methods, combining qualitative and quantitative methods, medical education, Native American society and culture, and cultural and social theory. His present research interests focus primarily on the philosophy and logic of research methodology; he also pursues investigations in cultural theory, diversity in educational settings, and how people learn to do qualitative research.

Janice M. Morse holds the Barnes Presidential Endowed Chair in the College of Nursing at University of Utah. Trained as an anthropologist, she founded and is former director of the International Institute for Qualitative Methodology at University of Alberta, where she taught for many years. She is author or editor of numerous volumes on qualitative research in health care and nursing and has been conducting mixed method research since the 1970s. Morse founded and edits the journal, *Qualitative Health Research,* and edits two book series for Left Coast Press, *Developing Qualitative Inquiry* and *Qualitative Essentials.*

Ronald J. Pelias is Professor Emeritus in the Department of Speech Communication at Southern Illinois University, Carbondale. He is the author of numerous books on performance studies and performance methodologies, including *Performance Studies: The Interpretation of Aesthetic Texts, 2e* (Kendall Hunt 2007), *Writing Performance: Poeticizing the Researcher's Body* (Southern Illinois University Press, 1999), *A Methodology of the Heart: Evoking Academic and Daily Life* (AltaMira Press, 2004), and *Leaning: A Poetics of Personal Relations* (Left Coast Press, 2011). In 2000, he received the Lilla A. Heston Award for Outstanding Scholarship in Interpretation and Performance Studies from the National Communication Association. In addition to numerous published articles and book chapters, he also publishes performance texts and poetry.

Christopher N. Poulos is Associate Professor and Chair of Communication Studies at the University of North Carolina-Greensboro. An ethnographer and philosopher of communication, he teaches courses in family and relational communication, dialogue, ethnography, film studies, and rhetoric. His work has appeared in *Qualitative Inquiry*, *American Communication Journal*, *Southern Communication Journal*, *Cultural Studies: A Research*

Volume, and in the books *9/11 in American Culture*, *Spirituality, Action, & Pedagogy: Teaching from the Heart* and *Spirituality, Action, and Teaching: Stories from Within.*

Elizabeth Adams St. Pierre is Professor and Graduate Coordinator of Language and Literacy Education at the University of Georgia. Her work has appeared in a range of scholarly journals, including *International Review of Qualitative Research*, *Educational Researcher*, *Qualitative Inquiry*, *Journal of Contemporary Ethnography*, and *International Journal of Qualitative Studies in Education*. She is also the editor of *Working the Ruins: Feminist Postructural Theory and Methods in Education* (Routledge, 2000; with Wanda Pillow).

Harry Torrance is Professor of Education and Director of the Education and Social Research Institute, Manchester Metropolitan University, United Kingdom. His substantive research interests are in the interrelation of assessment with learning, program evaluation, and the role of assessment in education reform. He has undertaken many applied, qualitative, and mixed-method investigations of these topics funded by a wide range of sponsors. He is an elected member of the UK Academy of Learned Societies for the Social Sciences.

Linda Tuhiwai Smith is Professor of Indigenous Education at the University of Waikato, New Zealand, where she also serves as Pro-Vice Chancellor. In New Zealand, she has been central to the development of a tribal university, *Te Whare Wananga o Awanuiarangi*, and to the nationwide movement for an alternative schooling system, *Kura Kaupapa Māori*. Her leadership represents the pioneering work of Māori scholars and activists, which inspires Indigenous and sovereignty work internationally. She is the author of the widely celebrated *Decolonizing Methodologies: Research and Indigenous Peoples* (Zed, 1999), which explores the intersections of imperialism, knowledge, and research. As part of the 2013 New Year Honours, she was made a Companion of the New Zealand Order of Merit, for services to Māori and education.